COUNSELLING PSYCHOLOGY

This is the first textbook to provide a complete overview of counselling psychology. Covering not only the underlying principles and philosophy of the profession, it offers a uniquely applied perspective in a concise, student-friendly format.

From the relationship between research and practice to key ethical and professional issues, the book is written by some of the most eminent academic and practising psychologists in the field. It initially defines what counselling psychology and a therapeutic relationship involves, before outlining the range of approaches that can be taken with clients, from CBT to psychodynamic perspectives, and the journey from training through to working as a counselling psychologist.

Supported by case studies and a range of features to illustrate how theory can be applied to practice, this is the ideal companion for courses in applied counselling psychology. The integrated and interactive approach covers the personal and professional issues which counselling psychologists face, making this the definitive introduction for any student of this growing field of study.

Victoria Galbraith is Registrar for the BPS Qualification in Counselling Psychology and former Programme Director for the Doctorate in Counselling Psychology at the University of Wolverhampton, UK. She has an independent consultancy and psychology practice.

COUNSELLING PSYCHOLOGY

Edited by Victoria Galbraith

Routledge
Taylor & Francis Group
LONDON AND NEW YORK

First published 2018
by Routledge
2 Park Square, Milton Park, Abingdon, Oxon OX14 4RN

and by Routledge
711 Third Avenue, New York, NY 10017

Routledge is an imprint of the Taylor & Francis Group, an informa business

British Library Cataloguing-in-Publication Data
A catalogue record for this book is available from the British Library

Library of Congress Cataloging-in-Publication Data
Names: Galbraith, Victoria, editor.
Title: Counselling psychology / [edited by] Victoria Galbraith.
Description: New York : Routledge, 2017.
Identifiers: LCCN 2017018026 (print) | LCCN 2017024051 (ebook) |
ISBN 9781315626499 (Ebook) | ISBN 9781317235170 (Adobe reader) |
ISBN 9781317235163 (ePub) | ISBN 9781317235156 (Mobipocket) |
ISBN 9781138648357 (hbk) | ISBN 9781138648364 (pbk)
Subjects: LCSH: Counseling.
Classification: LCC BF636.6 (ebook) | LCC BF636.6 .C6758 2017 (print) |
DDC 158.3—dc23
LC record available at https://lccn.loc.gov/2017018026

ISBN: 978-1-138-64835-7 (hbk)
ISBN: 978-1-138-64836-4 (pbk)
ISBN: 978-1-315-62649-9 (ebk)

Typeset in Bembo
by Apex CoVantage, LLC

CONTENTS

CONTRIBUTORS

India Amos, Lecturer in Counselling and Psychotherapy, University of Salford

Sophia Balamoutsou, Senior Lecturer at Institute for Counselling and Psychological Studies, Athens

Lewis J. Blair, Counselling Psychologist, NHS Forth Valley

Victoria Galbraith, Registrar for BPS Qualification in Counselling Psychology and Director of Galbraith Consultancy

Stelios Gkouskos, Programme Director of Professional Doctorate in Counselling Psychology, University of East London

Terry Hanley, Senior Lecturer in Counselling Psychology, University of Manchester

Isabel Henton, Senior Lecturer in Counselling Psychology, Regent's University

Nicola Hogan, Cpsychol, Registered Psychologist, Anamcara, Edinburgh

Ros Howard, Consultant, Counselling Psychologist, Director of Ros Howard Psychology Ltd.

Pamela E. James, Counselling Psychologist in Independent Practice

Lynne Jordan, Counselling Psychologist and Director of Jordan Consultancy

Elaine Kasket, Principal Lecturer and Head of Programmes for Counselling Psychology, Regent's University

Angela Ioanna Loulopoulou, Principal Lecturer/Programme Director of Professional Doctorate in Counselling Psychology, London Metropolitan University

Elena Manafi, PsychD, Programme Director, University of Surrey

Helen Nicholas, Counselling Psychologist, HCN Psychology and Senior Lecturer in Counselling Psychology, University of Worcester

Jane Simms, Counselling Psychologist at Northern Health and Social Care Trust, County Antrim

Faye Volker, Senior Psychologist, Hallam Street Hospital

PREFACE TO THE SERIES SECOND EDITION

Psychology is still one of the most popular subjects for study at undergraduate degree level. As well as providing the student with a range of academic and applied skills that are valued by a broad range of employers, a psychology degree also serves as the basis for subsequent training and a career in professional psychology. A substantial proportion of students entering a degree programme in Psychology do so with a subsequent career in applied psychology firmly in mind, and as a result the number of applied psychology courses available at undergraduate level has significantly increased over recent years. In some cases these courses supplement core academic areas and in others they provide the student with a flavour of what they might experience as a professional psychologist.

The original series of ***Texts in Applied Psychology*** consisted of six textbooks designed to provide a comprehensive academic and professional insight into specific areas of professional psychology. The texts covered the areas of ***Clinical Psychology, Criminal and Investigative Psychology, Educational Psychology, Health Psychology, Sports and Exercise Psychology***, and ***Work and Organisational Psychology***, and each text was written and edited by the foremost professional and academic figures in each of these areas.

These texts were so successful that we are now able to provide you with a second edition of this series. All texts have been updated with details of recent professional developments as well as relevant research, and we have responded to the requests of teachers and reviewers to include new material, and new approaches to this material.

Just as in the first series, each textbook is based on a similar academic formula that combines a comprehensive review of cutting-edge research and professional knowledge with accessible teaching and learning features. The books are also structured so they can be used as an integrated teaching support for a one-term or one-semester course in each of their relevant area of applied psychology. Given the increasing importance of applying psychological knowledge across a growing range of areas of practice, we feel this series is timely and comprehensive. We hope you find each book in the series readable, enlightening, accessible and instructive.

Graham Davey
University of Sussex, Brighton, UK
August 2014

PREFACE

Counselling Psychology is an applied psychology which involves both practice and research. It is broadly similar in nature to clinical psychology, as counselling psychologists work therapeutically with a variety of mental health conditions from the mild and moderate to the severe and enduring. Counselling psychology practice is rooted in empirical research and psychological theory, with professionals being competent in applying the most appropriate psychotherapeutic approach to an individual, couple or group, based on both scientific evidence and individual need.

The purpose of this book is to introduce undergraduate psychology students to the theoretical, practical, research and professional aspects of counselling psychology. Chapters are written by academics and practitioners who have considerable knowledge and professional expertise in their areas of specialism. The book has a mainly UK perspective, however many chapters would be relevant to most countries with international perspectives also being introduced in various sections. The book begins by initially setting the scene and providing the reader with an introduction to counselling psychology (Chapter 1), followed in Section 2 with an insight into the principles and perspectives of counselling psychology, the importance of assessment and formulation as opposed to diagnosis, and to the centrality of the therapeutic relationship (Chapters 2–4). Section 3 of the book then introduces the main theoretical approaches to practice, namely, the humanistic, existential-phenomenological, cognitive-behavioural and psychodynamic approaches (Chapters 5–8). Section 4 focuses upon the personal and professional issues of counselling psychology (Chapters 9 and 10), which include the ethics of practice and the importance of personal development and self-care. Section 5 introduces research and the scientist-practitioner vs reflective-practitioner (Chapters 11 and 12), with attention being paid towards the different types of evidence that can be considered. Finally, Section 6 considers the developments within the profession since its first inception and the importance of the professional body, the role and training of counselling psychologists and associated competencies (Chapters 13–15). Many chapter authors have provided examples from their own personal and/or professional experience(s), which adds richness to the text but also seeks to provide the reader with a sense of the profession as a whole whereby the sense of 'self' of the practitioner is central.

As with all books in the *Topics in Applied Psychology* series, this text is written as a support or a one-term or one-semester course in Counselling Psychology, and contains all the teaching and learning features appropriate to the series, including case histories, focus boxes, research and issues of theoretical, ethical or contemporary interest, and activity boxes that provide the student with the opportunity to engage in active learning. Each chapter also ends with extensive support for further reading, including relevant journal articles, books and websites, and this should enable the interested student to engage with a topic in some depth.

Finally, the over-arching aim of this book is to provide the undergraduate psychology student with a structured introduction to counselling psychology, covering both academic and professional issues. As such it aims to provide an insight into the philosophical underpinnings of counselling psychology, the main theoretical approaches of applied counselling psychology practice and the personal and professional issues which are pertinent to the profession. It is our hope that the reader will be inspired by the various distinct components of the profession.

Victoria Galbraith
British Psychological Society, Leicester and Galbraith Consultancy, UK
November 2016

SECTION 1
Background

1

WHAT IS COUNSELLING PSYCHOLOGY?

Pamela E. James

This initial chapter begins with a description of Counselling Psychology. The rationale for this approach is clear, as when considering the nature of the discipline, it is possible to think about its origins, form, function and future aspirations. Its emergence is reflective and informative as links with philosophy, psychotherapy and psychology are apparent.

Counselling psychology's form and function are included within Chapter 1, but elaborated much further in subsequent chapters. Forward-looking perspectives, for me, must be held in a cultural context. In fact, in a discipline that aims to relate with people where they are currently, then this aspect must always be in focus.

Describing and defining

This question invites the reader to consider a description of this discipline. It is one of the areas of psychology in application that has division status in the British Psychological Society (BPS), along with Clinical, Educational, Forensic, Health, Occupational, Sport and Exercise Psychology. This means that in the BPS, these disciplines each have a training syllabus that defines the material for learning when becoming a qualified psychologist who is eligible to become chartered by the BPS.

Counselling psychology is a helping profession, where the perspective or frame of reference of the *other* (i.e. the people receiving help) is of central value. The helping process occurs in relationship with the other; it is intended to be facilitative rather than giving directives.

Looking further reveals a multi-faceted discipline that reflects to some extent its name, i.e. a joining up of counselling and psychology. However, although this concerns the way in which psychological theories are applied to *enhancing well-being*, there are aspects of the discipline that need further exploration, elaboration and explanation.

Woolfe and Strawbridge (2010) describe counselling psychology as emerging in the context of a humanistic-valuing system. In addition, I am noting (James, 2016: 400) that in the UK the discipline can be seen in:

> the western perspective on the development of the self, acknowledging how learnt experience can affect responses to perceived distress;

the need to examine both old and current relationships between philosophy and psychology;
revisiting the philosophy that states that knowing about a person involves talking to them and hearing their perspective located in context;
sees the person in the context of their relationships in their family and community groups;
and finally, sees the person in the context of the historical perspectives of their current presenting issue, rather than accepting psychopathology.

(Douglas and James, 2014)

Counselling psychology is more than its component parts

If the component parts of psychology and counselling are taken separately, then counselling psychology is more than the sum of its parts. In the 'bringing together' and formation of the discipline taking place in the 1980s and early 1990s, the following are landmark dates:

> In 1982, the BPS Counselling Psychology Section and in 1989, BPS Special Group of Counselling Psychology were set up. In 1989: the BPS Diploma in Counselling Psychology with a training syllabus outlined the learning material for becoming a counselling psychologist who would be eligible for chartered status by the Society. In 1994, full Division Status was achieved. Sections, Special Groups and Divisions represent collections of colleagues; they represent a gradual increase in size and status in the Society.

Consider psychology

Looking firstly at the formation of the discipline of psychology, there were notable figures that carried influence. In the way that a river rises in the hills and picks up smaller streams or tributaries, so the early thinkers about nature of human beings brought their contributions to knowing about mind and behaviour. Reading about the history of psychology and its close association with philosophy, for example, Chung and Hyland (2012), will give a much fuller picture. However, at this point in the chapter, some salient writers are noted. In the 1850s Wilhelm Wundt's (1832–1920) view was that psychology was the study of consciousness. The resulting methodology was self-inquiry or introspection of feelings and experiences. William James (1842–1910) supported the centrality of inter-relationships in subjective experience. Philosophical thinking that accords with these beliefs, namely phenomenology and existentialism was pursued by Husserl (1859–1938); see for example, Polkinghorne (1983). This illustrates the close relationship with philosophy at the source of the river of psychology. Its enquiry or 'need to know' forms the basis of a human science, or human knowledge, where the word *science* comes from 'scio' in Latin, meaning 'I know'; the word *epistemology* means theory of knowledge.

Whilst these tributaries were arising in Europe, at nearly the same time in America, at the inter-face between psychology and sociology, symbolic inter-actionists Charles Cooley (1864–1929) and George Herbert Meade (1863–1931) were thinking about the formation of the self-concept. In this process, these writers both gave credence to place of inter-action with others, language, meaning and self-reflection.

By 1913, with the rise in technology and machinery in different parts of the world, a more mechanistic way of thinking about the nature of human being was developing. John B.

Watson (1878–1958) in America, and Ivan Pavlov (1849–1936), primarily a physiologist, in Russia, both focussed on the study of human behaviour. In bringing this contribution to the stream of psychology, behaviourism comes to the foreground, where the focus of enquiry is observable and measurable behaviour. Skinner (1904–1990) espouses that beliefs in human freedoms actually hold back the science of human behaviour, see Skinner (1971).

The methods of enquiry of natural science, employing positivism, the testing of theories and hypotheses formation, now flow to meet with phenomenology. The forming river of psychology now contains contributions from the study of both mind and behaviour. The reader may wish to pursue finding out the extent to which turbulence and confluence was caused in these earlier years in psychology. However, it is sufficient to note that these founding schools of thought coming from upstream would have their constant repercussions in thinking downstream as seen currently, both in psychology and in counselling psychology.

Turning away from behaviourism, and perhaps in reaction to it, about 40 years later, other notable American psychologists were in the foreground, namely Abraham Maslow (1908–1970) and Carl Rogers (1902–1987). They were speaking and writing about the need to value human beings holistically, not just as behavioural entities, but as sentient beings. These views reflect to some extent the European phenomenological schools of thought. Maslow and Rogers, however, bring *humanism* to the stream of psychology. Humanism is itself described as a philosophy; it upholds the value and agency of human beings. Rogers' (1951) 19 propositions underpin his client-centred theory. This base has been applied to the area of learning (Rogers and Freiberg, 1994); well-being (Rogers, 1961) and inter-personal communication. Although Rogers' work is often described as client-centred (later person-centred) counselling, he used the terms *counselling* and *psychotherapy* interchangeably.

Influence of humanism and other main approaches in the formation of counselling psychology

Rogers applied humanism and its *human valuing and prizing* to working with psychological distress; this begins the formation of the river that becomes counselling and psychotherapy *and* counselling psychology. Hence humanism flows from the main stream of psychology, furrowing its own path and bringing with it all the ideas from upstream. Other major contributions need to be noted as humanism is not the *only* influence in counselling psychology. Looking retrospectively, i.e. at the time of writing this chapter, the discipline has grown and expanded and included other approaches, whilst retaining its emphasis on the other's perspective, seen in context.

Sigmund Freud's (1856–1939) major contribution arising from working with distressed and 'neurotic' people puts forward his theory of personality; a drive theory where sex and aggression play prominent parts, as does the notion of the unconscious mind. Psychoanalysis and its subsequent transitions over recent years to various post-Freudian psychodynamic theories (including object relations theory) formed a major influence on the development of psychotherapy, a 'sister discipline' to counselling psychology.

In actual time, Freud precedes Rogers; both have theories of personality that have been applied to help people and form theories of psychotherapy. These exist in mainstream psychology, and emerge as theories that have their application in working with and to facilitate and help people who are distressed. However, looking back in time, upstream in the psychotherapy river from both Rogers and Freud, there are approaches and schools of psychotherapy that go back hundreds of years, often including more medical views, see Douglas (2014) where she discusses the history of psychotherapy.

Looking forward in time in mainstream psychology, cognitive theorists were beginning to stress their view that human beings' perception of their worlds influenced their thought and that interpretations were made on this basis. In the 1950s cognitive theories were abundant, perhaps as a reaction to or an emergence from behavioural approaches. When applied to helping people, Aaron Beck (1921 [Beck,1967]) and Albert Ellis (1913–2007) are prominent, and in the last decade, cognitive-behaviour therapy came into the foreground. In itself, this view was influenced by the philosophical thinking of Epictetus, in the first century, who said that people are distressed not by the event itself, but by the *view* that they take of this.

ACTIVITY BOX 1.1

Make a list of the major contributors discussed above, from Wundt to Ellis, in chronological order. Include a couple of sentences showing their viewpoints and emphases. Consider the origins and development of counselling psychology.

This spans the years1832–2007. Reflect on developments outside psychology at this time, including science and technology, conflict and war.

Forming and naming counselling psychology

Counselling psychology, currently, employs a broad theoretical basis, and can trace its main influences from mainstream psychology and psychotherapy. Yet how does this discipline actually find form and shape in the early 1980s? Ralph Hetherington (1983: 7), then President of the BPS, writes:

> The Section came into being at a time when . . . counselling as an enterprise has sadly lacked a coherent theoretical foundation and equally seriously has lacked systematic evaluation. There has been no lack of interest in the development of a large number of psychotherapies for people with problems which make them unable to cope with life unaided. These are the clients which doctors might be disposed to call 'neurotic', while for psychologists the important factor would be the client's inability to cope.

This illustrates an aspect of the nature of the Society's view; however the discipline's emergence is attributed to the thinking, discussing and reflecting of early counselling psychologists such as Strawbridge and Woolfe, and those others who had the reflective capacity and awareness to see that within psychology at that time, there was a tendency to view and work with people objectively. This approach almost disregarded the emphasis within psychology on consciousness and subjectivity. The relationship between mind and body, its potential for separateness and reconciliation, and its philosophical underpinning as seen by Descartes (1596–1650) has been threaded through psychology since its inception.

With the advent of the influence of humanism and its principles in the 1960s and 1970s, possibly here was an opportunity to take a more *holistic relational view* as to the nature of human beings. Looking back, the writer suggests that the ground was then prepared for forming a nucleus of like-minded psychologists who wanted to work and think in this way. The concept of psychology as an applied therapeutic science gradually now begins to emerge; the description *scientific practitioner* begins to be used. The chapter by Strawbridge and Woolfe (2003) is helpful in providing a fuller discussion of this development; see also Chapter 11 in this text.

However, its *naming* was a matter of considerable discussion at the time. It has been said in informal discussions that in choosing the word *counselling* in conjunction with psychology, that the potential for confusion began to occur. This debate has stayed with counselling psychology. It can be clearly seen from the above discussion, that this discipline arose from within mainstream psychology; it can also be seen that the contributions from psychologists were also psychotherapists. Whilst Rogers is usually seen as holding the primary influential position, Freud, Ellis, Beck and their subsequent associated theorists, are also representatives of the main schools of thought.

In the writers' view, it is argued that the origins of UK counselling psychology as a psychotherapeutic application of psychology have been influenced by its underlying European philosophers who were so formative in the development of psychology, and that the philosophy of humanism and its American influence from Rogers' practice of client-centred therapy has played a major part. The word *counselling* could be seen as a celebration of the major contribution from Rogers.

ACTIVITY BOX 1.2

Think about the naming of counselling psychology. What other name would you propose and why?

Explore, describe, reflect and evaluate, rather than compare and compete

Looking at the formation of UK counselling psychology, it is possible to see the rationale for the current training syllabus content. It is also possible to see how tensions and turbulence can arise in possible contradictions of approaches to which theory of helping is most beneficial and which has the evidence base to support the view. However, the writer would encourage the reader not to be lost in comparisons and competitions, but to think and walk more freely in the area of exploration and reflective thought, where different views can be tolerated whilst holding central a valuing of the other person's freedom and frame of reference. The most predominantly helpful in outcomes from a meta-analysis of research studies points to the therapeutic relationship (Wampold, 2015).

Philosophy, psychology and counselling psychology

It could be said that the philosophical approaches acted as the *catalyst* and as *glue* that provided a rationale as to how and why psychology has been applied in this way, how it could and should be brought together with psychotherapy.

ACTIVITY BOX 1.3

Reflect on the parts of the undergraduate psychology syllabus that have particular resonance with counselling psychology, as summarised below.

Counselling psychology arises from *within* the development of psychology, and also from *outside* psychology, namely from philosophy, sociology and psychotherapy. Yet in their combination and confluence come tensions as well as advantages. One point of view is that it heals the apparent rift between philosophy and a more positivist scientific psychology. However, today in psychology itself, there is gradual welcoming of a mixed methods approach to answering research questions, not just a strict, sole adherence to the experimental method. The rationale for the practice of counselling psychology is more rooted in human science; human beings are seen to exist in relationship. The rationale for the research methods of counselling psychology finds support in both phenomenology and positivism.

Overlapping and neighbouring disciplines

The origins and development of counselling psychology show the relationship with psychotherapy and counselling. Although there are marked differences, these disciplines share many theories in application and relational stance. The observable practice of some counselling psychologists is synonymous with some psychotherapists. Within the BPS there is a Register of Psychologists who specialise in Psychotherapy. Many counselling psychologists have counselling training and are accredited by the BPS *and* a counselling and psychotherapy profession, namely the British Association for Counselling and Psychotherapy (BACP), British Association for Behavioural Counselling and Psychotherapy (BABCP), and United Kingdom Council for Psychotherapy (UKCP).

There are also overlaps within the application of psychology itself, i.e. with clinical and health psychology. Whilst clinical and counselling psychologists share nearly all the same competences, (see BPS, 2016a, 2016b) the origins and development of counselling psychology are particular, its philosophical emphasis on relational aspects being central. These can be seen in approaches to the following factors.

The use of measurement, psychometrics; perspectives on symptoms and diagnosis; and the focus on relationships

Measurement: initially in the 1980s, psychometrics was seldom used when seeing clients with mental health issues. Measuring was viewed as seeing a person nomothetically, as an objective entity able to receive a score on a valid and reliable scale. Over the last 30 years, counselling psychologists now see the value of some psychometric tests; they can be used therapeutically, and also to obtain a score which may then result in the client being eligible for a resource. For example, clients' distress post-trauma can be assessed using the Impact of Events (R) scale. If the concept of diagnosis is employed, i.e. post-traumatic stress disorder, this can result in financial benefits. The use of psychometrics would always be in the context of the relationship and in the meeting time with the client.

FOCUS BOX 1.1

One particular area of psychometric measurement, arising from neuroscience, has contributed to understanding a person's cognitive functioning, most usually employed when there are functional difficulties. This is termed *neuropsychology*. Historically, counselling psychologists have not been active in this area, however, with the need to provide the most informed client assessment possible, more training and interest is emerging in relation to counselling psychology. Fairfax (2016) describes his training experience and points out that the application of this knowledge may include both psychometric tests and skilled observations of difficulties arising from, for example, Parkinson's or epilepsy. How the person *feels and thinks* about, and is affected by, their neurological conditions is an integral part of their holistic lived experience.

Diagnosis: this is one of the critical tensions, as seeing psychological distress as symptoms that can be categorised is not in keeping with a belief system about people that sees each as an individual to be appreciated in terms of their uniqueness, in their relational context; see Douglas and James (2014) for a fuller discussion. A preferred response is *assessment* and *formulation*. The BPS (2014a op. cit.: 20) now takes the following stance on diagnosis:

FOCUS BOX 1.2

4.6 When applying, or referring to, diagnostic terms, psychologists will recognise that these refer to disorder labels that have been assigned to the clinical features shown by service users and will be cognisant of the limitations in reliability and validity of diagnostic systems, especially in relation to functional psychiatric disorders. They will recognise the benefits that may accrue from a diagnosis for some people, such as access to specialist services, or from the 'understanding' that clients or others may derive from the diagnosis, but will also be mindful of the potential harm that can result from the use of diagnostic labels, particularly the risk of "pathologising" the individual.

The focus on relationship: this has philosophical significance as explained above. It also has theoretical meaning, as there is a belief that disturbance occurs in the relational domain. This can present both inter-subjectively and intra-subjectively. See Box 1.4 for an example of this.

ACTIVITY BOX 1.4

Mike had been in a job that he enjoyed for the past 12 years. There was a re-organisation at work and he found that he had two weeks' notice. He went into a deep depression and was aware of the following symptoms: early waking, irritability and loss of appetite. His GP prescribed anti-depressants; he also referred him to see a CBT therapist, who worked with Mike's symptoms of irritability. His core belief 'try hard and you'll get rewarded' had been challenged by his loss of job. Over a six-week period, Mike became less depressed, but he couldn't find the motivation to look for another job; he sometimes felt suicidal. He returned to his GP and went on a waiting list to see a counselling psychologist.

Following assessment, Mike's anger at his job loss was acknowledged, not only towards his employer (inter-subjectively), but also towards himself (intra-subjectively). He self-blamed and eventually said he was embarrassed that he had not seen this coming. He felt guilt and shame as in his family's eyes, he was the bread-winner.

This more in-depth work, unveiling the associated feelings resulted in Mike's being energised to seek another job. He had more self-understanding and insight; his symptoms lifted.

Although he could still become annoyed about what had happened, he said that he felt he had been acknowledged in the therapy.

Comment on the role that therapy played here.

Counselling psychology is an applied discipline

How is it applied?

This means that the discipline has a functional significance. Put more simply, it can be applied to help people towards psychological well-being. Principles of the manner of relating are transferable to different inter-personal situations; this discipline accepts a number of theories that can guide the therapeutic relationship. Theories provide frameworks, an evidence base and a rationale to guide the ways in which the therapeutic relationship is conducted. This can be described as 'being with' another person, empathically and unconditionally. One person (the therapist) can *sit with* or *be with* another person (the client). The concept of ontology has relevance here as the science of *being*.

ACTIVITY BOX 1.5

Comment on the meaning and relevance of ontology to counselling psychology.

The discipline of counselling psychology includes theories that also guide what the therapist *does*. In its quest for an informed evidence base for the therapeutic relationship, it does *not* uphold a manner or attitude of the therapist that might see or relate to the client as an *object*, and is not appreciative of the unique quality of a person's experience. Consequently, a person's thoughts, feelings and experiences are all of value, whether in the present or in the past.

Research methodologies

Evidence that supports the way in which the helping process is conducted comes from researching two main approaches: phenomenology and positivism. Phenomenology holds the view that knowledge about people comes from talking to them about their experiences (experiential). This standpoint then guides the way in which information is collected, which is described as its *methodology*. The experiential or phenomenological approach is one of the main parts of *the base* for the discipline of counselling psychology. It follows that human experience is valued in guiding both the therapeutic relationship and the research methodology.

Whilst phenomenological approaches are more akin to the philosophy of counselling psychology, the scientific method from the discipline of psychology encompasses a *positivist* perspective. This is not excluded by the counselling psychologist; it is appreciated *yet in tension*. Counselling psychology's research base contains outcomes from the testing of hypotheses (a positivist methodological approach) *as well as* from experiential studies. Consequently, a research evidence base has been formed which contains findings that are from different philosophical standpoints, informing both evidence-based practice and practice-based evidence. Corrie (2010) writes about the wide range of data that constitute an evidence base. The process of theory testing is a constant cycle of collecting evidence and refining theories. You will identify this process in other parts of your studies in psychology. It follows then that the therapies that are applied come from a theoretical base, supported by evidence.

What is applied?

This has led therapists to pose the question, which therapy shall I learn about and practice? *Therapy* leads on as a consequence of the *theory* or approach on which it is based. As the philosophy of counselling psychology supports the acceptance of a critical reflective stance, then a range of theories (and therapies) is permitted, providing that they have an evidence base. The counselling psychologist is a reflective-practitioner; client work is taken to regular supervision, both individually and in peer groups.

Most usually, underlying belief and value systems form the basis for resulting behaviours and action. Although value systems develop individually for each person, when considered collectively and in a professional context, these form *ethical codes*. These guide the applications of disciplines; counselling psychologists are bound by the codes of statutory regulation of the Health and Care Professions Council (HCPC), the British Psychological Society (BPS) and the BPS Division of Counselling Psychology Guidelines for Professional Practice in Counselling Psychology.

In Section 3 of this text, four main approaches are discussed, forming focal points around which theories and therapies cluster. Each approach holds an explanation of how people experience their life events and relationships, and the effect this has on them. The words *paradigm* and *approach* are used in texts that discuss and describe counselling psychology. Although these words have slightly different meanings, the wish is to convey a collection of knowledge. There are other approaches and therapies that are not included in this text, e.g. systemic family therapy and gestalt therapy. Integrating concepts from different therapies is also tolerated and recognised as inevitable. As therapists become more experienced, they find value in taking concepts from different theories and approaches and forming integrative therapies.

The underlying philosophy of counselling psychology provides the steer to give direction to the way in which different approaches and their therapies are useful in action. Epistemology (as for any discipline) is the philosophical analysis of the nature of knowledge and how it relates to connected notions such as truth, belief and justification. It refers to the compiling of a knowledge base and can give meaning to what counselling psychologists do and the way that they do it when working with people. Without this *steer*, a counselling psychologist in practice might find themselves in an epistemological wilderness, a place of not knowing why a particular therapy might be part of their (usable) knowledge base. The training syllabus to be a counselling psychologist is clearly an essential place where the learning material for the profession is stored; this is discussed and described later in this chapter.

Why is it applied and to whom?

The application of therapy is to facilitate a person's well-being. Counselling psychology is referred to as a helping profession. For someone to require (therapeutic) help in this way there is an assumption that they are in some state of need. The types of need refer to psychological distress, i.e. perceived mental distress. A typical case load could include people who have a range of issues, including anxiety, depression, relationship problems, work-place stress and the effects of trauma, loss, separation and bereavement. The range of experienced difficulty within each of these issues is sometimes described as being from mild to moderate and then severe. Chapter 15 in this text looks at this in more detail.

The 'hoped for' outcomes of therapy are that the person will have more insight into their issues and themselves as a part of the process of distress; their symptoms will be more manageable or no longer present; they will be clearer about what can be changed and what is not able to be changed, what kind of on-going support might be needed. These outcomes are in contrast to a more medical model approach that seeks a 'cure'.

FOCUS BOX 1.3

Differences in the use of language between the medical model and the therapeutic model:

> Language from a medical professional e.g. GP or psychiatrist is more likely to refer to symptoms that may lead to a diagnosis requiring treatment with the hope of working towards a removal of symptoms or cure.
>
> Language from a therapist, e.g. counselling psychologist is more likely to refer to distress and how it might be understood in relationship, leading to insight, self-empowerment, a knowledge of what might be changed and what might need to be managed in the future.

Symptoms may be assessed and measured using psychometric tests, for example, the Patient Health Questionnaire (PHQ-9).

Other types of need refer to being supported or coached when on a particular task. Interestingly, in 2000, a group of psychologists separated from the original core group of counselling psychologists to form the BPS Special Group in Coaching Psychology as a separate discipline.

Other applications of psychology refer to leadership, management and supervision which are discussed later in this chapter.

Pathways towards help

Let's consider the first of these, psychological distress which is experienced by a person as 'needing help'. Of course, many people experience distress and do not contact the professional services; they may prefer to talk with friends and family, or work the issues out themselves. In some cases, sitting alone with psychological distress can result in more upset in the long-term. For example, when a person has a road accident with resulting flashbacks and nightmares hopes they will eventually recede, only to find that these are getting more frequent.

The described pathways towards professional help are complex and varied. The starting point is often with the general practitioner (GP) who acts like a signpost towards a *talking* therapist. Presenting psychological distress in the current National Health Service (NHS) procedure is referred to a psychological therapist who will be probably located in an Improving Access to Psychological Therapy (IAPT) Service. The most common presenting issues are depression and anxiety. The waiting times are variable and could be up to six months.

Access to a counselling psychologist in the NHS is more likely when the distress that presents is moderate or more severe, as described by Douglas and James (2014). The NHS pathway to access a counselling psychologist is again variable and may depend on the availability of services in the particular Trust. For example, issues associated with eating or trauma or personality described as borderline would be referred to Adult Mental Health; issues with children and adolescents to Child and Family Mental Health Services (CAMHS); issues for people with learning disabilities would be referred accordingly.

However, outside the NHS, counselling psychologists are on professional body lists and directories, also with agencies that are accessible for insurance company funded referrals, and employee assistance programmes. The types of presenting issues forming the content of self or agency referral is open to the full range of presenting psychological problems. Counselling psychologists working outside the NHS are often independent practitioners. They see a wide range of presenting issues that come from individuals, couples and organisations. The NHS counselling psychologist, who works in a named part of the organisation, will meet and work with people who have similar reasons for their referral. In contrast, counselling psychologists working as independent practitioners are likely to receive referrals from a number of sources.

Each person's experience is unique and the philosophical and theoretical stance of the counselling psychologist guides their practice. Some people experience their difficulties in a way that results in their not being able to cope in the community and at this time, they may need to be in an in-patient psychiatric unit. For example, someone who is severely depressed and has suicidal intention would most probably need the support of psychiatric services. This means that the counselling psychologist must be aware of the need to refer to, liaise and work with other professionals in the care of the client.

ACTIVITY BOX 1.6

Comment on the potential difficulties of this complex pattern of pathways to help.

How many counselling psychologists are there?

At the time of writing this chapter, there are approximately 1,700 counselling psychologists in the United Kingdom who have the necessary statutory registration with the Health and Care Professions Council. Fifteen hundred of these psychologists also have chartered status with the British Psychological Society. Chapter 9 in this text describes this professional membership more fully. However, in this chapter it can be noted that according to recent surveys carried out by the Division of Counselling Psychology (unpublished), about half of the total number of counselling psychologists work either within or outside the NHS. In the current climate within the NHS where there are scarce resources, people with mild and moderate psychological distress (often expressed as anxiety and depression) are seen by mental health professionals whose salary is less than a psychologist. Consequently, more counselling psychologists are seeking employment (including self-employment) outside the NHS; they have different income streams as a result of having a mix of part-time strands to their work, as discussed in Chapter 15.

Training: what is the syllabus?

The reader will have had clues in the earlier parts of this chapter regarding what is to be included in the training syllabus: the BPS Accredited Standards for Doctoral Training (BPS 2016a) gives the full outline; training is discussed in Chapter 14 of this text. It is delivered at 13 UK Universities and also via the Society's Qualification (full details can be accessed from the BPS website).

The need for and purpose of an underlying philosophy and value-base has been discussed and also the theoretical approaches. The syllabus states a minimum of two theories to the standard of ability to practice. Acquiring further theoretical knowledge is clearly the remit of the counselling psychologist, whether in their original accredited training, or in continuous professional development (CPD). An ability to use appropriate skills (both spoken and unspoken) and to express these in a manner which values and respects the client in the therapeutic relationship is essential. At least 450 hours of supervised practice in a range of settings is required.

Training requires knowing how to assess clients describing their issues in a way that provides a psychological outline known as a formulation. This process strives to maintain a respectful valuing of each person. It may include using psychometric tests to provide a structured measuring of an expressed psychological state, for example, depression (Beck's Depression Scale) or post-trauma (IoE R Scale) or a neurological test (Wechsler Adult Intelligence Scale, WAIS) to assess intellectual ability. The trainee will learn to liaise with other colleagues in a multi-disciplinary environment. In keeping with current professional change, the concepts and skills required for leadership, supervision and management are now part of the syllabus. The ability to conduct and review research as well as being able to evaluate the process and outcomes of therapy are also essential. The trainee is also required to undergo their own personal therapy so that their personal dynamics and issues are known and are hence less likely to become entwined unknowingly into client work. As not every aspect of all situations can be encompassed, there is an emphasis on transferable skills so that when newly qualified, there is maximum opportunity for flexibility.

One of the particular elements of training is the capacity to tolerate situations where there is no clear answer, whether to clients' situations, differences of professional opinion or dilemmas that arise when contrasting views are expressed. This is the expectancy of a doctoral training, including an ability to critically evaluate evidence. Of particular emphasis is the need for a constant awareness of the diversity of each person along all dimensions of difference (for example, gender, sexuality, ethnicity, learning difficulty, religious beliefs, sexual orientation, etc.), so that non-discrimination is an intrinsic and extrinsic element of practice.

As the qualified counselling psychologist is likely over time to work in a range of settings, the training provides a sufficient knowledge base to begin employment. The preferred manner of practice is to *build on* many new learning experiences. These are found in discussion with professional colleagues, supervision, CPD and client work. This attitude to the professional role is described as reflective practice. Working in the scope and extent of competence is a necessary aspect of practice. For example, working with children or couples without some training input in this area might result in being *outside* competences. There is some tension here, as much of the counselling psychologists' skills and knowledge base is transferable across clients and situations.

Having adaptable, transferable knowledge and skills

An awareness of the adaptability of knowledge, skills, relational stance and research skills, combined with continuously following CPD that fits a meaningful framework, facilitates the counselling psychologist across employment settings. This repertoire can be transferred to management roles, teaching and training. Setting up in independent practice will require additional business skills to assist financial matters (e.g. tax, insurance and invoicing), drawing up contracts, making connections and tendering for potential income streams and possibly renting rooms.

Leadership competences are now part of the training syllabus and seen as the ability to articulate the discipline and speak in professional settings regarding client work as well as leading teams and managing services. Applying for management positions is sought by those who want to extend their job roles beyond therapy. The manner and attitude when managing people can be guided by the skills learnt when training as a therapist. To teach and train potential counselling psychologists it will be helpful and sometimes necessary to have a teaching qualification.

Counselling psychology: international perspectives

Counselling psychology exists as a discipline in different parts of the world. However, did it emerge in each country as an application of psychology or did one country influence another? The writer has considered an answer to this question which is discussed in James (2016). To look into each country across the globe would be too great a task for this chapter, but some themes can be noted. Western countries and those that have associations with the West, such as America, Canada, Ireland, Greece and Australia, have all applied psychology in a similar way to that described in the UK. Here, the concept of the self and its development, the belief that an individual's distress is helped by self-understanding, insight and self-actualisation is a shared theme. However, in Africa and Eastern countries, counselling psychology is more associated with helping distressed people by strengthening their community ties.

When counselling psychologists from Western countries have travelled to those areas of the East, after a disaster, e.g. after tsunamis and earthquakes, helping to re-build communities has been more helpful than individual therapy. It is particularly necessary to consider the culture in which the person was brought up as this will have an influence on beliefs about the nature of distress and the response to it. All human beings have relational ties, and when these are disrupted then distress occurs. It seems that the response to that distress can differ across the globe, regarding whether one-to-one and family talking therapies are helpful, or whether rebuilding community groups and their relationships is preferred.

These reflections will probably be further developed over future years, but for now, let's return to the UK and think about counselling psychology in this country. In the UK, the writer has discussed how the discipline has emerged and developed, bringing together not only humanistic valuing from the work of Rogers in America, but also the influence of European philosophers writing about the self.

As people we have an emotional response to what happens, whether sad, happy, angry or jealous. These feelings may or may not be disclosed, sometimes due to shame, guilt and embarrassment. The part played by emotion and its related thought cannot be over-looked by a helping profession and counselling psychology is well placed to take these concepts forward into research and practice in the years to come.

Future indications

- To work with and in the field of mental health, emphasising that disturbance is both inter- and intra-relational. This is in tension with those approaches in psychiatry that view mental health issues as medical and or physiological and seek a cure of symptoms;
- To keep psychology in touch with the study of both mind and behaviour;
- To keep in mind and work with other professionals on its appreciation of the perspective or *frame of reference of the other* as an essential aspect of all helping relationships.

Learning outcomes

When you have completed this chapter you should:

- Be able to describe and discuss philosophical approaches that have influenced and had impact on the formation of counselling psychology.
- Be able to describe and define counselling psychology.
- Be able to name and briefly describe the main theories in counselling psychology.
- Be able to discuss and describe the meaning of the therapeutic relationship in counselling psychology.
- Be able to define epistemology, ontology, phenomenology, positivism.
- Be able to distinguish between evidence-based practice and practice-based evidence.
- To know where, when, how and with whom counselling psychology is practised.
- Be able to distinguish counselling psychology from clinical psychology, coaching and mentorship.

Key concepts

- Assessment
- Be with
- Being

- Counselling
- Diagnosis
- Enhancing well-being
- Ethical codes
- Focus on relationship
- Formulation
- Frame of reference of the other
- Holistic relational view
- Human valuing
- Humanism
- Measurement
- Methodology
- Naming
- Other
- Positivist
- Prizing
- Scientific practitioner
- Sit with
- Theory
- Therapy

Sample essay titles

1. Describe and discuss the development of UK counselling psychology.
2. To what extent is the therapeutic relationship essential to the counselling psychology profession?

References

Beck, A. T. (1967) *The Diagnosis and Management of Depression.* Philadelphia, PA: University of Pennsylvania Press.

British Psychological Society (2016a) *Standards of Accreditation and Training in Counselling Psychology.* Leicester: British Psychological Society.

British Psychological Society (2016b) *Standards of Accreditation and Training in Clinical Psychology.* Leicester: British Psychological Society.

Chung, M. C. and Hyland, M. E. (2012) *History and Philosophy of Psychology.* Hoboken, NJ: Wiley-Blackwell.

Corrie, S. (2010) What Is Evidence?, in R. Woolfe, S. Strawbridge, B. Douglas and W. Dryden (eds.), *The Sage Handbook of Counselling Psychology*, 3rd edition (pp. 62–82). London: Sage.

Douglas, B. (2014) Chapter 1: Introduction, in B. Douglas and P. E. James (eds.), *Common Presenting Issues in Psychotherapeutic Practice* (pp. 1–18). London: Sage.

Douglas, B. and James, P. E. (2014) *Common Presenting Issues in Psychotherapeutic Practice.* London: Sage.

Fairfax, H. (2016) Chapter 21: Neuropsychology and Counselling Psychology, in B. Douglas, R. Woolfe, S. Strawbridge, E. Kasket and V. Galbraith (eds.), *The Handbook of Counselling Psychology* (4th edition, pp. 511–529). London: Sage.

Hetherington, R. (1983) Letter included in the Counselling Psychology Section January Newsletter, Vol. 1 (2), Published by the British Psychological Society.

James, P. E. (2016) Chapter 24: Counselling Psychology and Its International Dimensions, in B. Douglas, R. Woolfe, S. Strawbridge, E. Kasket and V. Galbraith (eds.), *The Handbook of Counselling Psychology* (4th edition, pp. 399–414). London: Sage.

Polkinghorne, D. E. (1983) Phenomenological Research Methods, in R. S. Valle and S. Halling (eds.) *Existential-Phenemenological Perspectives in Psychology* (pp. 41–60). New York: Plenum.

Rogers, C. R. (1951) *Client-Centered Therapy: Its Current Practice, Implications and Theory*. London: Constable.

Rogers, C. R. (1961) *On Becoming a Person*. London: Constable.

Rogers, C. R. and Freiberg, H. J. (1994) *Freedom to Learn*, 3rd edition. Upper Saddle River, NJ: Prentice Hall.

Skinner, B. F. (1971) *Beyond Freedom and Dignity*. Indianapolis, IN: Hackett Publishing Company Inc.

Strawbridge, S. and Woolfe, R. (2003) Chapter 1: Counselling Psychology in Context, in R. Woolfe, W. Dryden and S. Strawbridge (eds.), *The Handbook of Counselling Psychology* (2nd edition, pp. 3–22). London: Sage.

Wampold, B. E. (2015) How Important Are the Common Factors in Psychotherapy? An Update. *World Psychiatry*. 14(3): 270–277.

Woolfe, R. and Strawbridge, S. (2010) Chapter 1: Counselling Psychology: Origins, Developments and Challenges, in R. Woolfe, S. Strawbridge, B. Douglas and W. Dryden (eds.), *The Sage Handbook of Counselling Psychology* (3rd edition, pp. 3–25). London: Sage.

Journals and Journal articles

Applied Psychology (2011) G. C. Davey (Editor) Wiley-Blackwell: This text has on-line pages for Counselling Psychology: http://tinyurl.com/c3ztvtj.

BPS Publication: Counselling Psychology Review.

The European Journal of Counselling Psychology.

Special Issue: A Global Portrait of Counselling Psychology (2016) *Counselling Psychology Quarterly*: Volume 29, Issue 2.

SECTION 2

Principles of clinical practice

2

ASSESSMENT AND FORMULATION IN COUNSELLING PSYCHOLOGY

Jane Simms

Assessment and formulation skills are the hallmarks of competent and ethical practice. This chapter will explore the role of assessment and formulation in detail and show how it can be undertaken in a manner that upholds the humanistic ethos and philosophy of counselling psychology. An overview of these concepts and their definition will be provided. Whilst many modalities undergo assessment processes such as couples, children and the family, the focus of this chapter will be on the individual.

Introduction to assessment and formulation

The word 'assessment' comes from the Latin word *assessus* meaning 'to sit by' or 'to sit beside' (Ruddel, 1997). Yet, it is a term typically associated with judgement and opinion, and as such it has been quite a contentious issue in the field of counselling generally especially within the humanistic approaches (Foster, 2013; Simms, 2011; Bertolino & O'Hanlon, 2002; Ruddel, 1997). Similarly, assessment may seem at odds with the therapeutic practice of counselling psychology, as the core values of the profession are the prizing of client autonomy, personal meaning and subjectivity. However, assessment is an essential feature of counselling psychology practice and is a core competency that trainees are expected to demonstrate and qualified practitioners engage in routinely.

Formulation follows the assessment process. It is typically theory driven and is a method by which both client and therapist can try to make sense of the processes that have led to the client's particular difficulties in terms of how they began and what factors are maintaining them. Thus, information gathered at assessment is pieced together to gain an understanding of the client's difficulties and is informed by a particular theoretical framework that guides intervention. It helps the client and therapist create a coherent and holistic picture of the difficulties he or she is experiencing, for example, particular thinking patterns, negative life events, emotional and behavioural reactions and how these may interact. Furthermore, it serves as a blueprint or map in guiding therapy, and acts as a marker for change (Eells, 2007). Without an assessment and formulation framework, the process of therapy could be chaotic, confusing and in extreme cases, even harmful (Berman, 2015).

REFLECTIVE PAUSE

What do the terms 'assessment' and 'formulation' conjure up for you?

Understanding the process of assessment in counselling psychology practice

Counselling Psychologists in training must demonstrate their capacity to undertake client assessment. Assessment and the natural follow on, case formulation, are amongst the required learning outcomes during Doctoral training (BPS, 2015). For qualified practitioners registered with the Health and Care Professions Council, assessment and formulation are required standards of proficiency (HCPC, 2015).

Client assessment is the first part of the client's therapeutic journey and as such, it is a critical feature of the therapeutic process. It is the first opportunity the client has to meet the therapist, to be heard and understood. It may be the first time they have ever told their story and understandably may be feeling very anxious and uncertain as to the process that is about to unfold or they may be unsure if therapy is actually right for them. Attending to the client in an empathic manner and establishing trust at this stage is crucial as, without these features, it can lead to disengagement (Ruddel, 1997). Assessment is also a two-way process as the therapist has to gain as full an understanding as possible of the client's difficulties, which means that there is inevitably a degree of judgement required in the process. Churchill (2011) points out how we make judgements regardless of whether we realise it or not through the act of perception, which entails classifying information. Therefore, assessment will inevitably involve a degree of clinical judgement and in many instances it is essential. For example, part of the initial assessment process is assessing for risk. If the client is actively suicidal or severely depressed to the extent that their ability to think, comprehend and retain information is compromised; or they are abusing alcohol and turning up to appointments intoxicated, then a clinical decision has to be made as to their suitability for therapy and whether alternative sources of support may be available and more appropriate to meet the client's needs. To engage a person in therapy when they do not have the internal or external resources to cope or the motivation to engage may be confusing and harmful (Bennett, 2003).

The process of assessment serves a number of purposes. Firstly, information gathered helps both therapist and client to get a sense of how their difficulties have emerged. Clients often present with a sense of confusion as to why they are experiencing distressing thoughts, feelings and behaviours and an assessment can help them focus on what may seem like a bewildering, even frightening set of problems and their impact (Ruddel, 1997; Williams, Edwards, Patterson & Chamow, 2011). Secondly, assessment provides an opportunity for the client to piece together what may seem like disjointed and fragmented parts of their life history into a cohesive narrative that can provide a sense of clarity. Thirdly, it helps the client decide what help they are looking for and why now thus facilitating the client's self-awareness (Foster, 2013; Churchill, 2011). For the therapist, it enables various factors to be weighed up such as risk issues, motivation, suitability and type of intervention (Bager-Charleson & Van Rijn, 2013). In addition, it can enhance reflective practice as it can serve as a means to evaluate change. Furthermore, it is an opportunity to provide a safe, secure, welcoming, warm and empathic space that will set the scene for the development of a collaborative therapeutic relationship, strong working alliance and a clear idea for the client of what to expect in the coming weeks or months. Finally, the process of assessment enables the client to gain acknowledgement and validation of their experiences which, through being heard and understood, can have a profoundly therapeutic effect in its own right (Bertolino & O'Hanlon, 2002). It should provide a sense of hope that their distress can be alleviated and that change is possible. Research shows the importance of hope and expectancy in positive outcome (Assay & Lambert, 1999; Lambert, 1992).The importance of conducting an assessment skilfully, respectfully, empathically, whilst instilling hope cannot be overestimated as it acts as the doorway into therapy and can influence process and outcome. Therefore, the process of assessment and psychological therapy are inextricably linked (Goldman, 1971).

Assessment and counselling psychology values

Strawbridge and Woolfe (2010) define counselling psychology as being rooted in humanistic values and human potential, which advocates the role of self-determination and fulfilment of potential of the client, irrespective of the difficulties the person is experiencing. The subjective experience of the client is paramount and prized at all stages of the therapeutic journey and this is especially so at the initial stage of assessment. According to the authors, counselling psychology does not necessarily differ markedly from how other medical and psychological methods and approaches attempt to understand human problems. They contend that what makes counselling psychology unique is its emphasis upon a holistic and developmental view of the individual's life and the philosophical stance it embraces in attempting to understand the person, which inevitably includes the biological, social, economic and political context within which the individual resides. It is essentially relational and dialogical in its approach and emphasises the importance of *being with* the client and *being-in-relation* rather than focusing upon intervening or *doing something to* the client (Strawbridge & Woolfe, 2003). This implies that the self of the therapist is part of the process. Assessment marks the beginning of the therapeutic journey and as both client and therapist are fellow travellers both bring aspects of the self to the encounter (Yalom, 2001). They are what Calhoun and Tedeschi (1999) refer to as *expert companions*. Upholding these values and this ethos and philosophy of the profession is essential but can also be challenging as counselling psychologists work across a broad and diverse range of contexts, which bring with them competing philosophies, ethos and understanding of human distress and methods by which to make sense of it (Douglas, 2010).

Core assessment skills

Conducting an assessment requires a broad range of skills in its own right as it is both a fact-finding process, yet, at the same time, an opportunity to establish the therapeutic relationship. This requires a range of interpersonal and communication skills. An assessment is typically face-to-face and the type of structure will depend on the agency setting, the therapist style and theoretical orientation (Bager-Charleson & Van Rijn, 2013). The format can range from being highly structured, moderate or non-structured. Counselling psychologists would most likely work within a moderately structured format, which allows for key questions to be asked, specific areas to be explored but has a high degree of flexibility to accommodate the unique nature of the client's story and their subjective experience. This flexibility is crucial as

BOX 2.1 CORE ASSESSMENT SKILLS

Core skill	*Features*
Attending	Eye contact, vocal tone, attentive body language, verbal tracking, distance, silence.
Active Listening	Observing verbal and non-verbal behaviour, encouraging, paraphrasing, summarising, reflection of feelings, eye contact.
Questioning	Open, closed, socratic, probing.
Empathy	Paraphrasing, reflecting feelings, rephrase, perception check, caring, supportive.
Congruence	Non-defensive, warmth, without façade, internal thoughts and feelings match external communication.
Concreteness	Focus on facts and feelings related to client's issues, maintaining here and now focus, identifying and addressing specific concerns.
Respect	Eliminate negative and judgemental language, self-awareness of own views, do not interrupt, show interest and appreciation.
Self-attending	Self-awareness, centring, relaxing, non-judgemental attitude.
Cultural competency	Knowledge of diversity, anti-discriminatory practices.
Confrontation	Challenging, reframing,
Immediacy	Awareness of non-verbal behaviours, meaning behind what is spoken, attentive sensitive, acting on intuition.
Termination	Reviewing, reminding, understanding of meaning of ending,

it enables the client to participate in the process and promotes a collaborative relationship thus minimising any potential power dynamics (Churchill, 2011).

A core skill of assessment is being able to contain as well as listen and to strike the right balance between the two (Bager-Charleson & Van Rijn, 2011). Being able to manage time, keep the conversation focused, gather sufficient and relevant information, yet not delve too deeply into a particular issue or area so as not to overwhelm the client initially, and create a safe and trusting environment is crucial. Combined with this is having the capacity to be accurately empathic and to be able to communicate empathic understanding, to elicit and understand the client's personal meanings and to communicate unconditional positive regard (Hargie, 2011; Ruddel, 1997). Box 2.1 outlines a range of assessment skills which need to be adopted by the practitioner in order to conduct an assessment that is focused and containing for the client; for example, skills in questioning, explaining, probing, active listening, reflecting, paraphrasing and closure.

The task is to *'sit by'* the client and *'be with'* in order to gather the relevant information that will help guide the therapeutic journey. As highlighted, this *'being with'* stance is one that is regarded as a hallmark of counselling psychology practice and is what will make the client's assessment a therapeutic experience as opposed to an interview that could be experienced as cold, detached and mechanistic. This latter approach is what Ruddel (1997) highlights as being 'outside the client's frame of reference', which could potentially compromise the development of the therapeutic relationship. Therefore, the client's subjective experience and personal meanings are essential features of assessment.

Assessment as a therapeutic experience

The term 'therapeutic assessment' may be a more helpful way to consider assessment within counselling psychology practice, as the process of assessment, which if undertaken in a caring, empathic and compassionate manner, has the potential to be a positive and affirmative experience in its own right. Bager-Charleson and Van Rijn (2011) highlight how assessment can provide clients with an opportunity to reflect on their difficulties in a contained but supportive and empathic manner, which can bring a sense of relief. The assessment process with its emphasis upon containment can help the client feel that their difficulties are manageable and enable them to develop the capacity for insight as they begin to piece their story together in a coherent narrative. Focus Box 2.1 outlines a case example of a client referred with trauma symptoms, who, as part of the assessment process gained understanding into the impact of the many traumatic losses she had experienced during her life.

FOCUS BOX 2.1 DISCUSSION POINT: THE THERAPEUTIC USE OF ASSESSMENT

Cara was referred for psychological therapy by her GP. She had witnessed a burglary in a bank approximately 18 months ago. She and several other people were held up at gun point and one elderly man suffered a heart attack and died at the scene. The perpetrators were caught and charged. Cara had to give evidence in court, which in itself was very distressing. Since the event she had been experiencing flashbacks, panic-like symptoms, social withdrawal and low mood. She had been referred for psychological therapy for help in dealing with the trauma and to find ways to cope with the distressing symptoms. The psychologist undertook an initial assessment, which was guided by a generic assessment framework. As part of the assessment process, Cara relayed a number of traumatic losses in her life. The first related to the loss of her sister Emma when she was 10 years old. Cara had watched as Emma, aged 7 years old, got run over by a car. She stated that her mother was never the same after her death and that in many ways felt she had lost her too. Cara lost her best friend through suicide at age 15. At age 19 Cara had an abortion. Two years later she fell pregnant again and was looking forward to the birth of her child. Her baby girl, Joanna, was stillborn. Following this Cara had several miscarriages. Eventually Cara gave birth to a little boy, Gavin, who is now aged 6 and whom she describes as her reason for living. A year earlier, six months after the burglary in the bank, Cara's oldest sister Michelle was found dead in her apartment in London. Her death was classed as an accidental overdose but Cara and her family believe it was suicide, as her sister had a history of mental health and addiction problems and had made attempts in the past.

In addition to gathering information regarding the burglary, it was important for the psychologist to gather details pertaining to the various traumatic losses, as it also became clear that Cara had not processed her grief, which was evident in a number of behaviours she described such as visiting the graveyards every week. The psychologist gently and empathically acknowledged all these painful losses and the impact this had had upon Cara's mood, her behaviours relating to, for example, her frequent visits to the graveside, and her attitude towards life generally which was characterised by despair, hopelessness, bitterness, anger and futility . The psychologist took some time during the assessment to explain to Cara that she had suffered traumatic losses and that this had a profound impact on how she grieved. She described to Cara gently and simply the difference between normal grief and complex and traumatic grief reactions. The psychologist acknowledged how she had, yet again, in her lifetime witnessed another traumatic death by observing the gentleman in the bank experiencing a heart attack brought on by the burglary. Cara was surprised to hear that there was a difference in the types of losses and grief reactions that could be experienced. Cara stated that knowing this was a relief. Cara thanked the psychologist for sharing this information. Whilst the focus of the intervention going forward was to deal with the current trauma, it was essential that these losses were identified as they related to Cara's ability to deal with her current difficulties especially witnessing the death of the gentleman during the robbery.

Do you agree with the psychologist's decision to share this information relating to the traumatic losses and associated complex grief reaction with the client?

Can you think of reasons why it would not have been a good idea to share this information at this stage?

The psychologist shared with her information relating the differences between 'normal' bereavement and complex and traumatic grief, which helped the client feel less confused about her feelings and behaviours, and provided a sense of relief and validation.

Irrespective of the setting, there are key features of assessment in counselling psychology practice which enable practitioners to capture the relevant information in a manner that upholds the humanistic values and ethos that it espouses. This *generic assessment* process, conducted in a semi-structured style that is collaborative in its approach, enables the practitioner to get a broad view of the client's difficulties, life experiences and expectations. At the same time, providing an experience that is in its own right positive and affirming for the client and normalising of their difficulties. Box 2.2 displays the features of this *therapeutic generic assessment* process which would include capturing information on a broad range of areas.

All these areas may be covered and can provide an understanding of the many aspects that are worthy of exploration but this will depend upon the setting and therefore, should act as a guide on what to include rather than a definitive list. For example, a therapist working in an addiction setting will spend more time on capturing information relating to substance misuse. Bager-Charleson and Van Rijn (2013) also provide an outline of a generic assessment template. In addition, practitioners often incorporate questionnaires as part of the assessment process, such as measures of depression or anxiety. For example, The Patient Health Questionnaire (PHQ9) (Kroenke, Spitzer & Williams, 2001) and The Generalised Anxiety Disorder (GAD7) scale (Spitzer, Kroenke, Williams & Lowe, 2006) are psychometrically robust measures of mood and anxiety that can be used as screening tools to get a better understanding of the severity of symptoms. Questionnaires are also used as methods for evaluating change as they provide objective information that enables routine monitoring and evaluation at both an individual and service level. For example, the Clinical Outcome and Routine Evaluation (CORE) (Evans, Mellor-Clarke, Margison, Barkham, Audin, Connell & McGrath, 2000) is a measure

BOX 2.2 KEY FEATURES OF A THERAPEUTIC GENERIC ASSESSMENT

- Client personal details (name, contact details, address, DOB, GP, referrer details)
- Presenting issues(s) and impact
- Current situation
- Why therapy and why at this point in time?
- Family background
- Childhood and adolescence
- Trauma and/or loss
- Previous interventions and outcomes
- Medical problems, interventions and treatment
- Medication
- Risk (current and past to self and others)
- Occupational details and functioning
- Social functioning
- Social support
- Expectations
- Motivation
- Psychological mindedness
- Alcohol and drug history
- Relationships
- Sexuality
- Disability
- Culture
- Religion and spirituality
- Coping capacity and methods
- Resilience
- Strengths

of psychological well-being and is often used as part of the assessment and therapeutic process to monitor and evaluate change. Capturing objective information at pre- and post-stages of therapy can act as a means to enhance motivation and instil hope as the client and therapist can review from session to session any improvements that are being made. For example, scores on the PHQ9 can be plotted on a graph at each session and then reviewed to discuss any improvement or fluctuations in mood. Using this information in a collaborative manner assists the client in understanding their symptoms and any factors that are leading to changes. However, it is important to note that some agency settings will have adopted their own specific assessment protocol that psychologists will be required to adhere to. Nonetheless, counselling psychologists will always uphold their humanistic ethos and philosophy which is at the core of their identity and practice and as such will enable them to conduct an assessment in a manner that places the client at the centre of the process.

BOX 2.3 RISK FACTORS FOR CONSIDERATION DURING ASSESSMENT PROCESS

- Having a psychiatric diagnosis
- Being male
- Being male and unemployed
- Physical ill-health
- History of suicide attempts
- Having a family member who has attempted or committed suicide
- History of abuse
- Hopelessness
- No plans for the future
- Isolated and living alone
- Poor problem-solving capacity
- Substance misuse
- Recent experience of rejection or failure
- Attempts to seek revenge or influence another person

Another important area that is part of the assessment process is that of risk assessment. Risk is not static and is by no means an exact science, which is why gathering all relevant information is essential in order to help identify factors that elevate risk, factors that protect the person from risk and helps in the development of a safety plan (Reeves, 2010). These areas of risk include the client's risk to self through suicide or self-harm, the risk they may pose to others, information they share that indicates that others are at risk whether children or vulnerable adults, and ethical and legal issues such as reports of terrorist-related activities. Churchill (2011) provides an overview of the fixed and dynamic factors that increase the risk for suicide and are displayed in Box 2.3.

Assessment is of course an on-going endeavour. New information can come to light at any point in the therapeutic process and for many reasons. For example, a client may disclose abuse in later sessions as he or she may have needed more time to build up trust in the therapeutic relationship. Assessment is therefore not a one-off event but rather the foundation upon which therapy is built and should be flexible enough to enable the emergence of new material to be incorporated.

Underpinning the process of assessment is the therapist's personal and professional qualities. Assessment requires a range of skills but how this is undertaken is crucial because many helping professionals engage in assessment. However, counselling psychologists differ in how it is undertaken and a key element of this is the recognition of the role of the self of the practitioner (Strawbridge & Woolfe, 2010). Personal qualities such as empathy, compassion, respect for diversity, curiosity, flexibility, self-awareness, emotional stability, being hopeful, realistic and open-minded are essential.

Challenges in assessment

Assessment does not always run smoothly. Clients may not disclose all relevant information due to many factors such as not feeling safe or fear of being judged. Clients may not be good historians, have difficulty articulating and expressing their thoughts and feelings, lack insight and psychological mindedness. In some instances a client may focus on one issue in great depth and the psychologist can find it difficult to keep the focus. Some may find the assessment process confusing, not relevant and wish to get straight into talking about their problems. In some instances it may be necessary to suspend the assessment process temporarily if the client is distressed or communicates dissatisfaction. For example, in some mental health settings a client may have underwent a number of assessments with a broad range of mental health professionals and question why they should undergo a further assessment. It is therefore essential that the assessment process is flexible enough to withstand any challenges presented by the client.

FOCUS BOX 2.2 DISCUSSION POINT: CASE STUDY 'SORAYA'

Soraya has been referred by her psychiatrist for help in managing her self-harm behaviour and low mood. She has a diagnosis of borderline personality disorder. During the assessment process, she tells you that it has been a huge relief to know what is wrong with her. She tells you she has researched the diagnosis and found it helpful to read about all the symptoms she experiences and that she is not the only one who feels and acts this way. However, she tells you that her husband has been calling her names and telling her she is now 'officially crazy'. She tells you that when she is feeling low or does not want to socialise, he scrutinises her moods and behaviours which are then deemed abnormal reactions due to her 'mental illness'. This, understandably causes her a great deal of distress.

What are your thoughts regarding Soraya's diagnosis?
How would you help her deal with this situation?

Assessment and diagnosis

One of the key challenges with assessment has been its tendency to be associated with diagnosis, pathologising or labelling the client, all of which are sometimes deemed to be dehumanising experiences (Evans & Gilbert, 2005). It may also reinforce stigma or feelings of shame (Churchill, 2011; Ruddel, 1997).

Medical and psychiatric assessments are a particular type of assessment differing markedly from the *therapeutic assessment* undertaken by counselling psychologists (Strawbridge & Woolfe, 2010). In medical and psychiatric assessments the focus of information gathering is to elicit information pertaining to symptoms. The Mental State Examination carried out by a range of mental health professionals includes information gathering on mood, speech, appearance, behaviour, attention, concentration, delusions, memory, insight, orientation, obsessional traits, hallucinations, illusions, depersonalisation and derealisation (Curwen, 1997). Difficulties in any of these areas can inform the diagnostic process. Indeed, medical and psychiatric assessment often lead to diagnosis and having an understanding of the two diagnostic classification systems, the *Diagnostic and Statistical Manual of Mental Disorders (DSM-V)* (APA, 2016) and the *International Statistical Classification of Diseases and Related Health Problems (ICD-10)* (WHO, 2016), is important for counselling psychologist as the client's care may be shared within a mental health team requiring multidisciplinary support. Indeed, one of the core competencies to be met during Doctoral Counselling Psychology training is demonstrating a critical understanding of diagnostic frameworks such as *DSM-V* and *ICD-10*.

The medical model and psychological model emerge from different paradigms and do not necessarily blend well together but in routine clinical practice the two may co-exist (Hammersley, 2010). This includes also the use of psychotropic medications that are often prescribed for illnesses or conditions such as clinical depression, generalised anxiety disorder or bipolar disorder. Whilst medication and diagnosis imply illness or deficiency, which may be seen to be at odds with the ethos and philosophy of counselling psychology, it is essential that attention is given to the role of medication in the client's psychological care. To ignore it could be seen as harmful and unethical. Therefore, a basic understanding of the varieties of drugs prescribed is important (Hammersley, 2010).

The role of diagnosis

It is important to remember that it would be incorrect to assume that all clients dislike having a diagnosis. Some clients find having a label validating and it can provide a sense of relief regarding what may seem like a bewildering range of symptoms. For some it can be reassuring and can help them externalise their problems and view them in a more detached manner. It can reduce feelings of alienation, help others understand what they are experiencing and going through, thus eliciting support, which can help reduce feelings of guilt or shame. Yet, for other clients having a diagnosis or label can reinforce a sense of shame, embarrassment, lead to feelings of hopelessness, futility and lack of control (Christensen, 2013). A skilful and empathic assessment will enable the practitioner to gain insight and understanding into the meanings a client attaches to their symptoms and experiences. The BPS (2014) New Guidance on Diagnosis states that practitioner psychologists need to be aware of the individual impact of receiving a diagnosis. It stipulates that psychologists may seek to supplement or replace diagnosis, wherever appropriate, with evidence-based individual psychological formulations, models and theories as a way of informing their recommendations and interventions.

FOCUS BOX 2.3 DISCUSSION POINT: CASE STUDY 'KALI'

Kali is 27 years old and married with one child. During her assessment she relays a chaotic and unstable upbringing due to her father's drinking and her mother's mental health problems. She describes home as a prison and how at age 17 she joined the army to escape. She tells you she spent 7 months in the army and then returned home. At this point she becomes anxious and tearful. The psychologist pauses for a moment to allow Kali time to speak about what is clearly a distressing period of her life but Kali proceeds to talk about how life was upon her return. The psychologist, sensing that leaving the army was quite significant, asks Kali in a gentle manner if she can explain why she left the army. At this, Kali becomes irritated and states quite loudly that she does not wish to talk about it, that she has never talked about and never will. The psychologist accepts Kali's wish not to discuss what is clearly a very upsetting aspect of her life, and therefore, does not question any further. All other aspects of the assessment are completed.

Do you agree with the psychologist's decision not to probe further?
What would you do in this situation?
How does this missing information impact on the psychologist's understanding of Kali's issues?

Case formulation

As discussed so far, the purpose of assessment during routine clinical practice is to help the client and practitioner to define and understand the client's difficulties, which can include the use of multiple methods such as questionnaires and other sources of information (Bager-Charleson & Van Rijn, 2013). This information is then used to create a formulation or understanding of the difficulties informed by a particular theoretical orientation. It is also referred to as case conceptualisation. Sim et al. (2005, p. 290) provide the following definition:

> A case formulation summarises the salient features of the case in a nutshell and identifies important issues quickly, particularly complex cases with multiple problems . . . helps to organise and integrate the clinical data around a linchpin and allows the clinician to focus on the heart of the matter in each individual case.

Essentially, the task of case formulation is to turn the client's narrative or life story along with other data collected, such as questionnaires, into a coherent understanding of the difficulties, which can serve to inform the therapeutic process, intervention and goals (Henderson & Martin, 2014). A formulation of the client's difficulties can be a powerful affirming experience in that having their information captured and pieced together, then offered back to them in a synopsis that links all the past and present material, can be both illuminating and validating. It can offer a clarity to their situation, facilitate insight and self-awareness (Johnstone, 2006). However, developing a formulation or conceptualisation takes time and there is a temptation for practitioners to skip it and go directly to intervention (Berman, 2015).

There are many approaches and interventions to assist the practitioner in understanding the client's difficulties but most often, the practitioner will be informed by a particular model or theory. Counselling psychology is embedded in humanistic values and is client-centred in its approach; however this does not imply that all counselling psychologists work within a person-centred theoretical model as many will work across a diverse range of models. Section 3 of this text is dedicated to the most prominent therapeutic models used by counselling psychologists, namely humanistic, existential-phenomenological, psychodynamic and cognitive-behavioural therapies. For example, in Cognitive-Behaviour Therapy (CBT) formulation is a core clinical skill and a key feature of the therapeutic process (Johnstone & Dallos, 2006). Traditional Rogerian theory and practice have tended not to focus on case formulation (Rogers, 1961). The idea of including case formulation explicitly during the therapeutic process has been consistently rejected within this approach (Johnstone & Dallos, 2006; Eells, 2007). However, in recent years it has become a topic of debate (Simms, 2011; Gillon, 2009). Box 2.4 displays the main paradigms.

In addition to these four prominent therapeutic models, two alternative models that are often drawn upon to facilitate case conceptualisation are the Biopsychosocial Model and the Four Ps (Henderson & Martin, 2014). Both these frameworks will draw upon background biological and genetic factors, or pre-disposing factors, the social and psychological factors that are implicated in what precipitates problems, what maintains them, the protective features and how all these areas are interrelated. Michenbaum (2014) also provides a framework called the Case Conceptualisation Model (CCM) which provides an outline of the elements in a thorough formulation such as developmental, cultural, social, familial and contextual factors as well as risk and protective factors, impact on quality of life and identification of maladaptive behaviours.

BOX 2.4 MAIN THEORETICAL FRAMEWORKS

Theoretical paradigm	*Conceptualisation of problems informed by:*
Cognitive-Behavioural	Core beliefs, dysfunctional assumptions, automatic thoughts, irrational thinking patterns. Link between thoughts, feeling and behaviour.
Humanistic Person-Centred	Conditions of worth, core conditions, actualising tendency, personal growth, autonomy, locus of control, self-concept, self-awareness.
Psychodynamic	Early childhood and attachment relationships, unconscious forces, defence mechanisms, transference and counter-transference.
Existential	Meaning, subjectivity, purpose, choices, freedom, responsibility.
Systemic	Role of the family unit, belonging, separateness, individuality, dysfunctional patterns and interactions.

Many counselling psychologists will be eclectic in their approach, drawing upon a variety of methods and techniques to make sense of the information gathered at assessment in order to formulate an understanding of their client's difficulties (Strawbridge & Woolfe, 2010). This may actually be necessary given the complexity of issues a client can present with. Guidelines for training during counselling psychology as laid out by the British Psychological Society (2015) stipulate that practitioners in training and consequently qualified practitioners should be able to construct collaborative formulations drawing upon theoretical frameworks and the clients' subjective experience. This process is underpinned by an empathic understanding of their difficulties and should be explained in language that is accessible, culturally sensitive and non-discriminatory in terms of, for example, age, gender, disability and sexuality. It is does not stipulate any particular theory over another.

The purpose of a formulation

As a case formulation is essentially a synopsis of the client's presenting problems, informed by psychological theory and used to inform intervention, its purpose therefore is to link theory to practice (Johnstone, 2011). This ensures that an evidence-based practice and practice-based evidence approach to clinical work is maintained as it is used to review and evaluate client progress and change, as well as monitor the therapeutic process. However, it is important to note that it is not a prescribed set of rules, but rather as Johnstone (2011) states, it is a 'best guess' attempt at understanding what is going on and therefore is tentative, collaborative, reflexive and respectful. The challenge is to ensure that the practitioner does not engage in 'describing' and 'prescribing' which has a more directive stance and aligned to a medical model (Tudor & Merry, 2002). Ultimately, it is a conversation between two people, client and therapist, but it is the client telling the story and the therapist's task is to listen and make sense of it. Yet, it is a powerful experience in its own right if undertaken empathically and skilfully. As Johnstone (2011, p. 14) notes:

> Formulation can also be an intervention in itself. Sometimes the act of clarifying someone's difficulties, and in the process helping them to feel listened to, understood and accepted, is enough to allow them to move forward again.

Focus Box 2.4 sets out an outline of a fictional case study of a client called 'Jeff'. Two theoretical models have been drawn upon to illustrate the application of theory to practice issues and to demonstrate how each theory accounts for his problems and the interventions that can be used to facilitate change.

FOCUS BOX 2.4 DISCUSSION POINT: CASE STUDY 'JEFF'

Jeff is 28 years old, unemployed and lives with his parents. He went to University and graduated with a first class degree in engineering but has not worked since. During University he experienced a psychotic episode and bouts of recurrent depression. He believes this was brought on by the stress of studying and pressures of living away from home. Jeff is an only child and both his parents have been very overprotective of him. They were in their early 40s when he was conceived and regarded him as their 'miracle' baby as they had been told they would never have any children. When he was born, Jeff's mother gave up her nursing job and devoted her life to caring for him. His parents were highly affectionate and sacrificed a lot to provide him with an education. They ensured he kept to a rigid homework routine, encouraged him to work hard to get 'good grades' and minimised his time for socialising as they deemed it a distraction. Consequently, Jeff had few friends and as he got older, found it difficult to socialise, resulting in him becoming quite withdrawn and isolated. He never felt like he fitted in. Jeff's mother has arthritis that has resulted in a reduced mobility and his father was diagnosed with early stages of Alzheimer's disease. The deterioration in their health occurred when he went to University. Jeff deliberately chose a university that would require him to move away but his parents were angry and upset with him and he found it difficult to cope when he did move away. His parents rang him daily and with their deteriorating health, his difficulties socialising and the increasing workload, he became depressed. He took drugs briefly to cope but experienced a psychotic episode that left him feeling frightened. Jeff managed to complete his degree but when he returned home he found himself having to care for his parents' increasingly deteriorating health. He has tried on several occasions to get a job and move out but each time they become angry, aggressive and accuse him of not caring. Jeff feels overwhelmed, guilty, frustrated, hopeless and trapped. He has spoken to his GP who has referred him for psychological therapy. He tells his psychologist he is 'useless', 'mean' and 'uncaring' as he does not want to live with and take care of his parents. He states that he 'feels trapped' and 'is a bad son' and that he should be able to cope better, after all his parents 'sacrificed everything to give him the best opportunities in life' and that he should be 'grateful'. He states he is a 'failure' because he cannot overcome the 'depression'.

How would a psychodynamic or systemic approach account for 'Jeff's' difficulties and what methods would each of the approaches employ?

What are the limitations in these models?

Case conceptualisation of 'Jeff'

Two theoretical approaches to understanding 'Jeff' are provided below, namely CBT and Person-Centred. In CBT terms, we can formulate 'Jeff's' difficulties as stemming from his early childhood experiences whereby he has developed *core beliefs* around being a good, obedient, hard-working and high-achieving son. These have shaped 'Jeff's *intermediate belief system* or *assumptions* which he uses as a template to evaluate his interpersonal and intrapersonal world. For example, being a good and obedient son means he has developed rules around always having to be available for his parents and having to be responsible for their care. However, on a day-to-day basis he feels guilty as he feels trapped and frustrated resulting in *automatic thoughts* of 'I am useless', 'I am mean' and 'I should be grateful'. However, this sense of entrapment is at odds with other *core beliefs* instilled in early childhood in relation to achievement, success and independence, which he is unable to attain. This results in frustration for him causing him to feel depressed and despondent, which creates a further vicious cycle as it reinforces thoughts and feelings relating to being a failure and uncaring, which in turn reinforce his low mood. One approach to intervention with 'Jeff' within a CBT framework would be to challenge his *dysfunctional assumptions, irrational beliefs* and seek to assist him in making *behavioural changes* such as moving out, getting a job, developing a social network for himself and sourcing care and support for his parents. This active and directive stance would require him to be motivated and willing to make changes in order to improve his mood and general psychological well-being. He would be expected to be undertaking homework assignments between therapy sessions to *challenge his thinking*, improve *his problem-solving* capacity and *social skills.*

A Person-Centred theoretical formulation would provide insight and understanding into how 'Jeff's' developing *self-concept* emerged and how this has led to a state of *incongruence.* 'Jeff' has developed *conditions of worth* laid down in childhood due to his parents placing excessive demands upon him to achieve academically, emphasising his duty of care towards them as the only son, a child who was 'prized' and deemed a 'miracle'. His self-worth has been dependent upon their approval of him as being the dutiful son and his fear of detaching reinforced by their inability to let him go and live independently, despite them espousing that this is what they wanted for him. This has led to a state of *incongruence* for 'Jeff' as he struggles with dependency and autonomy: duty and care towards his parents on the one hand and desire for freedom and independence on the other. Their approval and affection it seems has been *conditional* upon him acting as the dutiful son. He has *introjected* values and beliefs relating to the importance of having a strong duty of care towards his parents and the importance of sacrificing one's own needs for others. He has *internalised* versions of his parents as being all-sacrificing, loving and dutiful, which he too believes is the correct *way of being.* However, it has resulted in a thwarting of his *actualising tendency* in that he has not achieved personal growth, autonomy and self-worth resulting in feelings of entrapment, guilt, shame and depression. Therapeutic intervention would focus upon *dissolving the conditions of worth* laid down in childhood and helping Jeff attain a state of *congruence.* The *therapeutic relationship* is regarded as the vehicle through which change occurs by offering a therapeutic environment that is rich in the *core conditions* of empathy, non-judgement and unconditional positive regard. In doing so, it is hypothesised that this would activate his *actualising tendency* in a healthy way and lead to *personal growth* and change.

Both approaches offer ways of understanding the factors that led to his difficulties, highlighting aspects that are maintaining them and offering ways to address his difficulties in order to feel better and attain an improved quality of life.

Conclusions

This chapter has focused on the essential role and skills of assessment and case formulation. Counselling psychologists working in routine clinical practice need to be able to assess and formulate clients' presenting issue(s) in a way that is collaborative, empathic and respectful. Practice is informed by a theoretical orientation, which serves as a guide to therapy and is used as a means to monitor and evaluate change. There are a number of challenges for clients and practitioners alike when conducting an assessment such as holding tension between medical and psychiatric models and diagnosis, and focusing on client meaning, which entails upholding the humanistic ethos and philosophy that counselling psychology as a profession espouses. However, aligning closely to this core humanistic value base is what sets counselling psychologists apart and is what ultimately makes the process of assessment and formulation a therapeutic experience in its own right which can be empowering for the client.

Learning outcomes

When you have completed this chapter you should be able to:

- Understand what is meant by the concept of assessment.
- Understand the process of assessment in the context of counselling psychology practice.
- Have an understanding of the core skills used in conducting an assessment.
- Understand the role of the therapeutic relationship in the context of assessment.
- Be aware of the challenges and debates relating to assessment and diagnosis.
- Understand what is meant by formulation and the varieties of formulation.

Key concepts and terms

- Assessment
- Case conceptualisation
- Cognitive-Behaviour Therapy
- Collaborative
- Diagnosis
- Formulation
- Humanistic
- Medical model
- Person-Centred Theory
- Reflective Practice
- Therapeutic Assessment

Sample essay titles

1. Describe the core features of assessment and formulation and why these aspects of practice are necessary.
2. Discuss how counselling psychology practice contributes to an assessment and formulation process that is an affirmative and positive for the client.
3. Describe the strengths and weaknesses of assessment and formulation.

Further reading

Bager-Charlson, S. & Van Rihn, B. (2011) *Understanding Assessment in Counselling and Psychotherapy.* Poole: Learning Matters.
Gillon, W. (2007) *Person-Centred Counselling Psychology: An Introduction.* London: Sage Publications.
Johnstone, L. & Dallos, R. (2006) *Formulation in Psychology and Psychotherapy.* London: Routledge.
Palmer, S. & McMahon G. (2009) *Client Assessment.* London: Sage Publications.
Simms, J. (2011) Case Formulation within a Person Centred Framework: An Uncomfortable Fit? *Counselling Psychology Review, June, 26(2).*

References

APA. (2016). *Diagnostic and Statistical Manual of Mental Disorders (5th Ed).* USA: American Psychiatric Association. www.psychiatry.org/psychiatrists/practice/dsm
Assay, T.P. & Lambert, M.J. (1999) The Empirical Case for the Common Factors in Therapy: Quantitative Findings. In M. Hubble, B.L. Duncan and S.D. Miller (eds.), *The Heart and Soul of Change: What Works in Therapy.* Washington, DC: American Psychological Association, pp. 33–5.
Bager-Charleson, S. & Van Rijn, B. (2011) *Understanding Assessment in Counselling and Psychotherapy.* Poole: Learning Matters.
Bennett, P. (2003) *Abnormal and Clinical Psychology: An Introductory Text.* Maidenhead: Open University Press.
Berman, P.S. (2015) *Case Conceptualisation and Treatment Planning: Integrating Theory with Clinical Practice.* Los Angeles: Sage.
Bertolino, B. & O'Hanlon, B. (2002) *Collaborative, Competency-Based Counselling and Therapy.* Boston: Allen and Bacon.
British Psychological Society (2014) *Diagnosis–Policy and Guidelines.* London: BPS. www.bps.org.uk/publications/policy-and-guidelines/general-guidelines-policy-documents/general-guidelines-policy
British Psychological Society (2015) *Standards for Accreditation of Doctoral Programmes in Counselling Psychology.* London: BPS. www.bps.org.uk/system/files/Public%20files/PaCT/counselling_accreditation_2015_web.pdf
Calhoun, L.G. & Tedeschi, R.G. (1999) *Facilitating Posttraumatic Growth: A Clinicians Guide.* New Jersey: Lawrence Erlbaum Associates Inc.
Christensen, E. (2013) Diagnosis and Treatment Planning. In D. Capuzzi and D.R. Cross (eds.), *Introduction to the Counselling Profession (6th Ed).* New York: Routledge.
Churchill, S. (2011) *The Troubled Mind: A Handbook of Therapeutic Approaches to Psychological Distress.* New York: Palgrave Macmillan.
Curwen, B. (1997) Medical and Psychiatric Assessment. In S. Palmer and G. McMahon (eds.) (2009), *Client Assessment.* London: Sage.
Douglas, B. (2010) Disorder and Its Discontents. In R. Woolfe, S. Strawbridge, B. Douglas and W. Dryden (eds.), *Handbook of Counselling Psychology (3rd Ed).* London: Sage.
Eells, T.D. (2007) *Handbook of Psychotherapy Case Formulation.* New York: Guildford Press.
Evans C, Mellor-Clark J, Margison F, Barkham M, Audin K, Connell J & McGrath, G. (2000) CORE: Clinical Outcomes in Routine Evaluation. *Journal of Mental Health, 9(3)*: 247–55.
Evans, K.R. & Gilbert, M.C. (2005) *An Introduction to Integrative Psychotherapy.* Basingstoke, UK: Palgrave Macmillan.
Foster, L.H. (2013) Assessment Practices in Counselling. In D. Capuzzi and D.R. Cross (eds.), *Introduction to the Counselling Profession (6th Ed).* New York: Routledge.
Gillon, E. (2009) *Person Centred Counselling Psychology.* London: Sage.
Hammersley, D. (2010) The Interface between Psychopharmacological and Psychotherapeutic Approaches. In B. Douglas, R. Woolfe, S. Strawbridge, E. Kasket and V. Galbraith (eds.), *The Handbook of Counselling Psychology (4th Ed).* London: Sage.
Hargie, O. (2011) *Skilled Interpersonal Communication.* East Sussex: Routledge.

Health and Care Professions Council (2015) *Standards of Proficiency Practitioner Psychologists.* www.hpc-uk.org/assets/documents/10002963sop_practitioner_psychologists.pdf

Henderson, S.W. & Martin, A. (2014) Case Formulation and Integration of Information in Child and Adolescent Mental Health. In J.M. Rey (ed.), *IACAPAP e-Textbook of Child and Adolescent Mental Health.* Geneva: International Association for Child and Adolescent Psychiatry and Allied Professions.

Johnstone, L.C. (2006) Controversies and Debates about Formulation. In L. Johnstone and R. Dallos (eds.), *Formulation in Psychology and Psychotherapy.* London: Routledge.

Johnstone, L.C. (2011) *Psychological Formulation: A Radical Perspective.* Middlesex University Research Repository. http://eprints.mds.ac.uk

Johnstone, L.C. & Dallos, R. (2006) *Formulation in Psychology and Psychotherapy.* London: Routledge.

Kroenke, K., Spitzer, R.L. & Williams, J.B. (2001) The PHQ-9: Validity of a Brief Depression Severity Measure. *Journal General International Medicine, September, 16(9)*: 606–13.

Lambert, M.J. (1992) Implications of Outcome Research for Psychotherapy Integration. In J.C. Norcross and M.R. Goldstein (eds.), *Handbook of Psychotherapy Integration.* New York: Basic Books.

Michenbaum, D. (2014) *The Role of a Case Conceptualisation Model and Core Task of Intervention.* Florida: Melissan Institute. http://melissainstitute.com/documents/Conf18-Meichenbaum-CaseConcept.pdf

Reeves, A. (2010) *Counselling Suicidal Clients.* London: Sage.

Rogers, C.R. (1961) *On Becoming a Person.* London: Constable and Robinson Ltd.

Ruddel, P. (1997) General Assessment Issues. In S. Palmer and G. McMahon (eds.), *Client Assessment.* London: Sage.

Sim, K., Gwee, K. P., Bateman, A. (2005). Case Formulation in Psychotherapy: Revitalizing Its Usefulness as a Clinical Tool. *Academic Psychiatry*, 29: 289–292.

Simms, J. (2011) Case Formulation within a Person Centred Framework: An Uncomfortable Fit? *Counselling Psychology Review, June, 26(2).*

Spitzer, R.L., Kroenke, K., Williams, J.B. & Lowe, B. (2006) A Brief Measure for Measuring Generalised Anxiety Disorder: The GAD7. *Archives International Medicine, May 22, 166(10)*: 1092–7.

Strawbridge, S. & Woolfe, R. (2003) Counselling Psychology in Context. In R. Woolfe, S. Strawbridge, B. Douglas and W. Dryden (eds.), *Handbook of Counselling Psychology (2nd Ed).* London: Sage.

Strawbridge, S. & Woolfe, R. (2010) Counselling Psychology: Origins, Developments and Challenges. In R. Woolfe, S. Strawbridge, B. Douglas and W. Dryden (eds.), *Handbook of Counselling Psychology (3rd Ed).* London: Sage.

Tudor, K. & Merry, T. (2002) *A Dictionary of Person Centred Psychology.* London: Whurt.

WHO. (2016) International Statistical Classification of Diseases and Health Related Problems, 10th Revision. http://apps.who.int/classifications/icd10/browse/2016/en

Williams, L., Edwards, T.M., Patterson, J., & Chamow, L. (2011). Essential assessment skills for couple and family therapists. New York, NY: Guilford.

Yalom, I.D. (2001) *The Gift of Therapy.* London: Piatkus Books Ltd.

3

COUNSELLING PSYCHOLOGY PERSPECTIVES

Faye Volker

This chapter describes the perspectives found in counselling psychology with a focus on the underlying values inherent within each of them. A perspective is a way of viewing, a lens, which allows us to make sense of the world. Perspectives always contain a set of values, assumptions, and beliefs, and this chapter encourages you to reflect on what these mean to you as a developing professional.

Values and counselling psychology

Although the concept of a value is difficult to define, therapy deals directly with values in some form or another (Patterson, 1989). In a seminal discussion of values in 1980, Bergin believed that therapists acted as moral agents and, therefore, their values were inseparable from the therapeutic encounter. We have professional values, therapeutic values, ethical values, and even the values that clients bring with them into therapy, as examples. It is incredibly important to reflect on these values because they shape the ways in which we engage with a therapeutic role, with other professionals and organisations, and with our clients influencing how we act, behave, and make decisions (Proctor, 2014). Counselling psychology is, arguably, distinct in its emphasis on encouraging professionals to critique their attitudes, beliefs, and values (British Psychological Society [BPS], 2015; Health and Care Professions Council [HCPC], 2015).

Training to become a therapeutic professional inevitably involves socialisation into a system of beliefs, which includes sharing myths, knowledge, language, discourse, and values (McLeod, 2013). A belief system consists of ideas about (a) what is true and (b) what helps us to make sense of the world, other people, and ourselves (Griffiths, 2014). This system helps us to manage each experience of life according to the thoughts we have about the nature of reality (Johnson, 2011). It may be easier to think about working with the belief system of our client, but we too have a system guided by personal and professional experiences. Moreover, each of the perspectives, outlined in this chapter, contain a set of values and beliefs that tell us something important about the ways in which we view the following:

- Human nature.
- The nature of distress.

- Ways of being.
- The purpose of therapy.
- Skills, techniques, and roles.
- Therapeutic outcome.

Pugh and Coyle (2000) provided some insight into why values may be so important to contemporary counselling psychology. They performed a discourse analysis on journal articles published in the *Counselling Psychology Review* (volumes dated from 1990 to 1996) and, in so doing, presented several themes on how counselling psychology in Britain was being constructed. One of their themes was titled "attributing a different value system to counselling psychology," and it alluded to the ways in which the profession demarcated itself from similar professions (such as clinical psychology or psychiatry) based on its values (Pugh and Coyle, 2000, p. 94). Reflection, sometimes also called reflexivity, was an important value for counselling psychologists contributing to a sense of professional distinctiveness (Pugh and Coyle, 2000) and, in light of this, the exercise in Activity box 3.1 facilitates the development of reflective skills that will be useful when interacting with the values found in counselling psychology.

ACTIVITY BOX 3.1

Before continuing with this chapter, think about how you conceptualise human nature; that is, what does it mean to be human? What are your beliefs about the nature of distress? Do you think that distress is a unique experience for each person or is it something that applies to all people? What does distress look like, sound like, and feel like? Given your views, what do you believe, at this moment in time, is the purpose of therapy and what is change or outcome? Contemplate what you would like your role to be. What skills and techniques would you like to develop?

Counselling psychology and its values

The BPS and the HCPC are arguably the best sources of knowledge regarding the professional values that guide counselling psychology. The BPS's Division of Counselling Psychology (DCoP) is a particularly salient resource for professionals affiliated with this subdiscipline of psychology. This chapter focuses on three prominent values in particular, which can be found in the DCoP (2005), the BPS (2015), and the HCPC (2015) guides (see Further Reading).

First, counselling psychology is inherently interested in understanding the lives of people, their subjective experiences, and their experiences of living in a relational world. The DCoP (2005, p. 1) suggests counselling psychology strives to "engage with subjectivity and intersubjectivity, values and beliefs." The BPS (2015, p. 15) expands on this, commenting that subjectivity "unfolds with the physical, social, cultural, and spiritual dimensions of living." Therefore, when thinking about subjectivity, counselling psychology seeks to take a holistic view of the person and their experience of life.

Second, counselling psychology is perhaps distinct in its endeavour to engage empathically with people resulting in a respect for the uniqueness and validity of every person's experience of life (DCoP, 2005; HCPC, 2015). Counselling psychologists achieve empathic understanding by using themselves in the therapeutic encounter, which requires not only creativity and artistry but also critical reflexivity (DCoP, 2005; BPS, 2015; HCPC, 2015). It is about recognising that if people define their own life, then no one definition can be superior. Another way to conceptualise this is in not privileging the truth; that is, the search for meaning uncovers multiple answers, none of which can be said to be more true or false than another (Cooper and McLeod, 2011).

Third, counselling psychology holds an "inquisitive, reflexive, and critical attitude that acknowledges diversity" (BPS, 2015, p. 15). The DCoP (2005, p. 1) suggests counselling psychology strives to "recognise social contexts and discrimination and to work in ways that empower rather than control." Therefore, counselling psychology seeks to promote social inclusion, to recognise power dynamics in different contexts, and to appreciate the diversity of our client group, especially in preventing stigmatising and discriminatory practices (DCoP, 2005; BPS, 2015; HCPC, 2015).

Counselling psychology and its perspectives

Counselling psychology has transcended its traditional humanistic routes, and there are some perspectives in counselling psychology that are emergent because they represent the evolving nature of societal thought. These perspectives embody ways of thinking that are new to the profession and ways of thinking that keep us in touch with the important values of today's society. The remaining sections will concentrate specifically on how counselling psychology perspectives view the human subject, and they have been grouped around several philosophical themes including (a) subjectivity and intersubjectivity, (b) shifting subjectivities, and (c) moving beyond the subject.

Subjectivity and intersubjectivity

Agents of meaning

Subjectivity, from a **humanistic perspective**, is the philosophical proposition that each person interprets the world, allowing them to have a unique understanding of what it means to be a living human subject (Mathieson, 1962; Crotty, 1998). **Objectivity**, in contrast, is the viewpoint that the world exists even in the absence of such interpretations; therefore, what is observed is not unique to the interpreting person but the object being interpreted instead (Mathieson, 1962; Crotty, 1998). The desire to know the internal life of an individual is called an **idiographic approach** (i.e., *idio* meaning "private"), and it is an approach that stays as close as possible to each individual's representation of life (Smith *et al.* 2009). Nevertheless, counselling psychology is located in a paradoxical position; it values recognising the subjective uniqueness of each person, but it also values an objective explanation applicable to all people (this is a **nomothetic approach**).

Cognitive-behavioural therapy, perhaps more so than other theories, holds an explanatory value; it involves understanding how a person's internal representations affect his or her sense of wellbeing. Beck (1996, p. 5), for example, postulated that depression consisted of a particular "system of personality" that offered an explanatory framework for understanding depression. The *Diagnostic Statistical Manual of Mental Disorders* (*DSM-V*) developed by the American Psychiatric Association (APA, 2013) also offers an explanatory framework. Take an individual who is addicted to substances; this person may want therapy to gain insight into how the addiction influences his or her life. Using a nomothetic approach, in the absence of the individual, we have a model that diagnoses this person as having a *substance-related disorder* explaining *impaired control* as well as issues related to *tolerance* and *withdrawal* (APA, 2013, pp. 485–486), yet do we know the meaning of these symptoms to the person?

There is a strong emphasis on *meaning* in counselling psychology. People act in ways that are imbued with meaning, and they can, therefore, be seen as the agents of meaning (Porta and Keating, 2008). When talking about research, Schwandt (2007, p. 160) believed that the task of inquirers was to "unearth meaning," but this is also applicable to therapy. Counselling psychologists are inquirers and clients are the agents of meaning, and there is a synergy in this interaction when, and only when, we avoid taking away agency, autonomy, or self-determination.

Perspectives that are grounded in subjectivism additionally recognise that we are "relational beings" living in a world of other subjects (Milton, 2010, p. xxiv) and, therefore, meaning is shared intersubjectively (Berger and Luckman, 1966, p. 34). Without **intersubjectivity**, people would be an island deprived of any connection (this is termed *solipsism* in philosophy). If meaning is located in the private mind of the individual subject, then we only have access to it when we connect, and this might explain why establishing a therapeutic relationship is not only necessary but also essential.

The temporal landscape and lifespan development

Crotty (1998) believes that the modern concept of **phenomenology** has shifted radically, and it has now become synonymous with experience. We will consider, here, how phenomenology embraces fluidity where meaning ebbs and flows with the passage of time. Time shapes subjectivity because each new experience brings a shift in values, beliefs, and ideas about life (Hess and Schultz, 2008), and counselling psychology is inherently interested in how we experience change over the course of time (Snyder, 1982). Adams (2014, p. 36), from an **existential perspective**, discusses a "lived time" where we live our lives in a temporal landscape of past, present, and future as well as present-past and present-future. **Mindfulness**, for example, encourages people to live in the moment and to reconnect with their sense of the here-and-now (Segal *et al.* 2013). The concept of lived time is crucial for understanding subjectivity because we only ever have access to meaning in the present moment. Jacobs (2012, p. 1), from a **psychodynamic perspective**, calls this the "presenting past" reminding us that our past only shapes us to the extent to which it is present to the moment; that is, our past is not deterministic of the present or the future (Snyder, 1982).

As can be seen, numerous perspectives all agree that therapy occurs in a temporal landscape, and if we are constantly changing with time, then it is also important to look at subjectivity as it develops. A **lifespan developmental perspective** complements counselling psychology because of the recognition that development is a process and not a state (Adams, 2014). According to the early lifespan theory of Baltes (1987, p. 611), later expanded on by Sugarman (2001), development is life-long (a simple idea that had been neglected in previous developmental theory). Development is both multidimensional and multidirectional and it involves both growth and decline (Baltes, 1987, p. 613). Because we are relational beings, development additionally involves an interaction between a person and their environment; it is historically, socially, and culturally situated (Baltes, 1987; Sugarman, 2001).

Human potential and strengths-based perspectives

The humanistic ethos, underlying counselling psychology, is historically entwined with the **human potential movement** of the 1960s, which was largely influenced by work carried out at the Esalen Institute in California (Kripal, 2007). It focused on the idea that people were intrinsically motivated to engage in a continual process of growth (Rowan, 1983) and, today, **positive psychology** presents us with a contemporary theory of human potential similar to humanism. The **strengths-based approach** of positive psychology, in particular, has received considerable attention; it has been enthusiastically adopted by the Criminal Justice System (CJS) to encourage people to develop prosocial skills (Ward, 2002; Ward and Marshall, 2004). Jones-Smith (2016, p. 566) believes strengths develop from a human tendency to meet our needs through adaptation to our circumstances, and adversity is seen as positive because it brings about resilience. Like human potential theorists such as Carl Rogers (1959), and Abraham Maslow (1971), Jones-Smith (2016) also believes in the innate human potential for growth.

Posttraumatic Stress Disorder (PTSD) is common in our everyday language, and the *ICD-10 Classification of Mental and Behavioural Disorders* developed by the World Health Organisation (WHO, 2006, p. 148) has introduced us to symptoms such as *emotional blunting* and *hypervigilance*. Although these symptoms help us to diagnose PTSD, they might serve to maintain a negative – symptom-only – focus (Amos, 2015). Posttraumatic Growth (PTG), alternatively, is an emerging outlook that acknowledges some people might have positive experiences following their trauma such as a greater sense of strength and resilience (Calhoun and Tedeshi, 2014). Nevertheless, van Deurzen (2015) argues that although growth is a natural part of being human, so too is despair. Like the lifespan theory of Baltes (1987), we need to recognise both growth and decline. In other words, counselling psychologists should become comfortable not only with growth and despair but also with knowing when focusing on one is more appropriate than the other (van Deurzen, 2015).

Shifting subjectivities

The social construction of subjectivity

So far, we have looked at subjectivity as it pertains to the mind of the individual, but instead of constraining human nature and the nature of distress to only a subjective or only an objective system of knowledge, **social constructionism** holds these two systems together (Crotty, 1998). It examines the ways in which our *knowledge* of reality creates reality, and it is primarily concerned with how we *use* knowledge in everyday life (this is termed *epistemology* in philosophy). The idea of subjectivity, from a social constructionist perspective, is a social construct, meaning that identity is embedded in society, culture, and politics (as opposed to the mind of the subject). It is increasingly acknowledged that therapy does not occur in a socio-political vacuum (Parritt, 2016) and, therefore, understanding the influence of history, society, culture, and politics is crucial for counselling psychologists (Strawbridge, 2016). Box 3.1 Research Methods offers an exploration of how social constructionism not only informs therapeutic work but also therapeutic research. The role of research is fundamental to counselling psychology and so too is the acknowledgement that there are many ways to understand human nature and the nature of distress.

BOX 3.1 RESEARCH METHODS

Counselling psychology is increasingly using social constructionism to inform research philosophy, design, and analysis. Instead of examining the subjective experiences of being an *immigrant*, for example, research might focus on the social label that serves to create a new category of person (i.e., a *foreigner*). Research might additionally examine the power that such labels hold both personally and socially. An immigrant is a social construct, yet it is saturated by political, economic, and social attitudes, beliefs, and emotions (see Hacking, 1999, for an interesting discussion). After all, an immigrant is really only a person that has *immigrated*. Social constructionism seeks to understand how the discourse of immigration shapes subjectivity not only as perceived by the individual but also by society. We can also apply the same interrogation to a *schizophrenic*, for example. Social constructionism is particularly useful for researchers that are interested in (a) developing a critical theory of psychopathology and (b) challenging taken-for-granted hegemonic practices (Burr, 1995; Gergen, 2015). Language and discourse are incredibly important to social constructionism because they are the tools by which social meanings are shaped and transmitted (Burr, 1995; Gergen, 2015). Try out this research stance by reflecting on a certain area of your life; think about what language is being used. What does this language portray? How is language being used to build your ideas? What function might this language serve and can you discern any power? If yes, who wields it? What are the politics of this language and what does society say? Try interrogating the language being used by maintaining an attitude of critique (i.e., strengths and limitations).

Postmodernism and multiple meanings

The emerging perspectives found in counselling psychology are more consistent with **postmodernism** and its focus on the dynamics of power, language, and discourse (Henton, 2016). A postmodern philosophy is committed to "ambiguity, relativity, fragmentation, and particularly discontinuity" (Crotty, 1998, p. 185), and what this means for therapy is that meaning is not only different for different people but also is different for the same person on different occasions (Loewenthal and Snell, 2003). Therefore, instead of looking at subjectivity as being stable and singular, postmodernism introduces us to the concept of **subjectivities**; that is, subjectivity shifts with language and discourse as well as history, society, and culture. If we work in a hospital setting, such as the NHS, alongside medical doctors and nurses, then at any one moment in time a person might be both a *patient* (as defined medically) and a *client* (as defined psychologically).

Discursive identities are multifaceted, discontinuous, and conflictual, and they are highly permeable to socio-political ideology (see Donohue and Moore, 2009, for an interesting discussion). Postmodernism is a liberating philosophy when used in therapy because a person experiencing depression, for example, will not always define his or her life by this grand narrative. Indeed, a **narrative inquiry** might regard depression as being one chapter of a story but not the whole story; it may be a story with one scene or numerous scenes and multiple characters. People have the ability to transcend classification, unlike a medical model where an individual without current symptoms may be in remission (APA, 2013), yet notice that language still dictates that depression exists.

McLeod (2001) compared humanistic and postmodern concepts of language use. In the former, language allows people to communicate their subjectivity and, in so doing, permits them to relate in an intersubjective space. In the latter, language is used for action; that is, it is active, it shapes, and it builds. Every social encounter brings with it new social meaning and, therefore, the idea of being the only author of our own life is contested in postmodernism (Loewenthal and Snell, 2003). Riessman (2008, p. 36) called this a process of *co-construction* where stories unfold in a complex interaction between a storyteller (e.g., a client) and an audience (e.g., a healthcare professional). Recently the BPS (2015, p. 15) stipulated that counselling psychologists' co-construct meaning with their clients, which is a positive step towards recognising that we are not passive listeners.

Embracing diversity

Pluralism (meaning more than one) has become fundamental to counselling psychology (Milton, 2010), and because it stems from the same branch of philosophy as postmodernism, they share common values (Henton, 2016). Pluralism recognises that we live in a diverse and global society, and it inherently values social inclusion, transparency, and egalitarianism, which allow us to recognise and to embrace multiple cultural views rather than one worldview (Cooper and McLeod, 2011, pp. 15–16). The essential feature of a multicultural perspective is the idea that we are all shaped by culture; each culture has its own construction of reality, each culture has its own set of values, and each person can transcend his or her cultural identity if they so desire (Laungani, 2005).

The prominent critique in recognising diversity is the tendency to be reductionist about it. In other words, **multiculturalism** is often thought to be synonymous with ethnicity and, as such, it is a concept confined to a handful of ethnocultural groups (Moodley, 2007); this might result in further categorisation such as *African American* or *White British* (Cornwell and Stoddard, 2000). To counter this critique, Moodley (2007) introduces us to the perspective of **critical** multiculturalism where practitioners are urged to interrogate cultural discourses; this critical stance converges with social constructionism. Broadening our ideas about culture allows us to recognise a plurality of cultural subjectivities including gender, race, ethnicity, class, sexual orientation, disability, religion, and age, for example. These cultural subjectivities interact, producing experiences of distress (Moodley, 2007, pp. 13–14). Activity box 3.2 encourages you to reflect on your own cultural subjectivities, allowing you to begin developing multicultural competency.

ACTIVITY BOX 3.2

Using a narrative approach, write a story about your cultural subjectivities. Think about your roles in life, the categories in which you fall or use to describe yourself, and the cultural groups or subgroups that shape you. You may want to structure this in terms of characters, storylines, or even genres. If you were writing a book about your cultural identity, consider what the chapter names would be. Consider how the characters or storylines interact.

Beyond the subject

Agents of social change and structures of power

Vera and Speight (2003) argue that if counselling psychology strives to commit itself to a multicultural agenda, then it too must commit itself to **social justice**. Social justice is a social responsibility, and counselling psychologists are progressively seeing their identity as the "agents of *social* change" (Prilleltensky and Nelson, 2002, p. 149). This change involves social action and advocacy, which mirror the legal notion of equity for all regardless of any cultural diversity (Fouad *et al.* 2006, pp. 1–3). Although the BPS (2015), the DCoP (2005), and the HCPC (2015) commit to tackling stigma, discrimination, and oppression, the agenda for social justice in the United Kingdom is not as coherent as that found in the United States of America (Cutts, 2013; Hore, 2013; Rupani, 2013). What is known about social justice, therefore, stems from this particular cultural paradigm. Nevertheless, in 2013, the *Counselling Psychology Review* released a special edition focusing on power and equality, and it was interesting to note the language being used as a "call to action" (Steffen and Hanley, 2013, p. 3). In this special edition, practitioners discussed the use of a social justice agenda within counselling psychology to tackle issues of oppression and discrimination.

Social justice is a noble ambition, but Rupani (2013) suitably argues that although we can work with experiences of stigma or discrimination, for example, the structures that maintain inequality continue to be unchanged. For example, in 2009, the Improving Access to Psychological Therapies Initiative (IAPT) sought to provide therapy to one of the most socially excluded groups of people in our society – offenders. There is much need for psychological intervention with this particular group of people, yet they are (a) stigmatised as dangerous and risky (Drake, 2011, 2012), (b) they experience service exclusion based on risk (O'Malley, 2004a, 2004b; Fossey and Black, 2010), and (c) paradoxically, stigma remains the main barrier to accessing support (Howerton *et al.* 2007; Bulten *et al.* 2009). In other words, it is fundamentally difficult to improve access unless we improve the structures that impede it, and it is perhaps for this reason that the heart of a social justice movement is *action* (Toporek and Williams, 2006, pp. 21–23). In a similar vein, Moodley (2007, p. 7) argued that the main failure of multiculturalism was its neglect of a critical attitude towards power inequity, resource disharmony, cultural hegemony, racism, sexism, homophobia, and economic oppression. Box 3.2 Beyond the Frontier discusses future developments within counselling psychology as related to the skill of critique.

Building relationships with the community

Bronfenbrenner, in 1979, was influential in his proposal of an **ecological systems theory**, which examined the interactions between people and their environment. In what he termed "nested, interconnected systems," Bronfenbrenner (1979, p. 8) believed that both proximal (e.g., individual and family) and distal (e.g., social and political) environments shaped the lives of people. It is now readily recognised that our social environment can contribute to and maintain mental health difficulties, and individualistic perspectives, such as humanism, often neglect this social terrain (Thatcher and Manktelow, 2007). Social neglect can lead to over-pathologising people and can result in blaming a person who already experiences substantial distress (Nelson and Prilleltensky, 2010). Nelson and Prilleltensky (2010) argue that

BOX 3.2 BEYOND THE FRONTIER

A "critical attitude" is a core competency for counselling psychologists, according to the BPS (2015, p. 15), and it involves committing oneself to transforming practices rather than maintaining the status quo (Guba and Lincoln, 1994). House and Feltham (2015) believe that critical engagement might help to facilitate an attitude that challenges oppression, and **critical psychology** is closely aligned to the social justice agenda for promoting social change (Parker, 2015). Critical psychology itself is interested in understanding structures of power and it shares a commitment to eliminating oppression (Prilleltensky and Nelson, 2002). What social justice and critical psychology, in combination, offer counselling psychology is a greater scope of practice, which includes challenging economic socio-political structures, promoting multicultural competencies, and combating racism, sexism, ageism, and homophobia, for example (Fouad *et al.* 2006). The future of counselling psychology, therefore, might involve practices that not only support the lives of individuals but also those that involve shaping (or re-shaping) society. Using a piece of paper, draw a mind-map of what you believe to be the scope of practice for counselling psychology. Think about the following domains to help you map out your ideas: First, whom might you build positive relationships with? Second, what can you influence as a professional? Third, how might you use your influence to transform current practices? Moreover, what skills and values might you need to achieve this?

therapeutic interventions often seek to change an individual's response to injustice, for example, but **community psychology** seeks to work in partnership with a social system to change injustice itself; a system that is more distal in its influence over an individual. Kagan (2015) suggests that community psychology helps counselling psychologists to be mindful of fostering healthy relationships with individuals and communities in ways that extend beyond an individualistic focus. Counselling psychologists are, arguably, in a unique position to achieve this because they value relational ways of working.

Despite the apparent contribution of social justice, critical psychology, and even community psychology to counselling psychology, there are limitations to their application, and as Moloney (2016, p. 369) suggests, these approaches are "not for the fainthearted." Guba and Lincoln (1994, p. 113) suggest a critical theory is one that engages in "confrontation, even conflict," and Moloney (2016) wonders how confrontational counselling psychologists are permitted to be. Committing oneself to a social justice agenda, in general, and a community psychology perspective, in particular, requires walking a fine line between being an activist and being a professional (Guba and Lincoln, 1994; Moloney, 2016). Further professional reflection, therefore, is needed to determine whether activism is ethically just when offset with issues of injustice itself. Returning to the ecological systems model, proposed so many years ago, it is crucial that we acknowledge the entire ecological landscape that shapes not only our individual identity but also our collective identity. Values, stemming from community psychology, such as community solidarity, partnership, and perhaps even innovation could enhance counselling psychology practices (Moloney, 2016).

Reconnecting with nature

With prominent discourses such as climate change, psychology is re-establishing its natural routes (Gatersleben, 2008). **Ecopsychology** reminds us of our connection to our natural ecosystem (Roszak, 1995); that is, people live in a natural world whether this landscape is manufactured or naturally occurring, and counselling psychology, in particular, is recognising this neglected terrain. Milton (2016, p. 382) proposes that relationships between people and nature are the heart of ecopsychology, allowing counselling psychology to move beyond only regarding "human-human" interactions. Higley and Milton (2008, p. 16) suggest that incorporating the natural environment into therapy allows us to develop an "ecological self," which is rooted in the phenomenology of natural experience.

Our relationship with the environment is not a new topic, yet it has been met with much dissonance and disconnection over the years (Milton, 2016). Ecopsychology itself is a broad area that might cover issues ranging from our changing environmental landscape, poverty, over-population, environmental stress, exposure to pollutants and toxins, to anxiety about environmental threats or concern over the fate of the natural world (Milton, 2009). *Environmentally aware therapy* and *ecotherapy* are examples of an ecopsychological perspective, as applied to therapy (Milton, 2016, p. 388).

In 2007, Mind proposed a *green agenda* for mental health following evidence that ecotherapy can have positive implications for physical health, lowering stress, improving self-esteem, and encouraging social inclusion. Subsequently, Ecominds (2013) was established with 12,000 people engaging in ecotherapy projects from 2009 to 2013, which included activities such as horticulture, animal-assisted interventions, conservation, care farming, and wilderness therapy often in combination with structured therapy. People involved in ecotherapy reported mood improvement and a greater sense of connection to their community (Bragg *et al.* 2013). What makes ecopsychology important to counselling psychology is that it can easily be integrated into traditional therapeutic practices; it is not a new type of therapy but rather a useful tool for addressing pressing "human-environment" issues (Milton, 2016, p. 389).

Summary

This chapter introduced some of the prominent perspectives found in counselling psychology and encouraged you to reflect on the values they impart. Counselling psychology, as a profession, holds a respectful attitude towards every person's subjective experience of life and, as such, it embraces diversity in meaning and in knowledge (DCoP, 2005; BPS, 2015; HCPC, 2015).

We have looked at how each perspective contains ideas about human nature and the nature of distress ranging from concepts like subjectivity to intersubjectivities. On the one hand, humanistic perspectives teach us about the value of the individual mind, allowing us to appreciate agency. On the other hand, postmodernism teaches us about the ultimate conflict that occurs between an agent and his or her social structure. Critical multiculturalism and its interest in promoting diversity, inclusion, and equality presented an interesting challenge for counselling psychology such as increasing our scope of practice effectively and ethically.

With a call to action, social justice and its commitment to social change may become increasingly important in our work (Steffen and Hanley, 2013). Challenging taken-for-granted practices and maintaining a critical stance were substantial values in social constructionism, critical psychology, and even community psychology (Burr, 1995; Gergen, 2015; House and Feltham, 2015). Moreover, emergent perspectives that are more pluralistic in orientation acknowledge that life is so much more complex than any one theory alone can explain (Cooper and McLeod, 2011). The final activity of this chapter, in Activity box 3.3, now encourages you to re-examine your values in relation to (a) what has been presented in this chapter and (b) what will be presented in the remainder of this book.

ACTIVITY BOX 3.3

Repeat Activity 3.1, but this time, think about how each perspective conceptualises human nature and the nature of distress. Compare and contrast each perspective and, then, compare and contrast this to your prior thoughts. Have your values shifted or were they reaffirmed? What fits with your own belief system and what is jarring? Keep this activity to hand when you go through this book, and repeat your process of reflection. Consider how your values may be shifting as you actively engage with the content of this book.

Learning outcomes

When you have completed this chapter you should be able to:

- Develop knowledge about the ways in which values influence therapy.
- Develop knowledge of the perspectives found in counselling psychology.
- Develop knowledge of your personal and professional values including the implementation of skills such as reflection and critique.

Key phrases, concepts, and terms

- Cognitive-behavioural therapy
- Community psychology
- Critical multiculturalism
- Critical psychology
- Ecological systems theory
- Ecopsychology
- Existential perspective
- Human potential movement
- Humanistic perspective
- Idiographic approach
- Intersubjectivity
- Lifespan developmental perspective
- Mindfulness
- Multiculturalism
- Narrative inquiry

- Nomothetic approach
- Objectivity
- Phenomenology
- Pluralism
- Positive psychology
- Postmodernism
- Psychodynamic perspective
- Social constructionism
- Social justice
- Strengths-based approach
- Subjectivities
- Subjectivity

Sample essay titles

1. Compare and contrast subjectivity and shifting subjectivities with emphasis on how each contributes to knowledge of human nature.
2. Critically discuss two counselling psychology perspectives with an emphasis on how they contribute to the knowledge of mental health.
3. In this reflective assignment, describe how the values found in counselling psychology may influence how you see (a) the therapeutic role and (b) the scope of practice for counselling psychologists.

Further reading

British Psychological Society. (2015). *Standards for the accreditation of doctoral programmes in counselling psychology*. Leicester: BPS.

Division of Counselling Psychology. (2005). *Professional practice guidelines*. Leicester: BPS.

Health and Care Professions Council. (2015). *Standards of proficiency: Practitioner psychologists*. London: HCPC.

References

Adams, M. (2014). Human development and existential counselling psychology. *Counselling Psychology Review*, 29(2), 34–42.

American Psychiatric Association. (2013). *Diagnostic and statistical manual of mental disorders: DSM 5*, (5th Ed). Washington, DC: American Psychiatric Publishing.

Amos, I. (2015). What is known about the post-traumatic growth experience among people diagnosed with HIV/AIDS? A systematic review and thematic synthesis of the qualitative literature. *Counselling Psychology Review*, 30(3), 47–56.

Baltes, P.B. (1987). Theoretical propositions of life-span developmental psychology: On the dynamics between growth and decline. *Developmental Psychology*, 23(5), 611–626.

Beck, A. (1996). 'Beyond belief: A theory of modes, personality, and psychopathy.' In: P. Salkovskis (Ed), *Frontiers of cognitive therapy*. New York: Guildford Press, 1–25.

Berger, P. and Luckman, T. (1966). *The social construction of reality*. Garden City, NY: Knopf Doubleday.

Bergin, A.E. (1980). Psychotherapy and religious values. *Journal of Consulting and Clinical Psychology*, 48(1), 95–105.

Bragg, R., Wood, C., and Barton, J. (2013). *Ecominds effects on mental wellbeing: An evaluation for mind*. London: Mind.

British Psychological Society. (2015). *Standards for the accreditation of doctoral programmes in counselling psychology*. Leicester: BPS.

Bronfenbrenner, U. (1979). *The ecology of human development: Experiments by nature and design*. Cambridge, MA: Harvard University Press.

Bulten, E., Nijman, H., and van der Staak, C. (2009). Psychological predictors of help needs in male Dutch prisoners. *International Journal of Forensic Mental Health*, 8(2), 71–80.

Burr, V. (1995). *An introduction to social constructionism*. London: Routledge.

Calhoun, L.G., and Tedeshi, R.G. (2014). *Handbook of posttrumatic growth: Research and practice*. London: Psychology Press.

Cooper, M., and McLeod, J. (2011). *Pluralistic counselling and psychotherapy*. London: Sage.

Cornwell, G., and Stoddard, E. (2000). *Global multiculturalism: Comparative perspectives on ethnicity, race, and nation*. Lanham, MD: Rowman & Littlefield Publishers.

Crotty, M. (1998). *The foundations of social research*. London: Sage.

Cutts, L.A. (2013). Considering a social justice agenda for counselling psychology in the UK. *Counselling Psychology Review*, 28(2), 8–16.

Division of Counselling Psychology. (2005). *Professional practice guidelines*. Leicester: BPS.

Donohue, E., and Moore, D. (2009). When is an offender not an offender? Power, the client and shifting penal subjectivities. *Punishment and Society*, 11, 319–336.

Drake, D.H. (2011). The 'dangerous other' in maximum-security prisons. *Criminology and Justice*, 11(4), 367–382.

Drake, D.H. (2012). *Prisons, punishment and the pursuit of security*. Basingstoke, Hampshire: Palgrave Macmillan.

Ecominds. (2013). *Feel better outside, feel better inside: Ecotherapy for mental wellbeing, resilience and recovery*. London: Mind.

Fossey, M., and Black, G. (2010). *Under the radar: Women with borderline personality disorder in prison*. London: Sainsbury Centre for Mental Health.

Fouad, N.A., Gerstein, L.H., and Toporek, R.L. (2006). 'Social justice and counselling psychology.' In: R.L. Toporek, L.H. Gerstein, N.A. Fouad, G. Roysircar, and T. Israel (Eds.), *Handbook for social justice in counselling psychology: Leadership, vision, and action*. London: Sage, 1–16.

Gatersleben, B. (2008). Humans and nature: Ten useful findings from environmental psychology research. *Counselling Psychology Review*, 23(2), 24–34.

Gergen, K.J. (2015). *An invitation to social construction*, (3rd Ed). London Sage.

Griffiths, E. (2014). *Towards a science of belief systems*. Basingstoke, Hampshire: Palgrave Macmillan.

Guba, E.G., and Lincoln, Y.S. (1994). 'Competing paradigms in qualitative research.' In: N.K. Denzin and Y.S. Lincoln (Eds), *Handbook of qualitative research*. London: Sage, 105–117.

Hacking, I. (1999). *The social construction of what?* Cambridge, MA: Harvard University Press.

Health and Care Professions Council. (2015). *Standards of proficiency: Practitioner psychologists*. London: HCPC.

Henton, I. (2016). 'Engaging with research.' In: B. Douglas, R. Woolfe, S. Strawbridge, E. Kasket, and V. Galbraith (Eds), *The handbook of counselling psychology*, (4th Ed). London: Sage, 132–148.

Hess, S.A., and Schultz, J.M. (2008). 'Bronfenbrenner's ecological model.' In: K.L. Kraus (Ed), *Lenses: Applying lifespan development theories in counselling*. New York: Houghton Mifflin, 52–82.

Higley, N., and Milton, M. (2008). Our connection to the Earth: A neglected relationship in counselling psychology? *Counselling Psychology Review*, 23(2), 10–22.

Hore, B. (2013). Is homelessness a matter of social justice for counselling psychologists in the UK? A review of the literature. *Counselling Psychology Review*, 28(2), 17–29.

House, R., and Feltham, C. (2015). 'Counselling psychology: Critical achievements, possibilities, and limitations.' In: I. Parker (Ed), *Handbook of critical psychology*. Hove, East Sussex: Routledge, 164–172.

Howerton, A., Byng, R., Campbell, J., Hess, D., Owens, C., and Aitken, P. (2007). Understanding help seeking behaviour among male offenders: Qualitative interview study. *British Medical Journal*, 334(7588), 303–309.

Improving Access to Psychological Therapy. (2009). *Offenders: Positive practice guide*. London: Department of Health.

Jacobs, M. (2012). *The presenting past: The core of psychodynamic counselling and therapy*, (4th Ed). Maidenhead, Berkshire: McGraw-Hill.

Johnson, A.P. (2011). Belief systems, metaphysical paradigms, and educational practices. *Encounter, Education for Meaning and Social Justice*, 24(3), 8–14.

Jones-Smith, E. (2016). *Theories of counselling and psychotherapy: An integrative approach*, (2nd Ed). London: Sage.

Kagan, C. (2015). Community psychological perspectives and counselling psychology. *Counselling Psychology Review*, 30(3), 12–21.

Kripal, J.F. (2007). *Esalen: America and the religion of no religion*. Chicago: University of Chicago Press.

Laungani, P. (2005). Building on multicultural counselling bridges: The holy grail or poisoned chalice? *Counselling Psychology Quarterly*, 18(4), 247–259.

Loewenthal, D., and Snell, R. (2003). *Post-modernism for psychotherapist: A critical reader*. Hove, East Sussex: Brunner-Routledge.

Maslow, A.H. (1971). *The farther reaches of human nature*. New York: Viking Press.

Mathieson, T. (1962). Subjectivism in sociological research. *Acta Sociologica*, 5(1), 1–14.

McLeod, J. (2001). *Qualitative research in counselling and psychotherapy*. London: Sage.

McLeod, J. (2013). *An introduction to counselling*, (5th Ed). Maidenhead, Berkshire: McGraw-Hill.

Milton, M. (2009). Waking up to nature: Exploring a new direction for psychological practice. *Ecopsychology*, 1(1), 1–13.

Milton, M. (2010). *Therapy and beyond: Counselling psychology contributions to therapeutic and social issues*. Chichester, West Sussex: Wiley-Blackwell.

Milton, M. (2016). 'Psychological practice in a time of environmental crisis: Counselling psychology and ecopsychology.' In: B. Douglas, R. Woolfe, S. Strawbridge, E. Kasket, and V. Galbraith (Eds), *The handbook of counselling psychology*, (4th Ed). London: Sage, 379–396.

Mind. (2007). *Ecotherapy: The green agenda for mental health*. London: Mind.

Moloney, P. (2016). 'Community psychology and the counselling psychologist.' In: B. Douglas, R. Woolfe, S. Strawbridge, E. Kasket, and V. Galbraith (Eds), *The handbook of counselling psychology*, (4th Ed). London: Sage, 364–378.

Moodley, R. (2007). (Re)placing multiculturalism in counselling and psychotherapy. *British Journal of Guidance & Counselling*, 35(1), 1–22.

Nelson, G., and Prilleltensky, I. (2010). *Community psychology: In pursuit of liberation and well-being*, (2nd Ed). Basingstoke, Hampshire: Palgrave Macmillan.

O'Malley, P. (2004a). *Risk, uncertainty and government*. London: GlassHouse.

O'Malley, P. (2004b). The uncertain promise of risk. *Australian and New Zealand Journal of Criminology*, 37(3), 323–343.

Parker, I. (2015). *Handbook of critical psychology*. London: Routledge.

Parritt, S. (2016). 'Working with difference and diversity.' In: B. Douglas, R. Woolfe, S. Strawbridge, E. Kasket, and V. Galbraith (Eds), *The handbook of counselling psychology*, (4th Ed). London: Sage, 198–211.

Patterson, C.H. (1989). Values in counselling and psychotherapy. *Journal of Counselling Psychology*, 5(3), 164–176.

Porta, D.D., and Keating, M. (2008). *Approaches and methodologies in the social sciences*. Cambridge: Cambridge University Press.

Prilleltensky, I., and Nelson, G. (2002). *Doing psychology critically: Making a difference in diverse settings*. Basingstoke, Hampshire: Palgrave Macmillan.

Proctor, G. (2014). *Values and ethics in counselling and psychotherapy*. London: Sage.

Pugh, D., and Coyle, A. (2000). The construction of counselling psychology in Britain: A discourse analysis of counselling psychology texts. *Counselling Psychology Quarterly*, 13(1), 85–98.

Riessman, C.K. (2008). *Narrative methods for the human sciences*. London: Sage.

Rogers, C.R. (1959). 'A theory of therapy, personality, and interpersonal relationships, as developed in the client-centred framework.' In: S. Koch (Ed), *Psychology: A study of science* (Study 1, Volume 3). New York: McGraw-Hill, 184–256.

Roszak, T. (1995). Where psyche meets Gaia. In: T. Roszak, M.E. Gomes, and A.D. Kanner (Eds), *Ecopsychology: Restoring the earth, healing the planet*. San Francisco: Sierra Club Books, 1–20.

Rowan, J. (1983). *The reality game: A guide to humanistic counselling and psychotherapy*, (2nd Ed). London: Routledge.

Rupani, P. (2013). Social justice and counselling psychology training: Can we learn from the US? *Counselling Psychology Review*, 28(2), 30–38.

Schwandt, T.A. (2007). *The SAGE dictionary of qualitative inquiry*, (3rd Ed). London: Sage.

Segal, Z.V., Williams, J.M.G., and Teasdale, J.D. (2013). *Mindfulness-based cognitive therapy for depression*, (2nd Ed). London: Guilford Press.

Smith, J.A., Flowers, P., and Larkin, M. (2009). *Interpretive phenomenological analysis: Theory, method, and research*. London: Sage.

Snyder, D.M. (1982). Some foundation of counselling and psychotherapy from a phenomenological perspective. *The Personnel and Guidance Journal*, 60(6), 364–367.

Steffen, E., and Hanley, T. (2013). The power of counselling psychology in an age of powerlessness: A call to action. *Counselling Psychology Review*, 28(2), 3–7.

Strawbridge, S. (2016). 'Science, craft and professional values.' In: B. Douglas, R. Woolfe, S. Strawbridge, E. Kasket, and V. Galbraith (Eds), *The handbook of counselling psychology*, (4th Ed). London: Sage, 20–38.

Sugarman, L. (2001). *Life-span development: Frameworks, accounts and strategies*, (2nd Ed). Hove, East Sussex: Psychology Press.

Thatcher, M., and Manktelow, K. (2007). The cost of individualism. *Counselling Psychology Review*, 22(4), 31–42.

Toporek, R.L., and Williams, R.A. (2006). 'Ethics and professional issues related to the practice of social justice in counselling psychology.' In: R.L. Toporek, L.H. Gerstein, N.A. Fouad, G. Roysircar, and T. Israel (Eds), *Handbook for social justice in counselling psychology: Leadership, vision, and action*. London: Sage, 17–34.

van Deurzen, E. (2015). Response to Steffen, Vossler, and Joseph – from shared roots to fruitful collaboration: How counselling psychology can benefit from reconnecting with positive psychology. *Counselling Psychology Review*, 20(3), 69–72.

Vera, E.M., and Speight, S.L. (2003). Multicultural competence, social justice, and counselling psychology: Expanding our roles. *The Counselling Psychologist*, 31(3), 253–272.

Ward, T. (2002). Good lives and the rehabilitation of offenders: Promises and problems. *Aggression and Violent Behaviour*, 7, 513–528.

Ward, T., and Marshall, W.L. (2004). Good lives, aetiology and the rehabilitation of sex offenders: A bridging theory. *Journal of Sexual Aggression*, 10(2), 153–169.

World Health Organisation. (2006). *The ICD-10 classification of mental and behavioural disorders: Clinical descriptions and diagnostic guidelines*. Geneva, Switzerland: WHO.

4

DEVELOPING A THERAPEUTIC RELATIONSHIP

Lynne Jordan

Introduction

This chapter will introduce the therapeutic relationship as central to the practice of counselling psychology. Common factors (or non-specific factors) research will be discussed, which indicates that the therapeutic relationship is one of the most essential ingredients for effective therapy. Concepts such as the use of self in a relationship and links to the theoretical concepts of congruence, transference and countertransference will be discussed. More recent developments of the pluralistic framework will be considered, paying particular attention to the collaborative relationship at its core.

Counselling Psychology, and some other therapeutic disciplines, hold the forming, maintenance and quality of relationship as central to all effective practice. Milton (2016: 184–197) reminds us in 'Forming a Relationship: A Phenomenological Encounter' in *The Handbook of Counselling Psychology* how 'we cannot *not* be in relationship' (page 185) due to the innate ability to attach and connect with others through empathic process and caring about and for others. It is the 'being in the world' of Heidegger (2010) quoted by Milton (page 185) that is without refute and places us in context to the wider social and political context of our world.

Everyday therapeutic relationships

When asked to write a chapter on 'developing a **therapeutic relationship**' my first thought was to make this as part of a perspective that encompasses relationships experienced as therapeutic in everyday life and in the caring professions in general, as well as in the formal therapy world. So the starting point for the chapter is to ask 'what makes a relationship therapeutic?' The concept of therapeutic value of relationships is a common theme within eastern and western society, even if experienced and constructed differently. For example, some societies have a more societal group identity and therefore the value of relationships will be far more focused on how the family or social group functions as it tends towards a group identity. Some societies in the western world are far more individualised and therefore the value of relationships will be more individualised. This is important to recognise in multicultural societies, as in the UK, whether in everyday relationships or in formal therapeutic relationships.

This chapter takes a broad perspective drawing from **attachment** insights as in Bowlby (1969, 1973, 1980a, 1988a and 1988b), Ainsworth and Holmes (2001), who looked at implications of attachment in clinical practice. Importance of attachments across the lifespan have direct and indirect effects on the way relationships work in ordinary life and in therapeutic settings. This provides a springboard to look at how therapy is often conducted via an integrative, eclectic or pluralistic (Cooper and Dryden, 2016) approach, even though a particular model's language may be the main reference point. Transtheoretical common factors in therapeutic practice have long been a source of fascination for discussion and research. First of all let us take a moment to reflect on what makes relationships vital and enjoyable to us in everyday life.

ACTIVITY BOX 4.1

Some questions to consider:

1. Consider the people that matter to you . . . what makes them important?
2. What emotional feelings come up for you?
3. How does that affect your general wellbeing?
4. If things go wrong in any of those relationships, how do you feel?
5. How does this affect your ability to concentrate and do the usual things of everyday and even creativity?

It is quite remarkable that whenever these kind of tasks come across my path, my time is suddenly under extra pressure of expectations from the most important relationships in my life. The irony did not escape me that I had set aside time to begin writing this chapter when my younger son, whom I do not get to see very often these days due to busy lives, had an unexpected day off and wanted to visit. I chose to spend time in that relationship rather than write about relationships in theory! In my example both my son and I enjoyed our time together and could say it was a 'therapeutic' time together. I certainly felt physically relaxed as it was a re-connection to one of the important people in my life, one of my closest attachments. Somehow other things in life find their perspective when we spend time with those we care about and with whom we also are cared for. Schore (2000) discusses how we can be soothed and settled by contact with those we are closely attached to, providing the attachment is secure enough.

ACTIVITY BOX 4.1 FOLLOW-UP

How do your close relationships affect you emotionally but also physiologically?

Merriam-Webster Dictionary (from 1828) defines 'therapeutic' as 'a good effect on body or mind' and also 'of or relating to treatment of illness'. 'Relationship' is defined in its most basic definition as: 'the way in which two or more people, groups, countries, etc., talk to, behave toward, and deal with each other; a romantic or sexual friendship between two people; the way in which two or more people or things are connected'. The English *Oxford Dictionary* defines 'therapeutic' as 'having a good effect on the body or mind; contributing to a sense of wellbeing'; and 'relationship' as: 'The way in which two or more people or things are connected, or the state of being connected'.

Arguably the first 'relationships' we ever form are those starting in utero (Schore, 2000). Those connections and that awareness that occurs as our neurological systems are developing allow us to begin to hear our mother's heartbeat and voice at around 20 weeks gestation of pregnancy. This early awareness begins our initial connection to the world around us and formation of relationships.

We can see that relationships in everyday experience can have varying degrees of therapeutic value in terms of how much they can be mutually beneficial. The focus of therapeutic benefit in formal therapy settings is clearly directed towards the person known as 'client' or 'patient'. This is also very different to everyday or more generic caring roles where the focus might be a lot more blurred. Clarkson (2008) quotes Holmes and Lindley (1989) as defining therapy as *'the systematic use of a relationship between therapist and patient – as opposed to pharmacological or social methods – to produce changes in cognition, feelings and behaviour'* (Clarkson and Wilson, 2008: 3).

Codes of ethics and conduct

There are ethical guidelines for any profession in the therapy world and Counselling Psychology is no exception. The ethical frameworks contribute to the development of the '**safe enough**' environment for both therapist and client. Therefore we can see that in contrast to everyday relationships, the main focus of the formal 'therapeutic relationship' is the person(s) coming for therapy, the therapist's wellbeing is also highly relevant due to the interplay in therapeutic encounters, whatever approach the therapist associates with. Therefore ethical guidelines guide the relationships we hold in various professional settings and whilst working in different therapeutic models. There is a power dynamic present in a helper/helped relationship that can subtly change how relationships operate. If there is a breach of ethical codes it can have serious consequences for client or indeed practitioner. Ethical principles inform working relationships within each practice setting, including clinical work with clients and supervision, research and teaching, or consultancy and service development, offering a framework for the formation of secure relationships that support work undertaken.

The British Psychological Society (BPS, 2009) in its *Code of Ethics and Conduct* covers the broad range of activities that any psychologists, including Counselling Psychologists, typically undertake. All these principles need to be interpreted carefully and often in consultation with senior colleagues. Please see Box 4.1 for an overview; further detail can be found in the References section.

FOCUS BOX 4.1 BPS CODE OF ETHICS AND CONDUCT

1. **Respect:** covering multiple issues but in essence to do with valuing 'dignity and worth of all individuals' and 'privacy and self-determination'.
2. **Competence:** maintaining high standards of competence and recognising 'the importance of preserving their ability to function optimally within recognized limits'.
3. **Responsibility:** valuing responsibility to 'clients, general public, and to the profession and science of Psychology' including 'misuse or abuse of their contributions to society'.
4. **Integrity:** valuing 'honesty, accuracy, clarity and fairness in all interactions with all persons'.

The *Code of Ethics and Conduct* is set alongside the BPS Division of Counselling Psychology's (DCoP) *Professional Practice Guidelines* (2005) in ethical decision making. The latter guidelines highlight management of and working with complex relational situations. Please see below for an overview of main points and further detail via the weblink provided in the Further Reading section.

FOCUS BOX 4.2 BPS DCoP PROFESSIONAL PRACTICE GUIDELINES (2005)

Obligations and Responsibilities

1. **To self and clients**
   a. Competence in awareness of both skill base and limitations.
   b. Fitness to practice re personal functioning, indemnity insurance, awareness of power dynamics.
   c. Contracting clarity.
   d. Confidentiality clarity.
2. **To self and colleagues**
   a. Supervision and consultative support.
   b. Clarity of roles and responsibilities in supervision.
   c. Practitioner as a trainer.
   d. Boundaries and dual relationship management.
   e. Researcher practitioner congruence between research models and Counselling Psychology values.
3. **To self and society**
   a. Awareness of context influencing therapy.
   b. Assessments to match context with client need and situation.
   c. Prioritise reflective practice in all activities.
   d. Expand knowledge base, especially in unfamiliar presentations.
   e. Awareness of societal influence, cultural difference.

The profession of Counselling Psychology is regulated by the Health and Care Professions Council (HCPC, 2016), and its *Standards of Conduct, Performance and Ethics* are also adhered to. These are very lengthy and broadly cover the same standards as the BPS general guidelines and the DCoP guidelines. HCPC standards are featured in Chapter 13 of this book so I will not discuss further here. However, it is important to raise awareness of the HCPC's role in the profession when discussing the 'Therapeutic Relationship' as these standards and the guidelines are protectors and facilitators in forming ethically sound relationships that provide a foundation for effective therapy, supervision, training and research. As we see in the guidelines specific to counselling psychology, there is an emphasis on the ethical management and priority of relationship within all aspects of counselling psychology practice. In the Further Reading section at the end of this chapter there is a weblink to the Health and Care Professions Council Standards document.

Relationships and theory

Clarkson's *The Therapeutic Relationship* (1995, 2000) and revised second edition with Wilson (2003, 2008) provides an excellent framework that encompasses the complexity of multiple perspectives in therapy models. She acknowledges that there are at least five relationships we may have with clients and others we are in a helping relationship with. These might co-exist in a therapeutic encounter or may transition over time from one to another or even be predominantly one style of relationship during a piece of work. Not all relationship kinds will be in existence in all therapy. In Box 4.3 the reader can find the five relationship model.

FOCUS BOX 4.3 THE FIVE RELATIONSHIP MODEL (CLARKSON, 1995, 2000; CLARKSON AND WILSON, 2003, 2008)

1. **Person to person:** real relationship based on two human beings in the here and now.
2. **Working alliance:** the relationship that allows the work to go on even when things are tough.
3. **Transferential/countertransferential:** the experience of transferred longings or fears onto and into the therapeutic relationship.
4. **Reparative/developmentally needed:** intentional provision by the therapist of a 'corrective, reparative or replenishing relationship or action' for someone with experiences in the outside world have been neglectful, abusive of suffocating.
5. **Transpersonal:** the aspect of the therapeutic relationship which is 'timeless and spiritual' as part of healing.

Clarkson's 'Five Relationships' model is easily incorporated into the more recently articulated 'pluralistic counselling' which is an approach developed by Mick Cooper and John McLeod in 2006 largely from the notion that all therapies have something useful to offer in helping people improve the quality of their lives. It was also developed in response to the tendency for 'dogmatism within the counselling and psychotherapy fields' (2016: 1) causing, in their view, an unnecessary differentiation between models and theories. This also was something that concerned Clarkson in her earlier writings (1995, 2000).

Clarkson's 'Five Relationships' have greatly informed my work over the years in my practice in therapy, supervision, teaching and training, and even as an examiner. This allows reference to various therapeutic models as the individual relationship types are usually seen to associate with different models. For example, the 'working alliance' is often seen as belonging to a cognitive-behavioural model but we cannot do any therapeutic work without some kind of alliance that allows the therapy to work in practical ways even if using a predominantly process-oriented insight-based psychodynamic approach. Psychodynamic approaches may refer to the relational aspects in therapy as predominantly 'transference/countertransference' relationships. In fact even in other therapies it could be asked: how can previous relationship experiences not map onto current ones? In cognitive models, schemas are seen to be formed from the basis of early relationships. This in turn maps onto the concept of 'Internal Working Models' in modern-day **Attachment Theory** (Holmes, 2001) and in Malan's (1999) triangle of insight taking into account each point of the triangle:

- Relationships outside therapy room in the historical or recent past.
- Relationships outside therapy room that are current.
- Relationship inside the therapy room with the therapist.

The reader will find more detail of CBT and Psychodynamic models of therapy in Section 3 of this book so this chapter simply flags their existence in the context of the varying uses of the therapeutic relationship.

Pluralistic theory as it is developing easily integrates with the multi-faceted Clarkson's model. **Pluralism** in action is a way of making more accessible to clients a whole range of theoretical insights and techniques that otherwise might not have been available to certain client groups or in certain settings. A definition of pluralism incorporates the philosophical belief of 'any substantial question admits of a variety of plausible but mutually conflicting responses' (Rescher, 1993: 79). In brief there are three pillars that provide a foundation for a pluralistic approach in counselling and psychotherapy as seen below in Box 4.4.

FOCUS BOX 4.4 PILLARS OF PLURALISTIC COUNSELLING (COOPER AND DRYDEN, 2016: 3)

1. **Pluralism across orientations:** open to various forms of distress presented and therefore to various ways of helping that distress. This 'poses a direct challenge to schoolism in counselling and psychotherapy'.
2. **Pluralism across clients:** 'recognising and celebrating diversity across clients'. Practitioners adapt the therapy offered to more closely suit the client.
3. **Pluralism across perspectives:** practitioners and clients are both involved in negotiating goals and therapy most relevant to client. Shared decision making and feedback informing therapeutic approaches are valued.

In my own practice I have found an integrative stance and an openness to various ways of working to be highly beneficial to clients. It allows for flexibility of approach depending on the individual client and particular context in which I am working.

A pluralistic approach seems very accessible to practitioners at any level as it allows for the use of knowledge, insight and experience to whichever stage they have reached both professionally and personally. It also acknowledges that perhaps some concepts cannot be 'integrated' in the classical meaning of the term. They can however, exist alongside one another being accessible for use when helpful either to a particular client or at a particular phase in the client's journey. Common factors research as seen in Hubble, Duncan, and Miller (1999) and Imel and Wampold (2008) would certainly support the ides that there is much common ground between models, in particular in relation to the quality of the therapeutic relationship, the motivation and readiness of the client to make changes and the goodness of fit between therapist and client.

One of my clients had this to say about her experience of the 'therapeutic relationship' and how she finds it helps her. We were talking about the therapeutic relationship and how it might be influencing our work together, and I had mentioned I was writing a chapter on the formation of therapeutic relationships. The use of this verbatim quote is made at her request to contribute to the chapter but I have used a pseudonym to protect her anonymity.

FOCUS BOX 4.5 EMMA

I've been thinking about that chapter you are writing and thought I would mention a few things that work for me in the "therapeutic relationship". . .

A major one for me is how you make me aware of the physicality of my body in its reactions to what I may be talking through. E.g. when discussing trauma related stuff you are quick to point out that I may feel cold and sometimes offer me a blanket. This really helps me stay in touch with my body and what I am feeling . . .

I have found your transparency in relation to anecdotes from your own therapy journey helps me relate to similar things I may be going through or have gone through. This helps me see you as equal in terms of power balance of the relationship. And helps me feel less ashamed of what I may have felt or feel.

You are always calm. Helping me stay calm.

And are careful to bring me back to the present before I leave our sessions.

Email or WhatsApp is excellent if stuff comes up for me and I'm alone or feel it's something too private to talk thru with others.

. . . hope that helps. Obviously this is just snippets of our work together and really words will never be enough to describe how life changing our work has been and continues to be. (sic)

Philosophical roots

Counselling Psychology has at its roots a two-fold perspective originating from humanistic perspectives but also from scientific enquiry, including quantitative and qualitative philosophies. **Humanistic psychology** has an optimistic stance on human beings, therefore relationships and human development, believing human beings will strive towards growth and development as a given. Maslow's (1943, 1968) **hierarchy of needs** and aspiration towards self-actualisation are also fundamental in the view of humans as being fundamentally good providing that at least basic and preferably higher-level needs are met. Subsequent chapters will deal with these approaches in more depth but see Box 4.6 for a summary.

FOCUS BOX 4.6 MASLOW'S HIERARCHY OF NEEDS (1954)

1. **Physiological needs:** air, food, water, clothing, shelter and sexual drive.
2. **Safety needs:** experiencing life as safe enough.
3. **Love and belonging:** being a part of a group, e.g. family or social network.
4. **Esteem:** feeling valued by others.
5. **Self-actualisation:** making the most of the self within context.
6. **Self-transcendence:** moving beyond the self to something beyond the self.

Basic human needs are encapsulated within Maslow's **Hierarchy of Needs** as above and also map across onto Rogers' **Core Conditions** as seen below.

FOCUS BOX 4.7 ROGERS' CORE CONDITIONS (1957)

1. **Empathy:** putting yourself in someone's shoes but without losing connection with yourself.
2. **Congruence:** being real, so being able to manage internal conflicts whilst still remaining connected to the client in an open way. Not necessary to disclose whatever is in your mind.
3. **Unconditional Positive Regard:** acceptance of the client as a human being but not necessarily agreeing with everything they say or do.

It is useful to recognise how both the needs of Maslow and these conditions of worth can be seen as core to safe enough relationships for professional therapeutic working but can also be seen to form the basics needed for other relationships in everyday life. In Mandy's story, which focuses on everyday relationships, the principles learnt can be translated to a therapeutic context where the counselling psychologist can be seen as providing a temporary **secure base** (Bowlby, 1969, 1988) that would support the work. So in Mandy's case we can see how the acceptance and perceived non-judgement of her husband met some of her basic needs and also allowed her to relax and develop herself emotionally and professionally.

FOCUS BOX 4.8 REFLECTION: MANDY'S STORY PART 1

Mandy is a health worker based in a youth crisis centre in of one of the UK's major cities in the north of England. The part of Mandy's story told here is from a time when she was also having a tough time in her personal life. She had three remaining children from other relationships who had also connected well with her husband (one child had died due to a rare genetic disorder). She also had one step-daughter from a previous relationship of his. Her marriage of 20-plus years looked like it was at an end as her husband had left her with no clear explanation. When he left she felt confused and rejected, wondering if what she believed her relationship to him was all a lie. When he left her she felt she had no secure base to stand on. His previous acceptance of her, or 'Unconditional Positive Regard' offered, provided in effect a 'secure base' to stand upon. This enabled her to have a sense of belonging and source of self-esteem and without him she felt adrift and without a platform to stand upon. Mandy had had an abusive but privileged childhood with little acceptance or empathy from either of her parents. She had a grandmother and a few other people in her life who, to some extent, made up for this. However, it was only when she met and married her husband that she felt that someone really treasured her, and her children, for who she was, and who they were, and offered acceptance and a secure base in spite of any shortcomings. After much discussion over a period of several months, Mandy became aware of how he might have decided overnight to leave saying he 'couldn't do this anymore' due to his own shortcomings predominantly, rather than as a direct reflection on her and the relationship. Initially it was completely confusing as he had shown no sign that he needed to leave the relationship or the family. She saw that her husband's empathy for her, that had seemed so strong, had become tainted as he gradually lost himself in her priorities so he, in effect, lost himself. Empathy can only be real when combined with congruence (a sense of being real with oneself about oneself) and over time he lost the ability to maintain this part of the 'core conditions'. Eventually his acceptance or unconditional positive regard (UPR) was undermined and empathy to her disintegrated and he felt overwhelmed, trapped inside his own lostness and left. She then questioned as to how genuine the empathy or UPR was that he had offered. We will revisit Mandy for part 2 of her story.

In professional therapeutic relationships where a relationship has the **Core Conditions** as a foundation for the work it could be seen to also provide a 'secure base' or safe enough relationship. According to attachment theorists this would allow for exploration needed in therapy as well as facilitate confidence and insight for change. The concept of a 'safe enough' relationship maps easily onto the concept of the 'good enough mother' or caregiver (Winnicott,1965) and also a 'secure enough base' experience that comes from attachment theory originally formulated by Bowlby (1988, Ainsworth and Bowlby (1991) and Ainsworth, Blehar, Waters, and Wall (1978); later expounded upon by de Zueletta (2006) and Holmes (2001)).

Attachment as underpinning for therapeutic relationships

Attachment Theory is not a model of therapy in itself, however it could be argued that utilising an Attachment Theory perspective can highlight relational aspects of any model and will therefore strengthen therapeutic work. It is well documented how it is the quality of the therapeutic relationship which is the most influential factor in therapy outcome. Holmes (2001) has taken Bowlby's (1969, 1988) original theories and developed them in a way that they can be integrated into therapeutic practice. He highlights the domains he sees as dimensions of attachments.

FOCUS BOX 4.9 ATTACHMENT DOMAINS (HOLMES, 2001)

- Secure base: external secure base and an internalised secure base.
- Exploration and enjoyment: capacity for playful, sexual or intellectual pleasure is central to secure base capacity.
- Protest and anger: an attachment regulator to maintain attachment bonds and secure base.
- Loss: central to much psychological distress. Attachment is only possible with negotiation of separation and real or potential losses.
- Internal Working Models: the shape of relationships, the 'who I am' and 'how I fit into the world' and 'how the world fits in with me'.
- Reflexive function and narrative competence: security of attachment is related to reflexive functioning, applicable for the narrative process of therapy in which clients learn to develop their reflexive functioning.

Internal Working Models are similar in concept to the schemata of cognitive psychology or mental maps operating as templates of relationship, the 'who am I and how I fit in with others'. Influence of technology and especially social networking sites is seen as greatly influential in relationship formation and maintenance across the board (Ozad and Uygarer, 2014). Younger people especially are familiar with using social media and online communications as an everyday resource for building and managing relationships. Inevitably this then has begun to map onto the world of therapy, supervision and research so it is useful to reflect on the way this can be effectual and what the differences might be from face-to-face work. There are online academic courses increasingly being introduced which also have a relational aspect to how students relate to the course leaders as well as other students in online discussion forums, for example. The Open University has to some extent been engaging in this for years. The technology field is sure to increase in value and versatility whilst managing privacy and security online to a much greater extent. Many professional conversations are routinely provided via email, Skype, message boards, texts and telephone. This has flagged new ethical criteria that needed to be developed for the therapy world as a starting point for discussion as per the 2005 and subsequent 2009 BACP Guidelines for Online therapy (Goss, Palmer, Jamieson, and Antony, 2005; Anthony and Goss, 2009).

FOCUS BOX 4.10 MANDY'S STORY PART 2: RESOLUTION

In spite of the lack of parental affection in childhood but due to others in Mandy's life who had supported her in the past and those who currently supported her and believed in her, she was able to reconstruct her life. Initially she was very upset, and then angry but eventually she found she was able to process the loss of her husband and have a sense of future through talking to supportive people, including a therapist. This shows how her ability to reflect upon events enabled her to place the traumatic memories of her husband leaving into the narrative of her whole life experience. In fact each of the attachment domains as above were activated as well as finding the core conditions of safe enough relationship met through others. Gradually her husband became more of the man he used to be in terms of empathy and interest in her wellbeing. She had continued to have close contact with him over the months of his absence, in spite of conversations being very fraught initially. They began to find their way back to each other but from a different perspective in realising that they both needed to be true to their own feelings and thoughts in order to genuinely find a middle ground and compromise that worked for them both at various points, without totally getting lost in the other's priorities and worlds. At last meeting they were well on their way to re-establishing themselves with an awareness of the above to hold in mind.

Mandy's situation demonstrates how even with a difficult start in life, if even just one person who believes in them and shows them acceptance or 'unconditional positive regard' (Rogers, 1957) and provides the basic needs (Maslow, 1954), that person can progress and find joy and satisfaction in life or at least a purposeful existence that gives them a sense that life is worth living. The 'secure base' experience (Bowlby, 1969, 1988; Holmes, 2001) can be seen to offer a platform on which a person can build and develop a rewarding life. This works via a trusted other as an attachment figure either in someone's personal life or as a therapist (Counselling Psychologist). It is certainly one of the most rewarding aspects of my entire working life when someone can trust enough to allow me alongside to facilitate their process of rebalancing their lives.

Cognitive-behavioural approaches and the National Health Service (NHS)

Cognitive-behavioural perspectives are often seen as the 'gold standard' within National Health Services (NHS) in particular and the National Institute of Clinical Excellence (NICE) which is attributed to the evidence base of Randomised Control Trials (RCTs). Cognitive-Behavioural Therapy (CBT) lends itself to measuring outcomes more easily than other therapies and therefore it is straightforward to get an evidence base for therapy. It is important to look at all kinds of evidence, some of which cannot be captured via RCTs. In terms of the subject matter for this chapter the therapeutic relationship formed between therapist and client in CBT therapy will mostly focus on the working alliance as it is action-oriented, with measurements and behavioural experiments to facilitate change. Ellis (1962) was less concerned with a relational aspect to the work than Beck and Steer (1993) who believed that a warm relationship was essential to the work. We can see below how this might work in a real-life therapy setting:

FOCUS BOX 4.11 JEREMY

Jeremy was a successful lawyer based in London, UK, who found immense satisfaction in his work. This was until a high-profile case he was dealing with was badly represented in the media and colleagues had also questioned his judgement; and as a result his job looked under threat. His doctor suggested having some CBT due to extreme stress and depression. He had received therapy numerous times in his 46 years, first seeing a psychiatrist as a boisterous 12-year-old with 'behavioural problems' and then as a teenager in social services' care when he was sent to speak to a psychologist about his tendency to lie and take his foster siblings' belongings. He saw a marriage counsellor when his brief marriage to Melanie broke down because of 'anger problems'. Therefore he was rather cynical as to how much it would help as previous experiences of therapy had left him feeling a failure and labeled as a problem person. Previous therapies had been enforced on him in some way which immediately alienated him from any opportunity to form a therapeutic alliance. Jeremy was aware he strongly resented being pushed into therapy so he probably did not make use of the therapies offered, as he was closed-off to the forming of the therapeutic relationship which would have potentially helped him to use the tools and strategies encouraged. This time he was more open to explore the option of therapy as it was an informed choice. When he first met Dr Josie he was struck by her warm, friendly manner and he relaxed a little. He received six sessions via the National Health Service (NHS) of CBT-based integrative therapy. This majored on the use of the therapeutic alliance as a tool to facilitate engagement in therapy and which ultimately engendered subsequent change. He began to understand and challenge the current relevance and usefulness of his underlying beliefs, patterns and responses, including how he had adapted his thinking to conform with his beliefs about himself, others and the world in general. He was able to really engage in the therapeutic relationship with Dr Josie, which was safe enough to allow him to do the work he needed to do at that time to improve his self-esteem and recognise alternative ways of responding to situations, which then improved his quality of life.

'New wave' cognitive-behavioural approaches as in Acceptance and Commitment Therapy (Hayes, 2004) together with 'Mindfulness' are becoming increasingly popular even in the NHS (Williams and Penman, 2011). Mindfulness is now considered a mainstream approach for a number of issues, for example, depression, anxiety and stress-based working (Silverton, 2012). Mindfulness is also part of the community-based preventative programmes for wellbeing and wellness promotion as well as the Mindfulness in Schools Project (MiSP, 2016). An example of this is in rolling out teaching programmes for mindfulness in primary and secondary schools. The reader can find out more detail about various therapy models throughout the book, but particularly in Section 3, and mindfulness is discussed further in Chapter 10.

Conclusions

Therapies continue to develop, differentiate and integrate; be defined, discussed and evaluated and yet as with all human endeavour arguably at the centre of excellence and effectiveness lies the relationship between people that strives at best to be therapeutic. The therapeutic relationship in its essence is a part of being human in the world in all its forms and with all its imperfections and yet rich complexity. Counselling Psychology is arguably one of the most rewarding and yet challenging professions in the caring professional world with its use of self in relationship (Wosket, 1999).

Learning outcomes

When you have completed this chapter you should be able:

- To gain a basic understanding of the centrality of the relationship between client and counselling psychologist in therapeutic endeavours.

- To understand the breadth of different aspects of the therapeutic relationship at work.
- To begin to understand how different models work in relationship.

Key concepts, terms and phrases

- Attachment
- Core conditions
- Counselling Psychology
- Ethics
- Hierarchy of Needs (Maslow, 1954)
- Humanistic psychology
- Pluralism
- Safe enough
- Secure base
- Therapeutic relationship

Sample essay titles

1. The therapeutic relationship appears to be complex. Discuss challenges and pitfalls of working in a close therapeutic relationship.
2. Describe, compare and contrast the five therapeutic relationships as discussed by Petruska Clarkson (2000).

Further reading

Ainsworth, M. D. S., and Bowlby, J. (1991). An ethological approach to personality development. *American Psychologist*, 46, 331–341.

Beck, A. T. (1967). *Depression: Causes and treatment.* Philadelphia: University of Pennsylvania Press.

Beck, A. T., Epstein, N., and Harrison, R. (1983). Cognitions, attitudes and personality dimensions in depression. *British Journal of Cognitive Psychotherapy.*

Bond, T. (2013). *Ethical framework for good practice in counselling and psychotherapy*. Leicestershire, UK: British Association for Counselling and Psychotherapy.

Butler, A. C., and Beck, J. S. (2000). Cognitive therapy outcomes: A review of meta-analyses. *Journal of the Norwegian Psychological Association*, 37, 1–9.

Carr, A. (2008). *What works with children, adolescents, and adults: A review of research on the effectiveness of psychotherapy.* New York: Routledge.

Cooper, M. (2015). *Existential psychotherapy and counselling: Contributions to a pluralistic practice.* London: Sage.

Cooper, M., Wild, C., Rijn, B. V., Ward, T., McLeod, J., Cassar, S., and Sreenath, S. (2015). Pluralistic therapy for depression: Acceptability, outcomes and helpful aspects in a multisite study. *Counselling Psychology Review*, 30(1), 6–20.

de Zueleta, F. (2006a). *From pain to violence: The roots of human destructiveness.* Second edition. Chichester: Wiley.

de Zueleta, F. (2006b). The treatment of psychological trauma from the perspective of attachment. *Journal of Family Therapy*, 28, 334–351.

Ellis, A. (1957). Rational psychotherapy and individual psychology. *Journal of Individual Psychology*, 13, 38–44.

Freud, S. (1953). Three essays on the theory of sexuality. In J. Strachey (Ed. and Trans.), *The standard edition of the complete psychological works of Sigmund Freud* (Vol. 7, pp. 125–245). London: Hogarth Press.

Heidegger, M. (2010). *Being and time.* Trans. J. Stanbaugh. Albany, NY: State University of New York Press.

Hofmann, S. G., and Barlow, D. H. (December 2014). Evidence-based psychological interventions and the common factors approach: The beginnings of a rapprochement? *Psychotherapy: Theory, Research, Practice, Training*, 51(4), 510–513.

Jordan, L. (2010). Relational Trauma. In R. Woolfe, S. Strawbridge, B. Douglas, and W. Dryden (Eds.), *Handbook of counselling psychology* (Third edition, pp. 235–255). London: Sage.

Kazdin, A. E. (June 2005). Treatment outcomes, common factors, and continued neglect of mechanisms of change. *Clinical Psychology: Science and Practice* 12(2), 184–188.

Kazdin, A. E. (July 2009). Understanding how and why psychotherapy leads to change. *Psychotherapy Research* 19(4–5), 418–428.

Lambert, M. J. (1992). Psychotherapy outcome research: Implications for integrative and eclectic therapists. In J. C. Norcross, M. R. Goldfried (Eds.), *Handbook of psychotherapy integration* (First edition, pp. 94–129). New York: Basic Books.

Lane, R. D., Ryan, L., Nadel, L., and Greenberg, L. S. (2015). Memory reconsolidation, emotional arousal and the process of change in psychotherapy: New insights from brain science (PDF). *Behavioral and Brain Sciences* 38, e1.

Luborsky, L., Singer, B., and Luborsky, L. (August 1975). Comparative studies of psychotherapies: Is it true that everyone has won and all must have prizes? *Archives of General Psychiatry* 32(8), 995–1008.

McAleavey, A. A., and Castonguay, L. G. (2015). The process of change in psychotherapy: Common and unique factors. In O. C. G. Gelo, A. Pritz, and B. Rieken (Eds.), *Psychotherapy research: Foundations, process, and outcome* (pp. 293–310). New York: Springer.

McLeod, J., and Cooper, M. (2015). Pluralistic counselling and psychotherapy. In S. Palmer (Ed.), *Counselling and psychotherapy: The essential guide* (Second edition). London: Sage.

Orlinsky, D. E., Grauwe, K., and Parks, B. K. (1994). Chapter 8. In A. Bergin and S. Garfield (Eds.), *Handbook of psychotherapy and behaviour change*. New York: Wiley.

Orlinsky, D. E., and Howard, K. I. (1986). Process and outcome in psychotherapy. In S. L. Garfield and A. E. Bergin (Eds.), *Handbook of psychotherapy and behavior change* (Third edition, pp. 311–381). New York: Wiley.

Paul, S., and Pelham, G. (2000). A relational approach to therapy: Chapter 6. In S. Palmer and R. Woolfe (Eds.), *Integrative and eclectic counselling and psychotherapy* (pp. 110–126). London: Sage.

Prochaska, J., DiClemente, C., and Norcross, J. (1992). In search of how people change: Applications to addictive behaviors (PDF). *American Psychologist* 47(9), 1102–1114.

Roth, A., and Fonagy, P. (2006). *What works for whom? A critical review of psychotherapy research*. Second edition. Edited by Anthony Roth and Peter Fonagy with contributions from G. Parry, M. Target, and R. Woods. New York: The Guilford Press.

Schore, A. N. (2001). The effects of a secure attachment relationship on right brain development, affect regulation, and infant mental health. *Infant Mental Health Journal*, 22, 7–66.

Schore, A. N. (2003). *Affect regulation and the repair of the self.* New York: W.W. Norton.

Schore, J. R., and Schore, A. N. (2007). Modern attachment theory: The central role of affect regulation in development and treatment. *Clinical Social Work Journal*, (2008) 36, 9–20.

Shaw, E., and Carroll, M. (2016). Towards ethical maturity in counselling psychology. In In B. Douglas, R. Woolfe, S. Strawbridge, E. Kasket, and V. Gailbraith (Eds.), *The handbook of counselling psychology* (Fourth edition, pp. 244–258). Los Angeles: Sage.

Smith, M., and Glass, G. (1977). Meta-analysis of psychotherapy outcome studies (PDF). *American Psychologist* 32(9), 752–760. doi:10.1037/0003-066X.32.9.752.

Weinberger, J. L., and Rasco, C. (2007). Empirically supported common factors. In S. G. Hofmann and J. L. Weinberger (Eds.), *The art and science of psychotherapy* (pp. 103–129). New York: Routledge.

Websites

British Psychological Society: www.bps.org.uk/system/files/documents/code_of_ethics_and_conduct.pdf

Definition of Therapeutic: www.merriam-webster.com/dictionary/therapeutic
Definition of Therapeutic: www.oxforddictionaries.com/definition/english/therapeutic
Health and Care Professions Council: www.hcpc-uk.org/assets/documents/10004EDFStandardsofconduct,performanceandethics.pdf

References

Ainsworth, M. D. S., Blehar, M. C., Waters, E., and Wall, S. (1978). *Patterns of attachment: A psychological study of the strange situation.* Hillsdale, NJ: Erlbaum.

Anthony, K., and Goss, S. (2009). *Guidelines for online counselling and psychotherapy 3rd edition, including guidelines for online supervision.* Rugby: BACP.

Beck, A. T., and Steer, R. A. (1993). *Beck anxiety inventory manual.* San Antonio: Harcourt Brace and Company.

Bowlby, J. (1969). *Attachment and loss, Vol. 1: Attachment.* New York: Basic Books.

Bowlby, J. (1973). *Attachment and loss, Vol. 2: Separation.* New York: Basic Books.

Bowlby, J. (1980a). *Attachment and loss, Vol. 3: Loss, sadness and depression.* New York: Basic Books.

Bowlby, J. (1988a). *A secure base: Parent-child attachment and healthy human development.* New York: Basic Books.

Bowlby, J. (1988b). *A secure base: Clinical applications of attachment theory.* London: Routledge.

British Psychological Society. (2005). *Professional practice guidelines.* Leicester, UK: Division of Counselling Psychology.

British Psychological Society. (2009). *Code of ethics and conduct.* Leicester, UK: Ethics Committee of BPS.

Clarkson, P. (1995). *The therapeutic relationship.* London: Whurr Publishers.

Clarkson, P. (2000). *The therapeutic relationship.* First edition printed 1995. London: Whurr Publishers Ltd.

Clarkson, P. & Wilson, S. (2003). *The therapeutic relationship* (2nd ed). London: Wiley-Blackwell.

Clarkson, P., and Wilson, S. (2008). *The therapeutic relationship.* Revised 2nd edition printed 2003. London: Whurr Publishers Ltd.

Cooper, M., and Dryden, W. (eds) (2016). *The handbook of pluralistic counselling and psychotherapy.* London: Sage.

Cooper, M. and McLeod, J. (2006). 'Establishing a counselling research clinic based on a pluralistic model of change'. 12th Annual BACP Research Conference, Glasgow.

Ellis, A. (1962). *Reason and emotion in psychotherapy.* New York: Stuart.

Goss, S., Palmer, S., Jamieson, A., and Antony, K. (2005). *Guidelines for online counselling and psychotherapy.* 2nd Edition. Los Angeles: Sage.

Hayes, S. C. (2004). Acceptance and commitment therapy and the new behavior therapies: Mindfulness, acceptance and relationship. In S. C. Hayes, V. M. Follette, and M. Linehan (Eds.), *Mindfulness and acceptance: Expanding the cognitive behavioral tradition* (pp. 1–29). New York: Guilford.

Health and Care Professions Council, (2016). *Standards of conduct, performance and ethics.* London: Health and Care Professions Council.

Holmes, J. (2001). *In search of the secure base: Attachment theory and psychotherapy.* Hove, England and USA and Canada: Brunner-Routledge.

Holmes, J., and Lindley, R. (1989). *The values of psychotherapy.* Oxford: Oxford University Press.

Hubble, M., Duncan, B. L., and Miller, S. D. (1999). *The heart and soul of change: What works in therapy.* Washington, DC: American Psychological Association.

Imel, Z. E., and Wampold, B. E. (2008). The importance of treatment and the science of common factors in psychotherapy. In S. D. Brown, and R. W. Lent (Eds.), *Handbook of counseling psychology* (Forth edition, pp. 249–262). Hoboken, NJ: John Wiley & Sons.

Malan, D. (1999). *Individual psychotherapy and the science of psychodynamics.* Second edition. Oxford: Butterworth-Heinemann.

Maslow, A. (1954). *Motivation and personality.* New York: Harper.

Milton, M. (2016). *Forming a relationship.* In B. Douglas, R. Woolfe, S. Strawbridge, E. Kasket, and V. Gailbraith (Eds.), *The handbook of counselling psychology* (Fourth edition, pp. 184–197). Los Angeles: Sage.

Mindfulness in Schools Project (MiSP). (2016). Retrieved from https://mindfulnessinschools.org

Ozad, B., and Uygarer, G. (2014). Attachment needs and networking sites. *Social Behaviour and Personality: An International Journal*, 4243–4252.

Rescher, N. (1993:79). *Pluralism: Against the demand for concensus.* Oxford: Clarendon Press.

Rogers, C. R. (1957). The necessary and sufficient conditions of therapeutic personality change (PDF). *Journal of Consulting Psychology*, 21(2), 95–103.

Schore, A. N. (2000). Attachment and the regulation of the right brain. *Attachment & Human Development*, 2, 23–47.

Silverton, S. (2012). *The mindfulness breakthrough: The revolutionary approach to dealing with stress, anxiety and depression.* Oxford, UK: Watkins Publishing Ltd.

Williams, M., and Penman, D. (2011, 2012, 2014). *Mindfulness: A practical guide to finding peace in a frantic world.* London, UK: Piatkus.

Winnicott, D. W. (1965). *The maturational process and the facilitating environment.* New York: International Universities Press.

Wosket, V. (1999). *The therapeutic use of self: Counselling practice, research and supervision.* London, New York: Routledge.

SECTION 3

Applications of theory to practice

5

HUMANISTIC APPROACHES

Person-centred approach

Sophia Balamoutsou

This chapter explores how different theoretical approaches are applied in therapeutic practice with the first chapter of the section presenting the person-centred approach. The chapter begins with a brief biography of Carl Rogers, the founder of the approach. The philosophical underpinnings of the person-centred approach, **humanism** and **phenomenology**, are then presented. Maslow's theory of motivation is also discussed. Subsequently, the basic qualities of the therapeutic relationship, as identified by Rogers, are discussed and post-Rogerian theoretical developments are presented. Finally, examples of research on the person-centred approach are summarised.

The person-centred or client-centred approach to Counselling Psychology has its origins in the work of one of the greatest American psychologists, Carl Ransom Rogers (1902–1987). Kirschenbaum (2007) describes Rogers as a withdrawn and intelligent child. He was the fourth child of six. His father was a civil engineer and his mother a homemaker. He was born in Oak Park, near Chicago. When Carl was 14 his family moved to a farm a few miles outside Chicago in order for the children to live a protected life away from non-Christian values. Both parents were strict Christians and the family attended church regularly. As a child he was interested in nature and enjoyed observing insects and crops growing. Subsequently many of the metaphors underpinning his theory came from agricultural images and procedures. Rogers went to study Agriculture at the University of Wisconsin. Soon, he became interested in religious studies and decided to study Theology in order to become a minister. An important event took place in Rogers' life; when he was 20 years old he was chosen amongst other young Christians to travel to China to attend an International Christian Conference. He was exposed to diversity as well as teachings from inspirational teachers and his view of God changed. According to Bozarth (2016) two main influences happened in Carl's life. First, he joined a self-directed seminar group of students where they explored important personal issues that affected their lives; and second, he was influenced by one of his instructors Goodwin Watson, who was an inspirational educator working closely with his students. These two encounters inspired Rogers to study psychological ways to help people at Columbia's Teachers College in 1926. He continued his studies, receiving his MA (1928) and PhD (1931) from Columbia University. He became Professor at the University of Chicago where he set up a counselling centre. He continued teaching at the University of Wisconsin and later in La Jolla, California, where he lived the latter part of his life.

Historical positioning of the person-centred approach

Phenomenology

The person-centred approach has its theoretical roots in phenomenology and humanism. Phenomenology is a philosophical movement deriving from the work of Edmund Husserl. It views the systematic reflection of conscious experiences as essential in how we acquire knowledge of ourselves. The way people experience their everyday life and the world around them provides a valid way of knowledge. This is very different from the Kantian objectivity that underpins behaviourist theories. According to McLeod (2013) an important aspect of phenomenology is the ability of humans to 'bracket-off' 'the assumptions one holds about the phenomenon being investigated, and striving to describe it in as comprehensive and sensitive a manner as possible' (p. 171). Counselling approaches influenced by the phenomenological approach consider areas of experience presented by the client as valid and worthy, without making interpretations or assumptions. The therapist is curious to enter the client's experiences and to make sense of them through the client's 'eyes'.

Humanism

Humanism is a philosophical movement that has its roots in the Renaissance. It postulates that the human being is capable of thinking critically and acting freely. There is an assumption that human beings have *agency*, in other words humans are able to reflect, choose and act. According to O'Hara (1996) in 1957 and 1958, Abraham Maslow and Clark Moustakas organised two meetings that took place in Detroit. A number of psychologists attended; they were interested to develop a professional association with a humanistic ethos. The topics discussed were the self, creativity, self-actualisation, individuality and meaningfulness. These key concepts formed the basis of a new approach to psychology with humanistic values. In another meeting that took place in Old Saybrook, Connecticut, in 1964, May, Maslow, Rogers and others formed the movement of Humanistic Psychology. The existing two dominant strands of psychology, behaviourism and depth psychology did not deal with the human aspect of individuals, instead they view the person as narrowly scientific. According to O'Hara (1996) humanistic psychology, the 'Third Force' in psychology has three main assumptions:

1. From birth to old age people try to actualize their potential while creating close relationships with each other.
2. All people, clients in therapeutic relationships included, have huge inner resources and qualities for self-healing and self-regulation.
3. To facilitate healing and self-actualization one has to enter relationships where the following qualities must be present: **empathy**, authenticity, respect, warmth, and acceptance.

Maslow's hierarchy of needs and the concept of self-actualization: a theory of motivation

Maslow was a prolific author and an important theorist of humanism. His work and ideas on *self-actualization* and the *hierarchy of needs* have influenced not only psychology but other disciplines such as business studies and sociology. Maslow (1943) saw humans as *organismic* in how they develop and that they have some basic needs that need fulfilment. These needs are physiological, safety, love and esteem. Once these are achieved, a person can seek growth needs, such as self-actualization. According to Maslow (1967: 281–4) self-actualized people have a number of characteristics:

1. 'They experience fully, vividly, selflessly, with full concentration and total absorption'.
2. 'At each point there is a progression choice and a regression choice. Self-actualization is an ongoing process, it means making each of the many single choices about whether to lie or be honest, whether to steal or not to steal and it means to make each of these choices as a growth choice'.
3. Humans are not *tabula rasa*, we have a temperament, and a biochemistry. 'Self-actualized people can like or dislike something based on their own feedback and not be influenced by others'.
4. Self-actualized people are honest and take responsibility for their actions.
5. 'Closely linked to the above self-actualized people dare to be different, unpopular, non-conformist'.
6. 'They use their intelligence' and realize their own potential.
7. They have 'peak experiences', moments of self-actualization and they know it. Many people have these peak experiences but they do not realise them. These moments cannot be 'bought, guaranteed or sought'.
8. Self-actualized individuals have defenses but 'they work towards identifying them and giving them up'.

Maslow's ideas were based on a small number of people that he was admiring greatly. They 'were older people, people who had lived much of their lives out and were visibly successful' (Maslow, 1967: 280). His work was criticised for lack of scientific rigour. Maslow was able to identify his limitations as a researcher, and was self-critical about his work and his limited sample. One could argue that his ideas provided a plausible narrative in a time when humanism was at its peak, thus providing a basis for the person-centred theory. His assumptions offered his contemporaries theoretical insights that were later systematically tested by psychologists such as Rogers and his followers.

Qualities of the therapeutic relationship

The therapeutic relationship is central in the person-centred approach in Counselling Psychology. It sees the therapist as a means of providing a reparative relationship, different from the ones the client has been usually engaging with. Clients experience distress because they have been surrounded by others who are non-genuine and impose **conditions of worth** on the client. They are not valued for who they are but for who the others would like them to be. A person in distress, a client, internalises those expectations and lives an inauthentic life. Rogers (1957: 96) in his seminal work 'The necessary and sufficient conditions of therapeutic personality change' defined the qualities of a therapeutic relationship. He argued that 'for constructive personality change to occur, it is necessary that these conditions exist and continue over a period of time' (see Focus box 5.1).

FOCUS BOX 5.1 NECESSARY AND SUFFICIENT CONDITIONS OF THERAPEUTIC PERSONALITY CHANGE

Rogers argued that if the following conditions are present in a therapeutic relationship, over a substantial amount of time, therapeutic personality change will occur. No other conditions are necessary.

1. Two persons are in psychological contact.
2. The first, whom we shall term the client, is in a state of incongruence, being vulnerable and anxious.
3. The second person, whom we shall term the therapist, is congruent or integrated in the relationship.
4. The therapist experiences unconditional positive regard for the client.
5. The therapist experiences an empathic understanding of the client's internal frame of reference, and endeavours to communicate this to the client.
6. The communication to the client of the therapist's empathic understanding and unconditional positive regard is to a minimal extent achieved.

No other conditions are necessary. If these six conditions exist, and continue over a period of time, this is sufficient. The process of constructive personality change will follow.

(Rogers, 1957: 96)

More specifically Rogers elaborated on these six conditions. The first condition suggests a minimal relationship, the bare minimum of **contact** with the other, while the rest of the conditions describe the qualities of a relationship that can result in therapeutic change. In the second condition Rogers explains that the client who is vulnerable or anxious is in a state of **incongruence**. He gives the example of a mother who develops an illness every time her son decides to leave home. Rogers explains that this mother wants her son to stay at home but this is inconsistent with her self-image resulting in a distorted manifestation of her desire where the good mother self-concept remains intact. Lack of self-awareness results in 'anxiety and disorganisation' (Rogers, 1957: 97). The third condition is that of the therapist's genuineness, where Rogers means a person who is 'freely and deeply' himself or herself and has a sense of self-integration and **congruence** when in this relationship. Rogers explained that therapists are by no means perfectly congruent in all aspects of their life. Instead a therapist is expected to be congruent during the therapy session. If issues of incongruence come to awareness the therapist, ideally, should become aware and place these issues aside (bracketing). Congruence requires an inner negotiation of where I am in relation to my now and to the therapeutic relationship. The fourth condition is **unconditional positive regard** or unconditional acceptance, where the therapist has no expectations or conditions for accepting the client. The therapeutic relationship allows a space for the client to be himself or herself. Rogers (1957: 98) illustrates this quality of the therapist in the following words from a client:

> [the therapist allows] fostering my possession of my own experience . . . that this is my experience and that I am actually having it, thinking what I think, feeling what I feel, wanting what I want, fearing what I fear: no 'ifs', 'buts,' or 'not really.'

The fifth condition is empathy; it is a way of experiencing the client's world in an *'as if'* quality. It is an experiential entering of the client's world of fear, anger, anxiety, sadness, loneliness without the therapist getting confused in his or her own feelings of fear, anger, anxiety, sadness or loneliness. Finally, the sixth condition, is about communicating to the client this genuineness, acceptance and empathy to a minimal degree. In other words the client should be capable of experiencing the therapist's qualities.

Rogers developed his ideas based on systematic research. Apart from the first condition which, according to Rogers had to be present, all subsequent conditions were measurable. Rogers used Q sort methodology (a combination of qualitative and quantitative methods) where he would give 100 cards to both client and therapist and they would rate how 'good' or 'how present' the therapist was in each condition. Rogers was one of the first psychologists to carry out process research and include clients' experiences of therapy in his research. The latter was in accordance with the humanistic ethos where the client is no longer an 'objectified patient' but an agent, capable to offer valuable information about therapy.

ACTIVITY BOX 5.1

How do you understand the conditions of therapeutic change?

1. In small groups discuss how you understand the Core Conditions for therapeutic personality change.
2. What is contact, congruence, empathy, unconditional acceptance?
3. Which condition is, for you, easier to experience and communicate?
4. Which condition is, for you, more challenging to experience and communicate?
5. Give example(s) from your life where you were able to support someone by showing one or more of the conditions.

Self-concept

Based on phenomenological and humanistic theories, Rogers believed that personality development is a reflexive negotiation between thoughts and emotions and how external objects are perceived. The world we live in is in a constant flux and, as a result, the self is seen as something changeable. McLeod (2013: 164) argues that the idea of **self-concept** is central in Rogers' theory. It is all the various ways that a person defines himself or herself in the form of an 'I' position for example, 'I am kind', 'I am sad', 'I am angry' and 'sometimes I feel vulnerable'. These are ways of experiencing oneself. To be kind, sad, angry and at times vulnerable are part of one's self-concept and as such there is congruence between what one experiences and what one expresses with words and actions. But if one enters a situation where a feeling of caring or nurturing is evoked she or he might not have a repertoire of inner feelings for this and thus there are no words to describe it. McLeod (2013: 164) gives the following example: 'someone who is not supposed to be nurturing may, for instance, become very busy "doing things" for someone who needs no more than companionship, comforting or a human touch'. When there is a distance between feelings and the awareness and symbolization of these feelings, there is said to exist 'a state of incongruence'. According to the person-centred approach clients bring to therapy issues of incongruence.

The organismic self

Rogers saw the self as having an inherent ability to grow. Influenced from his early life experiences and his love for nature, Rogers often explained his theory using lovely metaphors from nature referring to the human condition. In one of his papers, illustrating his conceptualization of the **actualising tendency**, Rogers (1963), describes his experience of observing seaweeds battered by the waves on a rock.

FOCUS BOX 5.2

Read the following excerpt and discuss how the actualising tendency relates with the organismic self.

> 'I watched the waves breaking over these large rocks in the distance, I noticed with surprise what appeared to be tiny palm trees on the rocks, no more than two or three feet high, taking the pounding of the breakers. Through my binoculars I saw that these were some type of seaweed, with a slender 'trunk' topped off with a head of leaves. As one examined a specimen in the intervals between the waves it seemed clear that this fragile, erect, top-heavy plant would be utterly crushed and broken by the next breaker. When the wave crunched down upon it, the trunk bent almost flat, the leaves were whipped into a straight line by the torrent of the water, yet the moment the wave had passed, here was the plant again, erect, tough, resilient. It seemed incredible that it was able to take this incessant pounding hour after hour, day and night, week after week, perhaps, for all I know, year after year, and all the time nourishing itself, extending its domain, reproducing itself; in short maintaining and enhancing itself in this process which, in our shorthand, we call growth. Here in this palmlike seaweed was the tenacity of life, the forward thrust of life, the ability to push into an incredibly hostile environment and not only to hold its own, but to adapt, develop, become itself'.
>
> (Rogers, 1963: 2)

ACTIVITY BOX 5.2

Where does personal growth take place?

Personal development is an important aspect in the continuous professional development of a psychotherapist. It can take place in many spaces and has different forms (personal therapy, group therapy, training, reading, spirituality, engaging with art, being in contact with the environment and many others).

1. Take some time and list where you feel more comfortable in achieving personal growth.
2. In a small group discuss experiences of personal growth.
3. In the small group explore the idea that personal therapy is a necessary path for the personal development of a therapist.

The qualities of the **actualizing tendency** are present no matter how challenging and un-nurturing the environment might be, the **organismic self** has this tendency 'maintaining, enhancing, and reproducing itself'. In psychotherapy, the therapist through the quality of the relationship, acceptance, congruence and empathy creates the environment for the person to consolidate what he or she already is, enhance and reproduce himself or herself.

Conditions of worth

We all grow up with conditions of worth. Parents, carers, other important people and institutions are expecting us to be patient, silent, nice to people, obedient, strong, hard-working, happy and so on. All these expectations are communicated either through clear messages or in other forms of narrative such as family stories, fairytales and other culturally available stories that contain values. As we grow up we put these values upon ourselves and we strive to perform these in our everyday life in order to be worthy and loved. In the person-centred approach to therapy these externally imposed values are identified and positioned where they belong (e.g. family values, religious values, broader cultural values). Some individuals grow with more and some with less conditions of worth. Those who grow up in environments with conditional positive regard experience themselves worthy only if they match those conditions. They feel worthy only if they are for example patient, silent, nice to people, obedient, strong, hard-working, happy. The aim of the therapist is to offer unconditional positive regard, a quality where the client is valued and honored for what he or she chooses to be and becomes. This offers the opportunity for the actualized tendency to flourish.

Ideal and real self

The ***real*** and the ***ideal self*** is central in the person-centred approach. The **ideal self** is what individuals perform in their everyday life whereas the **real self** is what one wants to become. According to Patterson (1977), the real self is the **self-concept** which one has about what he or she would like to be. The ideal self is what the person actually is. When the experience of what a person is and what she or he would like to be are in agreement, then the person is said to experience congruence in his or her life. When there is a discrepancy between the real and the ideal self the person is in a state of incongruence, anxiety, confusion and tension. Incongruence is a result of a conflict between the real and the ideal self.

FOCUS BOX 5.3 CASE STUDY

Sarah, a woman in her 30s holds a job as a nurse, has a partner and two children. Most people would describe Sarah as caring, patient, kind, focused and in control when in a crisis. When she is at work most of her colleagues see that identity of Sarah, and at home she is similarly, the ideal mum. She came for therapy because recently she had a few incidents of panic attacks. Initially, she thought there was something wrong with her heart, she had chest pains and experienced difficulty breathing. One night she visited the Accident and Emergency Department of the local Hospital. The doctor encouraged her to see her GP in order to refer her to a psychologist.

From a PCA perspective the psychologist would first engage in contact, and will create an environment where Sarah will feel un-rushed, accepted, understood and in a congruent relationship with the therapist; these will be the basis for therapeutic change to take place.

The therapist would be interested to explore Sarah's *self-concept* and *her sense of anxiety*.

The therapist could explore Sarah's sense of *ideal self*, how she comes across in her day-to-day encounters, and her sense of her *real self*, what is not seen in public, perhaps a more vulnerable sense of self that is frail, worried, lonely and in need. Then, as and when Sarah becomes aware of her *real self needs* this will be further explored.

A therapist may explore Sarah's *conditions of worth*, the expectations, that were put upon her in order to be her *ideal self* and how her *real self*, this more silent sense of self, seized being present in her relationships.

Ideally, Sarah will decide to make changes in her everyday life and the role of therapy is to support her in this path. It might involve a series of challenging changes, such as confrontations with important people in her life and learning how to self-care. The aim of therapy is for Sarah to start living *aware* of her real self, attending to her values, needs and longings. The therapist walks next to Sarah in this journey of self-awareness and growth offering companionship, presence and hope.

Post-Rogerian developments in person-centred therapy

A number of themes of Rogers' theory have developed over the years, each emphasizing different aspects of the theory. Some call them tribes (Sanders, 2004; Lago and Charura, 2016) and differentiate these tribes into focusing-oriented therapy, experiential person-centred therapy, existential approaches to person-centred therapy, expressive arts, pre-therapy, emotion-focused therapy and others. I would prefer not to refer to these developments as tribes. I follow Bazzano's (2014) argument that 'tribe' is a metaphor that separates and positions its members different from the others. The 'tribe' metaphor views 'Otherness' as alien and strives to reinforce tribal superiority, thus lacking critical reflection within its group. In addition to that, a tribe in its effort to assert superiority, does not see similarities with and allegiances to other groups. Above all, the 'tribe' metaphor does not fit within the person-centred approach as theorists from various post-Rogerian ideas are both critical and reflexive. Furthermore, an approach such as person-centred, which has at its heart the 'organismic' metaphor, would view new ideas as inherent in this 'organismic growth process'. Various developments within the person-centred approach can be seen as 'narrative shifts' that emphasise or downplay different aspects of Rogers' initial values and ideas.

Configurations of self

Influenced by a social constructionist paradigm of the self, Mearns and Thorne (2000) opened a new space for the person-centred approach with their concept of **configurations of self**.

> A '**configuration**' is a hypothetical construct denoting a coherent pattern of feelings, thoughts and preferred behavioural responses symbolised or pre-symbolised by the person as reflective of a dimension of existence within the Self.
>
> *(Mearns and Thorne, 2000: 102)*

The client is seen as having a multiplicity of voices, I-positions, that form a 'coherent pattern' which reflects an aspect of one's existence inside the broader sense of self. This is different from the notion of mere parts which can be seen as fragmented and not integrated into the Self. Another important characteristic of a **configuration of self** is that it can be within the awareness of a person (symbolised) or on the edge of awareness of a person (pre-symbolised). This allows space in the person-centred approach for unconscious material to be explored. Mearns and Thorne, 2000) referred to 'rehearsed material' which are aspects of the Self that are rehearsed in common social exchanges and that are rather superficial ways of presenting oneself. As the client trusts the therapist and the therapeutic process, and as relational depth is built, the client discovers other less surface and more silent aspects of himself or herself. Sometimes these **configurations** are competing or conflictual.

Cooper (1999: 107) noticed that the concept of self can have 'violent fluctuations' suggesting that individuals can shift between the plurality of **self concepts**. Cooper (1999) goes on to suggest that individuals choose which configuration to fashion with different relationships in order to achieve higher self-regard. For example, as a teacher I am self-assertive with my students, but as a partner I am self-sacrificial. One aim of therapy may be to shed light on all aspects of the self, explore which configurations are at the edge of awareness and which configurations are more often manifested in social occasions. Furthermore, a therapist could explore which configurations are results of conditions of worth and introjects in the client's life. Also, it would be worth exploring configurations that are 'growthful' (Mearns and Thorne, 2000) supporting the actualizing tendency. A therapist should value all configurations of the client and explore the purpose of their existence.

Note that although the concept of configurations of self has been influenced by a postmodern/social constructionist theoretical paradigm, in the concept of Configurations there is a Self that has agency and decides which configuration he or she will be at any given point in time. However, the person-centred concept of an agentful coherent Self is at odds with social constructionism where self is seen as fragmented and saturated.

Pre-therapy

Prouty (2001) was innovative in his way of working with persons who were 'low-functioning', in this category he included people diagnosed with schizophrenia, people with 'retardation' and geriatric patients who were withdrawn. According to Rogers (1957) the first of the conditions for therapeutic change is two people being in contact. Rogers claimed that this is a condition that is either present or not. In fact this was the only condition that he did not research. Prouty's theory developed further the concept of contact; he asserted that contact can be varied and can also be demonstrated in various forms and ways. There are five main contact reflections: Situational, Facial, Word-for-Word, Bodily, and Reiterative Reflections. The therapist is expected to use the techniques of reflection with empathy, acceptance and genuineness and compassion for the implicit selfhood even when working with people who seem 'to regress'.

Fragile process

Closely related to the work of Prouty, the work of Margaret Warner focuses on clients who have a '**fragile**' style of processing experiences. Warner (2016) defines 'difficult or **fragile processes**' as current experiential changes or longer-term issues that relate to a person's experience of self. A person who has a fragile style of processing experiences the important issues either at very high or very low levels of emotional intensity. In this category are clients diagnosed as having borderline, narcissistic or schizoid personality disorders and are said to be using 'archaic defences' such as projective identification and splitting. Fragile processes can also be experienced by persons who suffer post-traumatic stress disorder or have experienced complex trauma. Although Warner refers to fragile processes as a unified phenomenon, she points out that people may experience varied degrees of fragile processes. In addition to that, one can experience fragile processes for some aspects of their experiences and not for others. Many clients who seem to be functioning well in their everyday life might have aspects of their self dissociated or fragmented and she suggests that therapists work with empathy and stay with what the client presents. A therapist might be able to see aspects of self that the client is not yet capable to integrate into their sense of self. As a result, interpretations or even the therapists own understanding of what the client says might be very painful and scary and may undermine the client's sense of self. Warner suggests that a therapist who works with clients who experience overwhelming experiences (fragile processes) should first make contact and stay in contact with what the client presents. This might involve simply repeating the client's presented experience. This work can be very challenging for a therapist. Sometimes therapists can feel scared when working with dissociated parts, while it may feel difficult to work so slowly with a client. Yet, Warner emphasises that although existing work is about managing dissociated parts and bringing them to awareness, her work is the opposite, it is about letting these experiences emerge when the client feels ready. When the client experiences a therapeutic relationship that is safe enough to contain all these parts, then the client is ready to present them and eventually look at these or integrate them into his or her sense of self.

Focusing

Gendlin and his colleagues developed further **congruence** and **presence** in Rogers' work. Gendlin was a young student of Rogers and a philosopher. He was a fervent supporter of Rogers' theory. **Focusing** was originally meant by Gendlin as a process of listening to the body and its constant changing of experiencing. For Gendlin (2000) 'the person suffuses every part of the body' giving emphasis to the embodied aspect of the human condition. A number of clients enter therapy knowing, intellectually, what the problem is, they may define it as anxiety, depression, sadness, despair, conflict and so on. A focusing-oriented therapist invites the client to attend to the body and the **felt sense** and provide information from there. Therapist and client explore that felt sense and draw meaning from it. Focusing has been wrongly thought of as a series of techniques but its basis is deeply rooted in person-centred phenomenological epistemology. The six steps in focusing are the following:

1. Clearing the space: the client is invited to attend to what goes on inside his or her body.
2. Felt Sense: allowing the body to come and offer a new experience, maybe new information.
3. Handle: finding one metaphor, maybe a word, a phrase or an image that captures the felt sense.
4. Resonating: does this image really fit the felt sense? Is there resonance between the felt sense and the word?

5. Asking: what is it about this difficulty or issue that brings this image? How do these relate? Stay with the felt sense and wait for a 'shift' in awareness. Ideally this will be accompanied by a sense of relief.
6. Receiving involves accepting what has come.

The process ends here but the person can go through this again. Through these steps the therapist invites the client to attend to his or her bodily sensations and provide information on what is 'between' the client and the problem. The emphasis is on listening to the body. The therapist encourages the client not to think of the problem but to focus towards the bodily felt sense of the problem when the client recalls the problem. This can be an image, a word or even a phrase that captures the bodily felt sense. In this process the notion of *pause* is central.

Grafanaki (2013) explores further the concepts of congruence and incongruence conducted through systematic research. She analysed video-recorded real therapist and client sessions. She then analysed moment by moment client and therapist experiences of good and bad moments in psychotherapy; she concluded that congruence and incongruence are shifting phenomena and they are profoundly affected by the quality of the therapeutic relationship. Grafanaki continued becoming a trainer in focusing and later developed with William Hernandez the pause movement (www.pausemovement.org/). They train groups on the essence of pause and they have done tremendous applications in a number of areas such as community development, anti-bullying projects, team building, peace building, family and couple relationships, and social and human development projects.

Emotion-focused therapy

Emotion-focused therapy was initially named 'process experiential therapy' in the late 1980s (Greenberg et al., 1993, cited in Elliott and Greenberg, 2016). While focusing emphasised the experiential part of the person-centred approach, emotion-focused therapy emphasised the role of emotion in therapy. It is an approach that is extensively researched and has its basis in humanistic and constructivist assumptions. Emotion is 'seen as a foundational in the construction of the self and is a key determinant of self organization' (Greenberg, 2010: 1). While people experience emotions they process these in order to give meaning to these emotions. Emotion-focused therapy postulates six basic principles, **client markers**, which contribute to emotion processing and give therapists a map of interventions; these are as follows:

1. Problematic reactions are those such as dilemmas about emotions or situations. The therapist has the opportunity to stay with these emotions and explore their meaning.
2. Unclear ***felt sense*** are feelings that the client is not able to verbalise and has no clear sense of this experience. The therapist may invite the client to practice a focusing technique to get a clearer bodily felt sense and a shifting of the experience.
3. Conflict splits are parts of the self in conflict or critical of each other. The therapist can invite the client into two-chair work, a technique used widely in Gestalt psychotherapy. In so doing, the two parts enter a dialogue which can end in a resolution or at least some clarity.
4. Self-interruptive splits are markers in clients' discourse where a part of the client stops an emotion from being expressed. The therapist may invite the client to challenge that part and express blocked emotions.

5. Unfinished business usually involves unresolved strong feelings towards an important person in one's life. Again, the therapist would invite the client to enter a dialogue with the other person through two-chair work. The aim of this is for a resolution to take place, through forgiving, understanding or taking responsibility.
6. Vulnerability is an emotional state where the client feels very shameful, scared or frail. The person who feels vulnerable would benefit from a therapist who responds with empathy and strengthens the client's sense of self.

Emotion-focused therapy in its practice has elements of attachment theory, theory of pluralism (Cooper and McLeod, 2011) and life-span development. It has been criticised from purist person-centred therapists for being too directive and mixing too many approaches. However, the empirical grounding and the vast amount of research by Elliott and Greenberg and their colleagues support that emotion-focused therapy produces change in clients.

Research in the person-centred approach

It is said that the person-centred approach has not been researched enough. However, this is not true. Rogers was one of first psychotherapists to conduct systematic research with recordings of counselling/psychotherapy sessions. During the later years of Rogers' life he did less research and developed his theory more theoretically. According to Elliott this was a problem as the person-centred approach remained 'silenced'. Any therapeutic model in order to remain in dialogue with other approaches should show empirical evidence.

As one can see from discussions above, the person-centred approach is very broad and has many different expressions. It is an approach that is difficult to manualise and research. However, Truax and Carkuff (1967) developed structured training programmes in the use of person-centred qualities such as empathy, warmth and genuineness. The problem here is that an effort to make person-centred qualities observable and measurable reduced the 'forms of personal knowing' (Barrett-Lennard, 1993, cited in McLeod, 1999) to a set of communication skills. Barrett-Lennard (1981, 1986) developed a relationship scale of 40 items where empathy, regard and congruence is measured. It has been used widely to measure qualities of a relationship such as therapist-client, teacher-student, partners in a relationship, parent-child.

An example of humanistic research is the work of Rennie (1990, 1992, 1994a, 1994b, 1994c, 2012) and Levitt, Lu, Pomerville, and Francisco (2015) who offered a major contribution to person-centred experiential psychotherapies. His earlier research was process research focusing on clients' experiences in psychotherapy. His seminal paper (1994a) on client deference argues that clients, even when they disagree with the therapist, defer to his or her authority in order to continue to position him or her as the expert. Furthermore, based on his research Rennie (1994c) emphasised that the client is an active agent, reflecting during the therapy session. For example, Rennie (1994c) suggested that through storytelling clients create space from the therapist in order to reflect on what is happening in therapy, to distance themselves from painful moments and to give the therapist a positive image of themselves.

Angus et al. (2015) conducted a review of 25 years (1990–2015) of humanistic psychotherapies (HP) research. They reviewed qualitative and quantitative research findings of humanistic psychotherapy evidence-based treatments for a variety of psychological difficulties. They concluded the following:

1. Core concepts such as empathy and the role of the therapeutic relationship should be revisited and should be endorsed as fundamental in a number of psychotherapy areas.
2. Humanistic psychotherapies should be included in the development of clinical practice guidelines for depression and other client presenting problems, as they meet criteria for evidence-based practice.
3. Humanistic psychotherapy researchers have been innovative in developing methodologically pluralistic approaches (qualitative, process/outcome) consistent with the underlying values and principles of the humanistic approach.
4. Reviewed research in humanistic psychotherapies offered new understanding of humanistic principles as they relate to clients' experience of change.
5. Finally, there is strong empirical support that humanistic practice principles are fundamental in the training of psychotherapists and as such should be included in taught clinical programs.

Angus et al. (2015) argue that mental health treatment can only be influenced by systematic research studies with evidence. Person-centred research could benefit if practitioners develop research networks and if systematic research can be disseminated.

Conclusion

The person-centred approach to counselling and psychotherapy has changed since the times of Carl Rogers. Bazzano argues that now the conflict lies not between different therapeutic orientations but different worldviews (Bazzano, 2016). Today, the battle that lies within the PCA approach is between a neo-liberal discourse where the person and therapy is seen as measurable and controlled. The other perspective appreciates therapy as complex and difficult to explain, and control is seen as unethical. For Bazzano being-in-the-world is essentially 'unknown'. The philosophy of therapy should openly refuse to abide to 'dominant neo-liberal narratives' and instead embrace the unknown. The aim of this kind of person-centred therapy is to 're-write' the human experience embedded in the person-centred values.

Rogers and his followers have contributed greatly in the practice of Counselling Psychology. Rogers' vision of the human was optimistic and hopeful; he believed that 'people are just as wonderful as sunsets if you let them be. When I look at a sunset, I don't find myself saying, "soften the orange a bit on the right hand corner." I don't try to control a sunset. I watch with awe as it unfolds' (Rogers, 1969: 236). In this quote and in all his work there is humility and respect for the human condition.

Learning outcomes

When you have completed this chapter you should be able to:

- Define the theoretical underpinnings of the person-centred approach to counselling psychology.
- Understand the basic principles of person-centred approach to therapy.

- Apply the basic concepts of therapy, taking into account the view of the person, in a fictitious case scenario.
- Evaluate the contribution of the post-Rogerian developments in counselling/psychotherapy.

Key terms, phrases and concepts

- Client markers
- Conditions of worth
- Configurations of self
- Congruence
- Contact
- Emotion-focused therapy
- Empathy
- Felt sense
- Focusing
- Fragile process
- Humanism
- Incongruence
- Maslow's hierarchy of needs
- Organismic self
- Phenomenology
- Real Self vs Ideal Self
- Self-concept
- Unconditional Positive Regard

Sample essay titles

1. Can a therapist experience unconditional positive regard with a client throughout the course of therapy?
2. Are there three or six conditions? Often the person-centred approach has been reduced to three conditions: *Empathy, Congruence and Unconditional Positive Regard*. However, Rogers (1957) referred to 'six necessary and sufficient conditions for personality change' to take place. Discuss.
3. Identify the strengths and weaknesses of the person-centred approach in comparison with another therapeutic approach.
4. 'When I look at the world I am pessimistic but when I look at people I am optimistic'. Discuss this quote by Rogers drawing from person-centred theory.
5. Purist person-centred therapists have argued that emotion-focused therapy is directive whereas emotion-focused therapists believe it is deeply rooted in person-centred qualities and values. To what extent is this true?

Further reading

Books

Kirschenbaum, H. (2007). *The Life and Work of Carl Rogers*. Ross-on-Wye: PCCS Books.

Lago, C. and Charura, D. (Eds). (2016). *Person-Centred Counselling and Psychotherapy: Origins, Developments, and Contemporary Applications*. Berkshire: Open University Press.
Mearns, D. and Thorne, B., and McLeod, J. (2013). *Person-Centred Counselling in Action* (4th edn.). London: Sage.
Rogers, C. R. (1961). *On Becoming a Person: A Therapist's View of Psychotherapy*. Boston, MA: Houghton Mifflin.

Journal articles

Rogers, C. R. (1957). The necessary and sufficient conditions of therapeutic personality change. *Journal of Consulting Psychology*, 21 (2): 95–103.

References

Angus, L., Watson, J. C., Elliott, R., Schneider, K., and Timulak, L. (2015). Humanistic psychotherapy research 1990–2015: From methodological innovation to evidence supported treatment outcomes and beyond. *Psychotherapy Research*, 25 (3): 330–347.
Barrett-Lennard, G. (1981). The empathy cycle-refinement of a nuclear concept. *Journal of Counseling Psychology*, 28: 91–100.
Barrett-Lennard, G. (1986). The relationship inventory now: Issues and advances in theory, method and use. In L. S. Greenberg and W. M. Pinsof (Eds) *The Psychotherapeutic Process: A Research Handbook* (pp. 439–476). New York: Guilford Press.
Bazzano, M. (2014). On the person-centred approach. *In Counselling Directory*. Retrieved August 10, 2016 from www.counselling-directory.org.uk/counsellor-articles/on-the-person-centred-approach#disqus_thread
Bazzano, M. (2016). The conservative turn in the person-centered therapy. *Person-Centered and Experiential Psychotherapies*, 14: 1–17.
Bozarth, J. D. (2016). The phenomenological, cultural, and historical antecedents to the person-centred approach. In C. Lago and D. Charura (Eds) *Person-Centred Counselling and Psychotherapy: Origins, Developments, and Contemporary Applications* (pp. 3–14). Berkshire: Open University Press.
Cooper, M. (1999). If you can't be Jekyll be Hyde: An existential phenomenological exploration on lived plurality. In J. Rowan and M. Cooper (Eds) *The Plural Self: Multiplicity in Everyday Life* (pp. 51–70). London: Sage.
Cooper, M. and J. McLeod (2011). *Pluralistic Counselling and Psychotherapy*. London: Sage.
Elliott, R. and Greenberg, L. (2016). Emotion-focused therapy. In C. Lago and D. Charura (Eds) *Person-Centred Counselling and Psychotherapy: Origins, Developments, and Contemporary Applications* (pp. 212–222). Berkshire: Open University Press.
Gendlin, E. (2000). "Eugene Gendlin Introduces Focusing (Pt.1 International Conference Toronto)" [Video file]. Retrieved 20 August 2016 from www.youtube.com/watch?v=j7PEC5Mh5FY
Grafanaki, S. (2013). Experiencing congruence and incongruence. *Person-Centered and Experiential Psychotherapies 12*(3): 183–186.
Greenberg, L. (2010). Emotion focused therapy: A clinical synthesis. *Focus: The Journal of Lifelong Learning in Psychiatry*, 8 (1): 1–11.
Kirschenbaum, H. (2007). *The Life and Work of Carl Rogers*. Ross-on-Rye: PCCS Books.
Levitt, H. M., Lu, E. C., Pomerville, A., and Francisco, I. (2015). Pursuing the question of reflexivity in psychotherapy and qualitative methods: The contributions of David L. Rennie. *Counselling and Psychotherapy Research*, March, 15 (1): 3–11.
Maslow, A. H. (1943). A theory of human motivation. *Psychological Review*, 50: 370–396.
Maslow, A. H. (1967). Self-actualization and beyond. In J. F. T. Bugental (Ed) *Challenges of Humanistic Psychology* (pp. 278–286). New York: McGraw-Hill.
McLeod, J. (1999). A narrative social contructionist approach to therapeutic empathy. *Counselling Psychology Quarterly*, 14 (4): 377–394.

McLeod, J. (2013). *An Introduction to Counselling* (5th edn.). Berkshire: Open University Press.
Mearns, D. and Thorne, B. (2000). *Person-Centred Therapy Today: New Frontiers in Theory and Practice.* London: Sage.
O'Hara, M. (1996). Psychotherapy: Humanistic, experiential and relational approaches. In *The Encyclopedia of Alternative and Complementary Medicine* (pp. 1–10). London: Creative Enterprise Publications.
Patterson, C. H. (1977). *Foundations for a Theory of Instruction and Educational Psychology.* New York: Harper and Row.
Prouty, G. F. (2001). The practice of pre-therapy. *Journal of Contemporary Psychotherapy*, 31 (1): 31–40.
Rennie, D. L. (1990). Toward a representation of the client's experience of the psychotherapy hour. In G. Lietaer, J Rombauts and R. Van Balen (Eds) *Client-Centred and Experiential Psychotherapy in the 90s* (pp. 155–172). Leuven, Belgium: University of Leuven Press.
Rennie, D. L. (1992). Qualitative analysis of client's experience of psychotherapy: The unfolding of reflexivity. In D. L. Rennie and S. G. Toukmanian (Eds) *Psychotherapy Process Research: Paradigmatic and Narrative Approaches* (pp. 211–233). Thousand Oaks, CA: Sage.
Rennie, D. L. (1994a). Clients' deference in psychotherapy. *Journal of Counseling Psychology*, 41: 427–437.
Rennie, D. L. (1994b). Storytelling in psychotherapy: The client's subjective experience. *Psychotherapy: Theory, Research, Practice, Training*, 31: 234–243.
Rennie, D. L. (1994c). Clients' accounts of resistance in counselling: A qualitative analysis. *Canadian Journal of Counselling*, 28 (1): 43–57.
Rennie, D. L. (2012). Qualitative research as methodical hermeneutics. *Psychological Methods*, 17: 385–398.
Rogers, C. R. (1957). The necessary and sufficient conditions of therapeutic personality change. *Journal of Consulting Psychology*, 21 (2): 95–103.
Rogers, C. R. (1963). The actualizing tendency in relation to 'motive' and to consciousness. In M. Jones (Ed) *Nebraska Symposium on Motivation* (pp. 1–25). Lincoln: University of Nebraska Press.
Rogers, C. R. (1969). *Freedom to Learn: A View of What Education may become.* Columbus, OH: Charles Merrill.
Sanders, P. (Ed). (2004). *The Tribes of the Person-Centred Nation: An Introduction to the Schools of Therapy Related to the Person-Centred Approach.* Ross-on-Wye: PCCS Books.
Truax, C. B. & Carkhuff, R. R. (1967). *Toward effective counselling and psychotherapy: Training and Practice.* London: Aldine Publishing Company.

6

EXISTENTIAL-PHENOMENOLOGICAL PERSPECTIVES

Elena Manafi

> *What path do I want to pursue in my life and for what purpose? How do I navigate myself in a shared world full of multiplicity? Who is this me I think I am? How do I know that my choices are mine rather than other people's expectations? What do I hold on to when everything that was taken for granted is lost? Who do I become at the face of adversity, disappointment, betrayal and rejection? Why should I commit to anything when I know that nothing lasts? Can I get a grip on life without denying my emotions or being swayed by them? How can I use my passion and despair without feeling overwhelmed or scaring those around me? What is the meaning of (my) life? And why on earth is all this suffering in the world?*

I could have ended the chapter here, having greeted you all as fellow travellers with openness and wonder but with no answers let alone explanations; life is a riddle to be lived rather than solved. It would have been a truly existential moment, an honest, vulnerable, and exposing dialogue between human beings who had the courage to raise questions pertaining to their existence. The editor would probably consider this act as a bad joke and I would probably smile with embarrassment and try again – embracing the same uncertainty and possibility of yet another failure. Recognising the paradox in my experience reminds me that I am on the right track because life is a paradox. Despite the uncertainty and anxiety of the situation I am in (i.e., writing a very complex chapter), I cannot fail to notice that I *care* and that the possibility of failing is less terrifying than not trying at all!

Introduction

As the name implies, existential-phenomenological perspectives to therapeutic practice are inevitably philosophical in nature. *Philosophical!* As I am writing down this word, I wonder whether you will fall prey to the general view that sees philosophy as an obsolete field that has nothing to offer. This wouldn't come as a surprise because the discipline of philosophy has become a theoretical subject that is divorced from our everyday concerns and concrete existence; however in ancient times, philosophy (i.e., love for wisdom) was a passionate and concrete way of life. A *reflective* and *inquisitive* attitude that is better understood as *a verb* rather than a noun, and that focuses on a clarification of what it means to live a life that is worth living. Existence is also a verb rather than a noun; it has its roots in the Greek word *ek-stasis* (i.e., to stand outside oneself) and the Latin *ex-sistere* (i.e., to stand out) – both terms denote a *movement*, which is also evident in our ability to reflect upon our selves and life as a whole (i.e., we live *forward*, moving from the actual to the conceptual). This is the kind of existence that human beings share and so we are also a *verb* rather than a noun; a *process* rather than a static entity; an *action* that reveals and illuminates the world and our relations with other people. It follows that awareness is at the centre of our existence; we apprehend the world in a *critical* way that allows us to act through reflection rather than mere instinct. This ability to be critically aware of the situation we are in brings about *temporality*. Rather than being imprisoned in an one-dimensional present, we emerge *from* time; we can *transcend* (i.e., surpass) our immediate situation to reach back to our past and extend to our future. In his journals, Kierkegaard (1847/1967: 167) – the great Danish existential philosopher – wrote, "it is perfectly true, as philosophers say, that life can only be understood backwards. But they forget the other proposition, that it must be lived forwards". We are historical beings that need to withstand the tension between actuality (past) and possibility (future).

There are many ways of understanding human predicament and *no* way should be considered as *the* way. Like every perspective, existential phenomenology embraces a particular view of human nature and a particular understanding of distress and well-being. One needs to remember that at the heart of all understanding lies an interpretation rather than a claim for absolute truth or certainty. With this attitude in mind, I will attempt to clarify the main ontological and epistemological premises[1] upon which the approach rests. Although I promise to do my best and limit my reference to philosophical 'jargon' down to the bare minimum, I need to warn you that you are about to expose yourself to a whole new vocabulary for a reason. The reason being that existential phenomenology emerged at a time when 'ontological dualisms' predominated; dualisms that during the 17th century became even sharper with Descartes' separation of the mind (*res cogitans*) from the body (*res extensa*). This so-called Cartesian dualism, apart from alienating human beings from their environment and other people also created the still-unresolved epistemological problem of explaining how the ideas in our mind can be true and valid representations of external reality (Kuhn, 1962). It is these ontological and epistemological divisions that the approach set out to overcome by reconfiguring human existence in a way that challenges our mainstream ideas regarding knowledge acquisition and human nature. As a result a whole new language is introduced which at times might feel bizarre but deserves your curiosity and most likely perseverance!

Spinelli (2001, 2015) has argued at great length how the English language is the epitome of this dualistic, Western heritage that continues to bedevil our ways of understanding subjectivity, otherness, and the relationship between the two. He brings to our attention the consequences of expressing ourselves through a language that is constructed mainly in dichotomous terms and a series of binary oppositions (e.g., self/other, inner/outer, mind/body, emotion/intellect, passion/reason, etc.). I concur with his view that existential phenomenology, instead of eradicating dualisms, 'bridges the gap' that they create and does so by introducing a perspective, which presents a paradox; we need order **and** chaos; passion **and** reason; freedom **and** determinism. The paradoxical position is *dimensional* and *complementary* in nature; rather than being categorical (i.e., either/or stance), paradox introduces the **both/and** stance of **co-existence** and **co-creation**.

Finally you will notice that I will be making references to dead philosophers whose wisdom continue to be of great relevance and an immense source of inspiration that became the impetus for the development of existential phenomenological practice. Although you do not need to become a philosopher in order to embrace an existential phenomenological attitude to therapeutic practice, I highly recommend Deurzen (2009), Macquarrie (1972), and Warnock (1970) as three excellent introductory texts.

A sketch of the historical origins[2] (and definition) of the approach

Walter Kaufmann (also dead), a German/American philosopher and translator of a great number of philosophical works, argued that at the heart of existentialism is "a refusal to belong to any school of thought, the repudiation of the adequacy of any body of beliefs, and especially of systems, and a marked dissatisfaction with traditional philosophy as superficial, academic, and remote from life" (1975: 12). One cannot fail to witness the attitude of defiance that springs out of these lines or the invitation to engage with life. Existential phenomenological approaches are concerned with an elucidation of *individual, concrete* human existence: what it means to live one's life in the most deliberate way possible and with the awareness of the inherent limitations, tensions, and contradictions that life entails.

It is in this sense that we could all embrace the term 'existentialist'; the question is not so much whether we will accept the label or not, but whether we are prepared to passionately engage with the limited time we have been given on this earth and to transform this accident called life into a meaningful journey towards our inevitable demise. It follows that well-being is inextricably linked to our ability to withstand the tension created by existential polarities such as certainty/uncertainty, continuity/discontinuity, meaning/meaninglessness, life/death and create meaning and purpose. It is with this attitude in mind that I deliberately started the chapter the way I did; these questions lie at the heart of the kind of being that we are, a being whose Being[3] is an *issue*. This Heideggerian (1927) attitude of *concern* (or *care*) brings to our attention that how we live our lives *matters* to us; it also creates an intrinsic and inescapable sense of *anxiety* or *angst* which comes with the recognition that we are free to choose and are responsible for our choices.

When we try to define the approach, we are confronted with a certain elusiveness that needs to be embraced, as one needs to remember that to define something is to limit it! For an approach that attempts to illuminate rather than explain the human predicament and that does so through celebrating the multiplicity of human existence, an attempt at a definition defeats the purpose. There are however key features that constitute the existential phenomenological attitude to therapeutic practice. At its heart lies an exploration of the ways in which each one of us responds to the givens of existence – also known as the 'ultimate concerns' of death, meaninglessness, isolation, and freedom (Cohn, 1997; Yalom, 1980, 2001). It is an exploration that embraces the paradoxes, tensions, contradictions, and dilemmas that are inherent in living and are reflected on the physical, personal, social, and spiritual dimensions of our lives (Deurzen, 2012). It is also an exploration that requires humility and a stance of 'un-knowing' based upon the existential principles of 'relatedness', 'uncertainty', and 'existential anxiety' as we all construct a unique worldview that becomes the interpretative lens of all understanding (Spinelli, 2015). As I have already argued (Manafi, 2010a, 2010b) existential/phenomenological practice is based on the premise that human beings are active agents of their fate; despite being *thrown* into a world that they have not chosen and a life that is full of inescapable facts, they are capable of choosing *how to respond* and are responsible for their choices.

The attitude

Given the above brief sketch, it should not come as a surprise that therapeutic practice becomes collaborative and dialogical in nature. For any dialogue and collaboration to be constructive certain qualities need to be present – the most important of which is *respect* for the Otherness of the Other. Facilitation of a person's understanding of their difficulties in living pre-supposes an attitude of openness and wonder, as well as trust, care, genuineness, and acceptance that invites people to examine their ways of being in the absence of unnecessary labelling and alienating interpretations that emerge out of a position of authority and pre-set frameworks of meaning. It follows that practitioners need to be prepared to recognise that their valuable knowledge *about* the human condition emerges out of a commitment to their own and their clients' *lived experience* rather than an *unquestioning reliance* on pre-existing constructs (Manafi, 2010b). My emphasis on 'unquestioning reliance' is not accidental as my aim is not to introduce a polemical attitude that discards (theoretical) knowledge; instead I want to highlight the importance of exploration and in-depth understanding as opposed to eradication and control of the inherent *paradoxes, dilemmas, uncertainties, complexities*, and *insecurities* that lie at the heart of the human condition.

The relationship therefore becomes the *sine qua non* of therapeutic practice – together with the phenomenological method (see Deurzen and Adams, 2011; Langdridge, 2007; Spinelli, 2001b, 2005) – they lie at the heart of the existential attitude and its focus on an exploration and clarification of clients' dilemmas and distress. Rather than conceptualising distress as a mere deficiency or an illness that can be reduced to one's physiology (say chemical imbalances or brain disease) and upbringing (e.g., childhood trauma), suffering is viewed as inextricably linked to the human condition and as *relational, situational*, and *dynamic* in nature. It follows that (severe) emotional difficulties, rather than being a meaningless manifestation of a 'thing-like' disorder that can be objectively classified into specific categories of symptoms, become vulnerabilities that need to be understood from the vantage point of our clients' *subjective* account, relational patterns, and concrete situation. Construction of *meaning* **is/becomes** the work: understanding rather than eradicating or curing 'difficulties in living' therefore lies at the heart of the therapeutic endeavour.

Understanding distress as part and parcel of the human condition is most evident in the work of Jaspers (1913/1997, 1951), who argued that the concept of distress is inextricably linked "to the *incompleteness* and *vulnerability* of human beings and their *freedom* and *infinite possibilities*" (1913/1997: 8). Essentially, what he argues is that the possibility of well-being and distress is inextricably linked to our fundamental *lack* (i.e., absence of a concrete essence to define us). Moreover it is this fundamental incompleteness that brings to the fore our capacity for self-awareness, freedom of action, possibility and ability to create meaning as well as avoidance, deception, manipulation, and (self) destruction. From this angle, human distress becomes inevitable, meaningful, and purposeful – the purpose being one of avoidance of something that inflicts more pain and dread than the 'symptom' itself. Jaspers' (1951) concept of *limit situations* is particularly pertinent for therapeutic practice. Death, uncertainty, anxiety, guilt, chance, aloneness, and meaninglessness (to name but a few) are *givens* of existence that cannot be avoided and yet "in our day-to-day lives we often evade them, by closing our eyes and living as if they did not exist. We forget that we must die, forget our guilt, and forget that we are at the mercy of chance" (Jaspers, 1951: 20). It is a forgetfulness that deserves compassion, as it tries to evade the inherent vulnerability of the human condition – known as *ontological insecurity*; sooner or later however we come face to face with a limit situation that overwhelms and paralyses us. Facilitating our clients to understand and *confront* the limitations of the human condition is at the heart of the aforementioned non-pathologising attitude and its claim that the possibility of resilience and courage are created **because** of suffering not despite it. Let me be clear! I am not glorifying pain, instead I am highlighting that distress 'forces' us into a state of awareness which when worked through (be it in therapy, alone, or with trusted others) can transform a *breakdown into a breakthrough* (Deurzen, 2015) as insight slowly turns a 'crisis into an opportunity' (Manafi, 2010b: 174).

Nothing exists in a vacuum – the box below provides you with the ontological and epistemological premises that sustain everything that has been argued so far.

FOCUS BOX 6.1 MAIN PHILOSOPHICAL ASSUMPTIONS

- Human existence is conceptualised as a verb rather than a noun or static entity.
- The distinctive principle of the approach is *relatedness*; a view that stresses a co-constituted understanding of the world, 'self', and others that is in direct opposition to dualistic understandings that are founded upon dichotomies and binary oppositions.
- The self ceases to be an autonomous, self-contained, and isolated entity and becomes a 'relational act or process' that is embedded, embodied, and temporal in nature.
- Living is a paradox, a dynamic co-existence of opposites: it is dimensional (i.e., both/and) rather than dichotomous (i.e., either/or).
- Meaning and purpose lie at the heart of our attitude in living; this attitude of *care* is inevitably the source of existential angst as it comes with consequences and responsibility.
- Human suffering is inherent in living: the aim of therapy ceases to be one of cure or treatment and becomes a dialogical investigation that focuses on understanding and clarifying the client's concrete, lived experience.
- Therapeutic practice is dialogical in nature; understanding is achieved *with* the client, not *for* them.

The primacy of lived experience or the 'phenomenal' over the 'real'

Twenty years ago I was an undergraduate psychology student; I remember the sleepless nights during the exam period when I was surrounded by books focusing on psychology as a natural science. I hopelessly tried to predict the possible exam questions and memorise (I had given up on understanding) the answers to topics that seemed so remote from what I thought psychology was about. Behaviourism, cognitivism, experimentation, and quantification dominated the curriculum of the mid-1990s, which relentlessly divided the outward behaviour of human beings (actions) from the inward and therefore unfathomable processes of memory, perception, thoughts, and emotions. For three years I was torn between the *behaviour–experience* polarity and the *objective–subjective* divide trying to figure out what is real and what can be trusted!

Then one day, prompted by a friend of mine – to whom I obviously owe a lot – I secretly joined a different class; the module was called 'continental philosophy' and the topic was phenomenology or the study of appearances (i.e., phenomena) as they are presented to our *immediate experience*. I owe my long-term affair with existential/phenomenological psychology (see Valle and Halling, 1989) to my accidental meeting with a charismatic professor who showed us that certain problems exist as a result of particular questions that have been asked from particular angles. He argued that if the questions are asked differently the problem ceases to exist – not by way of magic – but because it never emerges in the first place! He was alluding to Descartes (1596–1650) who by asking the epistemological question '*what can I know with certainty*?' set out to discover ultimate and objective truths. Descartes' method of doubt led him to question everything, including the existence of his own body. The only thing that survived his methodological scepticism was his existence as a thinking and knowing being (*res cogitans*) expressed in his famous dictum *cogito ergo sum* (I think therefore I am). This ontological understanding of human beings as disembodied and disembedded self-constituting, autonomous, and rational entities is known as Cartesian solipsism (Manafi, 2010a).

Changing the angle

What if instead of *'what can I know with certainty?'* we asked *'how do I experience whatever it is that is presented to me?'* be it an object, a feeling, the view from my window, or the absence of the person I used to share my life with. Let's take absence as our phenomenon of investigation. From this angle we are interested in understanding the *meaning* that absence has for me and *how* I experience it. Focusing on my experience immediately brings to my awareness the *horizon of my existence* – a horizon that encompasses the givens of my *embodiment, temporality, embeddedness,* and *relatedness*. All these I cannot doubt let alone deny. They are part and parcel of how I experience and understand absence. I feel it in my body through this sense of tightness in my stomach; I connect it to the past (when the absence was presence) and to the future (where longing and apprehension live). I notice that it restricts my engagement with space as there are certain places that I tend to avoid and that it also influences my ways of relating to people (through conversations that I choose or ignore) and to myself as single in my early 40s. I also become aware of a *mood* that attunes me to the world and others; a mood that is sometimes coloured by sadness and others by relief and a sense of freedom.

Staying with my experience immediately illuminates the sense of who I am and the totality of my situation. If you were genuinely interested in understanding this experience of mine without imposing *your* views and explanations of how I feel through reference to pre-existing theories and causal links, you would try to stay as close as possible to *my* understanding and you would ask me questions that would further elucidate the quality of *how* my experience of absence is *lived*. You would use questions such as 'what is it like?,' 'how does it feel?,' 'what does it mean to you?,' 'can you tell me a bit more?' 'has it always been like this?' etc. All these questions are *phenomenological* in nature because they are asked with an attitude of invitation and openness and with the aim of describing, clarifying, and exploring further the meaning of absence as experienced by Manafi. Staying with the experience of another person is easier said than done and yet so important when we are sitting with our clients who are in distress and in a state of utter confusion. Thankfully there is a method!

The phenomenological method as the centre of the existential attitude to practice

> *Phenomenology may be characterized initially in a broad sense as the unprejudiced, descriptive study of whatever appears to consciousness, precisely in the manner in which it so appears.*
>
> *(Mooney and Moran, 2002: 1)*

The phenomenological method has its own historical origins as well as ontological and epistemological foundations. The space is limited, but I hope that I will capture your attention so that you will immerse yourself in further reading through secondary (Deurzen and Adams, 2011; Gallagher and Zahavi, 2012; Langdridge, 2007; Spinelli, 2005) and primary sources – i.e., the works of Edmund Husserl and Martin Heidegger. Further reading will enable you to clarify important distinctions between transcendental and existential turns in phenomenology. Knowing the epistemological consequences of these two branches is essential, especially if you choose to engage with qualitative research (see Willig, 2013).

Consciousness as an embodied and embedded intentional act

It all started with Franz Brentano (1838–1917) in Germany at the end of the 19th century; he focused on the development of a *descriptive* psychology that will manage to establish itself *outside* the natural scientific approach. As Gallagher and Zahavi (2012) argue, traditionally 'consciousness' is seen as a *terra incognita* – a mysterious container of ideas that resides *within* our minds and can only be known through introspection. In phenomenology however consciousness assumes a very different character that breaks through 'dualistic ontology' and proposes a **co-constituted** understanding. Specifically, it becomes *intentional* in nature. By intentional is here meant **directional**. Consciousness ceases to be a static entity and instead becomes a reflective, *directional act* that has an object (i.e., a point of focus). In simple terms we are always conscious **of something.** Intentionality therefore brings to the fore the *'aboutness'* of the conscious act: for example every act of avoidance is avoidance *of something*. This emphasis on directional action presupposes the world, other people, and a body. We therefore talk about an *embodied* and *embedded* consciousness and so the aforementioned Cartesian dualism is the problem that never arises in the first place!

Later on Edmund Husserl (1859–1938) took the concept of intentionality as the basic structure of consciousness and developed a philosophical method devoted to a descriptive (as opposed to explanatory or causal) understanding of lived experience. His dictum was *'back to the things themselves'* – an attitude that essentially demands an understanding of phenomena outside pre-existing categories, theories, and meanings. This embodied and embedded, intentional act is the foundation upon which the concept of **inter-relatedness** rests. Consciousness and the world are a correlational *a priori*; they are inter-dependent and co-constitutive in nature. The real world *exists* **but** this world can only be understood through our own conscious reflections upon it: it is an *interpreted world* (Spinelli, 2005).

Pre-reflective and reflective consciousness[4]

Our brief exploration of the 'phenomenological land' would be incomplete in the absence of these two modes of consciousness that are central to our understanding and therapeutic practice. Earlier on when we attempted to understand my experience of absence, we took absence as the (intentional) object of my conscious act. In the process of our phenomenological investigation, I **became** *reflectively* aware of the phenomenon and my experience of it. Notice the word 'became'; prior to this reflective exercise absence was still present in my life but in a *pre-reflective* manner. This does not mean that I was unconscious of it; instead it means that I was *pre-reflectively* aware of it as a *'background'* to my experience. When I reflect on something I bring it to the **foreground** of my experience, which in turn allows me to examine its qualities; it follows that reflective awareness **thematises** an otherwise concept-free/abstract experience. From an existential/phenomenological perspective my everyday mode of being is pre-reflective in nature. I go along, engaging with the world (i.e., the ground of my existence) attending only to the projects that concern me (e.g., writing this chapter). Moreover I do so without being explicitly 'self aware' – in fact I don't need to be self-aware in order to live my everydayness and write this chapter. Self-awareness is a reflective mode of consciousness where 'self' becomes the 'object' of my intentional act.

The centrality of the phenomenological method[5] to therapeutic practice

The phenomenological method lies at the heart of counseling psychology theory and practice, which focuses on an "exploration, clarification, and understanding of clients' world-views, underlying assumptions, and emotional difficulties that emerge out of our interaction with the world and others" (CoP Standards, 2015: 16). When the world we are living in is an 'interpreted world', assumptions, biases, and all sorts of evaluations become inevitable as they are inherent to all understanding – an understanding that is part of a 'relational totality' that is historical, cultural, political, and social in nature. We can never speak of 'facts' or 'objective truth' and it is not accidental that Heidegger (1927) used the Greek word *αλήθεια* (*alítheia*) instead of 'truth'. Etymologically the word is a synthesis: the privative affix – a, is the key here because the second part of the word is *λήθη* (*líthee*) which means oblivion! So *alítheia* is something that has been brought to light out of a state of forgetfulness. This process of illumination and unveiling lies at the heart of our attitude to practice. Our aim is to strengthen our clients' **reflective awareness** so that they can examine the meaning of their distress within the context of their situation, relationships, and horizon of their existence. With this in mind let's take a closer look to what this attitude is about; forgive my prescriptive style – in action the style is yours and *yours only*.

- Centre yourself, watch your pace, and *notice*. Carefully attend in other words to the ways in which your client communicates with you. Focus on the 'what' (i.e., content) and the 'how' (i.e., process – the manner in which they present themselves).
- While you are listening become reflectively aware of your *biases* and *assumptions* and try to suspend or 'bracket' them. It is impossible to do so in an absolute fashion; the aim is to become *reflexively aware* so that you do **not** impose your pre-existing understanding (theories included!) onto your client.
- Describe, clarify, and explore rather than explain your client's predicament; the aim is that of elucidation of your client's *immediate experience* as it is lived.
- Try not to jump to conclusions (at least not too fast!); instead treat everything with the same importance (equalise them in other words). This is difficult when in the presence of distress as we usually try to alleviate our client's (and our own) anxiety and uncertainty by jumping into explanatory, causal links that narrow the focus of our investigations.

- A note on the use of interpretations: they are present all the time! The question is what kind of interpretations. Illumination of one's world necessitates a hermeneutic rather than reductive attitude.[6] Hermeneutic interpretations take into account the aforementioned 'referential totality' (be it social, cultural, and/or political) as well as your client's personal history and understanding. Their aim is making the **implicit explicit** by facilitating creation of meaning as it emerges from experience rather than pre-existing theoretical constructs.

ACTIVITY BOX 6.1 FORM A THERAPIST/CLIENT DYAD

The one who chooses to be the therapist needs to attempt to embrace the phenomenological attitude described above and to elucidate the experience that the client shares. The aim is to *stay with* the experience and to explore it in depth with openness and attention to subjective meaning.

From the recesses of the mind to an investigation of existence as a human landscape

I Am therefore I Think

Martin Heidegger (1927)

Such was Heidegger's reversal of the Cartesian dictum. The focus becomes existence rather than Descartes' isolated 'mind' that is separate from the world and others. As Cohn (1997) argues rather than conceptualising human essence as part of a theory of mind or personality that can be categorised or divided into different compartments and subagencies (e.g., ego, superego, and id), existential phenomenology understands agency as inextricably linked to existence as a whole. As a result human essence becomes dynamic in nature; an open-ended, dialectical movement that is always in flux, and with enormous plasticity when it comes to experience. There is no **fixed** essence in other words; *our essence lies in our existence* rather than inner traits and personality characteristics. We are the species that have the capacity to be (self) aware and go beyond (i.e., transcend) the immediacy of our situation by reflecting upon life and claiming it as our own.

Here come the first two 'philosophical jargons': *Dasein* and *Mitsein* (Heidegger, 1927). *Dasein* replaces the notion of a self as an isolated, inner/fixed entity; in colloquial German it means 'everyday human existence' and is translated in English as *being-there* or *being-in-the-world*. Cohn (2002) argues that the emphasis on *there* should not be interpreted only as a *spatial* relationship (i.e., in the world) but also as the *manner* in which we exist. 'Being-there' stresses our *embodied* engagement and involvement with the world and other people; it brings to the fore the fundamental principle of existential phenomenological theory and practice – meaning *relatedness*. This mode of inter-realtedness brings us to the concept of *Mitsein* (i.e., *being-with-others*). The hyphens you notice in all translations are **not** accidental; they indicate a **unitary phenomenon:** self-world-other *co-constitute* one another.

A number of scholars (Boss, 1963; Cohn, 1997, 2002; Deurzen, 2012, 2013, 2015) have interpreted Dasein as *'embodied possibilities'* that we realise or put them aside (our growth in other words is not a given; it requires work and cultivation). As already mentioned our lives *matter* to us; like a 'ray of light' we **illuminate** our involvement with the world and others by creating meaning, interpreting, and realising our potential. We do so because the basic structure of our existence (our essence) is that of care and concern. Heidegger (1927) used another term – namely **bodying-forth** (notice the emphasis on *future action*) – to indicate that we live and inhabit our bodies as 'vehicles of understanding' of our (inter) subjective experience. The 'self' in existential phenomenological theory therefore becomes a *meaning making and interpretative activity* that is *always* in flux. Moreover, Dasein is always **in relationship** and in relationship we evolve, change, create, and re-create ourselves. It follows that there is no concrete, inner, or true self to rely on, instead we are inherently **incomplete** beings that are always in the process of becoming.

Our uniqueness, the 'mineness' of our being, the *'deliberate I'* that we all cherish, is inextricably linked to the 'Other', our situatedness, and life as a whole. It is an 'I' that **emerges out** of the relational matrix that sustains us and which is absolutely necessary for our survival and for this 'I' to exist at all. To put it bluntly, I am first being defined by others (including culture, society, politics, economic status, etc.) and only *after* I define myself (usually at a cost as individuation is holding hands with anxiety). The 'I' therefore becomes a dialectic with inherent tensions that – unless carefully negotiated – can result in feelings of *alienation* (by being too different) or *anonymity* (by merging with others and society as a whole). This conceptualisation of 'mineness' offers a different slant to the mainstream understanding of yet another cherished concept, namely *authenticity*. Dasein has been *thrown* into the world (a concept also know as *falleness*) from which it cannot be extricated; this state of throwness is our primordial mode of being and is inherently inauthentic as we exist in the so-called *they mode* which is nothing but the anonymity of the crowd. As Heidegger argued, "the self of everyday Dasein is the '*they-self*' " (Heidegger, 1927/1962: 167). It is important to notice that there is **no** negative judgement placed on that *falleness* and *inauthenticity* as both are part of our *structure of existence*. This is a radical re-conceptualisation of authenticity that is usually understood as something that resides *within* an individual (i.e., his/her true self). From an existential phenomenological perspective authenticity ceases to be a goal in itself and instead becomes a "gradual process of self-understanding that is never fully achieved" (Deurzen, 2013: 205) and a mode of being that reflects "an openness to existence, an acceptance of what is given, as well as our freedom to respond to it" (Cohn, 1997: 127). As a result authenticity and inauthenticity become a dance and a dialectic which departs from the mainstream understanding of 'genuineness' and 'falseness' and introduces the concept of **resolution** which signifies "letting oneself be *summoned* out of one's lostness in the 'they' " (Heidegger, 1927/1962: 345, emphasis added). As Deurzen (2015) argues, owning my life and living it deliberately without breaking away from the 'relational ground' that sustains me necessitates a fragile development of *mastery* (Deurzen, 2015); it is fragile because it is not a given, instead it is an ability that we need to develop so that we can negotiate the inherent tensions, conflicts, and contradictions that co-existence entails. The whole process of living therefore becomes a dialectic that is experienced in time and on the continuum between the polarities of birth and death:

Birth □ *living* □□□ **Death**

Temporality is therefore at the centre of our awareness and understanding. Our lives and narratives are arranged around time, which we know is limited regardless of whether we reflect upon it or not. We are temporal beings (i.e., *beings-in-time*) who live their present by simultaneously looking back and anticipating the future. From an existential phenomenological perspective time is a *unified* rather than *linear* concept: the present moment (which is our starting point) contains the past and at the same time anticipates the future (Cohn, 1997, 2002). Any attempt to create a 'pure present' is futile as our 'lived time' is always informed by past experiences and guided by future expectations. Unlike other approaches that tend to focus on the past, the existential approach places equal importance to the future dimension as our temporal existential structure necessitates an understanding of where we have been but also where we are heading!

ACTIVITY BOX 6.2 THE 'WEB' OF TIME (WORK ON YOUR OWN ALLOWING 10 MINUTES)

Reflect upon your choice to study psychology and ask yourself the following question: *What brought me here and what are my expectations in the future?* Notice how your past has informed your decision and what kind of projects you intend to actualise in the years to come.

Birth and death are two sides of the same coin; life is constituted by a number of polarities that are to be found in all dimensions of existence (i.e., physical, personal, social, and spiritual – see Figure 6.1 below).

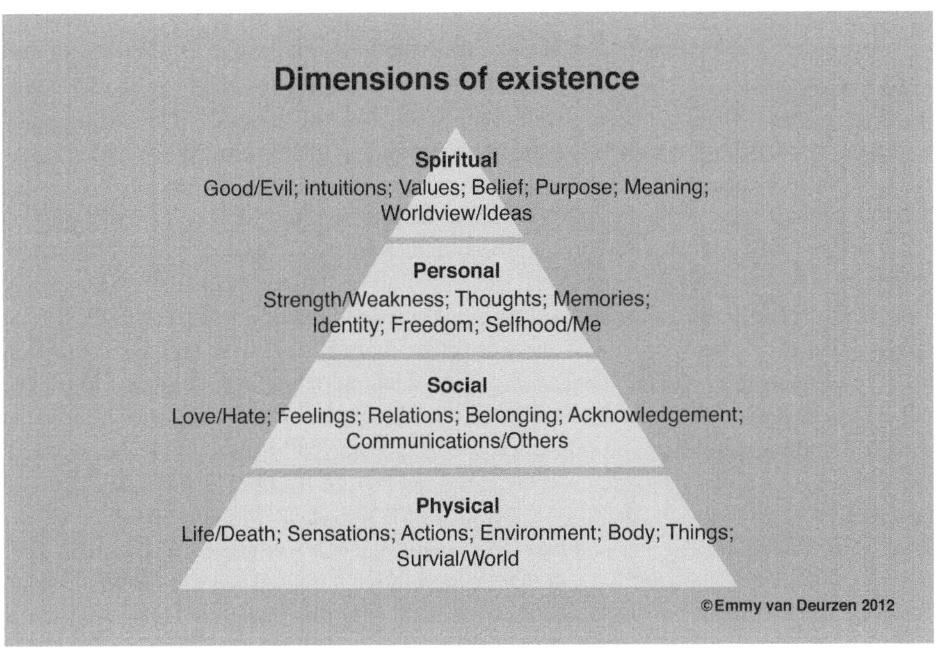

FIGURE 6.1 Dimensions of existence

The emphasis on an examination of the human condition relocates human distress from *within* a person to the *realm of living* and our interactions with the world, other people and life as a whole. Distress is co-constituted in other words. The aforementioned dimensions that are interwoven present us with a number of challenges that require *constant* negotiation. As shown in the diagram, the *physical dimension* exposes us to strength and weakness; health and illness; desire and scarcity. The *social* to intimacy and separation; trust and distrust as well as belonging and isolation. On the *personal dimension* we need to navigate between authenticity (i.e., openness and fluidity) and inauthenticity (i.e., rigidity and closeness) as well as creativity and rigidity and on the *spiritual* – the dimension of values – we oscillate between purpose and futility as well as logic and absurdity (Deurzen, 2012). When we try to isolate one polarity from the other, we step out of the paradox of living and find ourselves cut off from the interrelatedness of existence.

Living is participatory in nature; it is a synthesis of opposites, a paradox (i.e., both/and position), and a balancing act (Manafi, 2010a). Nietzsche (1882/1974: 270) claimed *happiness and unhappiness are twins that grow up together.* We often fail to see the value in the 'negative' polarity and we set out to eliminate it; in the process of elimination we cease to live life to the full by restricting our being through concretisation. Learning to live with the tension and the anxiety that the dialectic of polarities produce is one of the most essential achievements in living as breaking the dialectic leads to (self) estrangement, alienation, and stagnation (Manafi, 2010b).

Encountering the abyss

Nothingness lies coiled in the heart of being – like a worm.

Jean Paul Sartre (1943/1998: 56)

I will leave you with this brief but vital encounter. Nothingness is a source of creativity **and** *angst* – a term that denotes the ontological status of anxiety as an inescapable given rather than pathology (Cohn, 1997; Deurzen, 2015; Yalom, 1980). *Existential angst* is to be distinguished from fear; it designates our experience of apprehension that emerges out of life's uncertainty and our inherent incompleteness. We are *all* gazing into the abyss of our existential predicament because we are beings, whose essence is **not** to have an essence (i.e., set properties) (Sartre, 1943/1998). We are a paradox, a process, a dialectic, and a balancing act. This is how life was described in previous sections and the repetition here is not accidental. As Heidegger (1927) argued, our *essence lies in our existence* – the human condition in other words. It is an existence that entails the awareness of non-being (i.e., finitude and death) and the recognition that we can never have absolute control and understanding of our being and that of others. Rather than having a solid nature (or self) to rely on, we live our lives in the space in between being and nothingness. This is an inherently *insecure* position to be in but, as is the case with all paradoxes, the nothingness that we are gives rise to the freedom that we also are and together they become the driving force and impetus to all creation. In the words of Nietzsche (1884/1961: Prologue), *'one must still have chaos in oneself to be able to give birth to a dancing star'.* Sooner or later life will nail us! We will find ourselves totally unprepared and we will have no choice except to embrace or deny the situation we are in. In times like this the groundlessness of our existence becomes so apparent that it fills us with dread. It is important to remember the paradox of living and to trust that "only to the extent that we expose ourselves over and over to annihilation can that which is indestructible be found in us" (Chödrön, 2016: 8). Holding on to something or someone that no longer exists temporarily creates the illusion of security and maintains our desire for continuity; however, as Spinelli (2015: 85) argued, "to exist is to change", by embracing the uncertainty and the inevitable anxiety it evokes, we allow the perpetual interplay of existential polarities to unfold and we learn to withstand the tension they create without concretising our existence.

> *Whoever has learned to be anxious in the right way has learned the ultimate.*
> *Sören Kierkegaard (1844/1980:155)*

Learning outcomes

When you have completed this chapter you should be able to:

- Understand the main premises of existential/phenomenological theory and practice.
- Conceptualise the approach as an exploration and clarification of lived experience.
- View existence and the notion of the self as verbs and processes rather than static entities.
- Have an understanding of the phenomenological method and its centrality to therapeutic practice.

Key concepts and terms

- Awareness and the Act of (Self) Reflection
- Biases and Assumptions
- Care
- Consciousness as an Intentional Act, not a Container
- Dasein and Mitsein
- Dialogical, Inquisitive, and Non-Pathologising Attitude
- Embodiment, Temporality, and Embeddedness
- *Existential Dimensions:* Physical, Personal, Social, and Spiritual
- Freedom, Choice, and Responsibility
- Human Existence as a Verb: a Dynamic Movement
- Inauthenticity *and* Authenticity
- Intersubjectivity
- Meaning and Purpose
- Nothingness
- *Paradox:* Co-existence/Co-creation/ Co-constitution
- *Phenomenological Method:* Description, Clarification, and Exploration of Lived Experience
- Polarities of Existence
- Possibilities and Limitations
- Reflective and Non-Reflective Consciousness
- Reflexivity
- Relatedness
- Self as a Verb: a Process not Static/Inner Entity
- *Ultimate Concerns* or *Limit Situations:* Death, Meaninglessness, Isolation, Chance
- Uncertainty and Angst

Sample Essay Titles

1. Evaluate the statement "existence and self are verbs rather than nouns or static entities".
2. Discuss the existential phenomenological view of human distress and its relevance to well-being.
3. Discuss the centrality of the phenomenological method and its relevance to therapeutic practice.
4. Discuss the concepts of Dasein and Mitsein.
5. Discuss the concept of existential anxiety.

Useful Journals and Recommended Reading

Journal of the Society for Existential Analysis
The Indo-Pacific Journal of Phenomenology
Journal of Phenomenological Psychology
Research in Phenomenology
Phenomenology and Practice
Deurzen, E. van (2009). *Everyday Mysteries: Existential Dimensions of Psychotherapy*. London: Routledge.
Deurzen, E. van and Adams, M. (2016). *Skills in Existential Counselling and Psychotherapy*. London: Sage.
Laing, R. D. (2010). *The Divided Self*. London: Penguin.
Spinelli, E. (2015). *Practising Existential Therapy. The Relational World*. London: Sage.

Notes

1 Ontology is the study of being (i.e., what exists), and epistemology is the study of knowledge (i.e., how we know what we know).
2 The reader is referred to the seminal book *Existence* (1958), edited by Rollo May, Ernest Angel, and Helen Ellenberger. New York: Basic Books.
3 The capital B denotes existence as a whole rather than a particular individual predicament.
4 For those interested in further reading I highly recommend Zahavi (2004).
5 For an in-depth explication refer to Deurzen and Adams (2011) and Spinelli (2005).
6 See Cohn (1997) for a detailed account of the two.

References

Boss, M. (1963). *Psychoanalysis and Daseinsanalysis*, (transl. L. B. Lefebre). New York: Basic Books Inc.
Chödrön, P. (2016). *When Things Fall Apart*. Boulder: Shambhala.
Cohn, H. W. (1997). *Existential Thought and Therapeutic Practice*. London: Sage.
Cohn, H. W. (2002). *Heidegger and the Roots of Existential Therapy*. London: Continuum.
Deurzen, E. van (2009). *Everyday Mysteries: Existential Dimensions of Psychotherapy*. London: Routledge.
Deurzen, E. van (2012). *Existential Counselling and Psychotherapy in Practice*. (3rd Edition). London: Sage.
Deurzen, E. van (2013). 'Existential Therapy' in W. Dryden and A. Reeves *The Handbook of Individual Therapy* (pp. 155–178). London: Sage.
Deurzen, E. van (2015). *Paradox and Passion in Psychotherapy: An Existential Approach*. (2nd Edition). Chichester: John Wiley & Sons.
Deurzen, E. van and Adams, M. (2011). *Skills in Existential Counselling and Psychotherapy*. London: Sage.
Deurzen-Smith, E. van (2009). *Everyday Mysteries: Existential Dimensions of Psychotherapy*. (2nd Edition). London: Routledge.
Gallagher, S. and Zahavi, D. (2012). *The Phenomenological Mind*. (2nd Edition). London: Routledge.
Heidegger, M. (1927). *Being and Time*, (transl. J. Macquarrie and E. Robinson). Oxford: Basil Blackwell, 1962 Edn.

Heidegger, M. (1953). *Introduction to Metaphysics*, (transl. G. Fied and R. Polt) (2nd Edition). New Haven, CT: Yale University Press, 2014 Edn.

Jaspers, K. (1913). *General Psychopathology. Volume 1*, (transl. J. Hoenig and M. W. Hamilton). New York: Johns Hopkins University Press, 1997 Edn.

Jaspers, K. (1951). *The Way to Wisdom*, (transl. R. Manheim). New York: International University Press.

Kaufman, W. (1975). *Existentialism: From Dostoyevsky to Sartre.* New York: A Plume Book.

Kierkegaard, S. (1844). *The Concept of Anxiety*, (transl. R. Thompte and A. B. Anderson). Princeton, NJ: Princeton University Press, 1980 Edn.

Kuhn, T. (1962). *The Structure of Scientific Revolutions.* Chicago: University Press.

Langdridge, D. (2007). *Phenomenological Psychology: Theory, Research, and Method.* London: Sage.

Macquarrie, J. (1972). *Existentialism.* London: Penguin.

Manafi, E. (2010a). 'Existential-Phenomenological Contributions to Counselling Psychology's Relational Framework' in M. Milton *Therapy and Beyond: Counselling Psychology Contributions to Therapeutic and Social Issues* (pp. 21–39). London: Wiley-Blackwell.

Manafi, E. (2010b). 'Existential Contributions to Pluralistic Practice' in M. Milton *Therapy and Beyond: Counselling Psychology Contributions to Therapeutic and Social Issues* (pp. 171–187). London: Wiley-Blackwell.

May, R., Angel, E., and Ellenberger, H. F. (1958). *Existence.* Jason Aronson, 1994 Edn. New York: Basic Books.

Mooney, T. and Moran, D. (2002). *The Phenomenology Reader.* London: Routledge.

Nietzsche, F. (1882). *The Gay Science*, (transl. W. Kaufman). New York: Vintage Books, 1974 Edn.

Nietzsche, F. (1884). *Thus Spoke Zarathrusta*, (transl. R. J. Hollingdale). Harmondsworth: Penguin, 1961 Edn.

Sartre, J. P. (1943). *Being and Nothingness*, (transl. H. Barnes). London: Routledge, 1998 Edn.

Spinelli, E. (2005). *The Interpreted World: An Introduction to Phenomenological Psychology.* (2nd Edition). London: Sage.

Spinelli, E. (2015). *Practicing Existential Therapy: The Relational World.* (2nd Edition). London: Sage.

Valle, R. S. and Halling, S. (1989). *Existential-Phenomenological Perspectives in Psychology.* New York: Plenum Press.

Warnock, M. (1970). *Existentialism.* Oxford: Oxford University Press.

Willig, C. (2013). *Introducing Qualitative Research in Psychology.* (3rd Edition). London: Open University Press.

Yalom, I. (1980). *Existential Psychotherapy.* New York: Basic Books.

Yalom, I. (2001). *The Gift of Therapy: An Open Letter to a New Generation of Therapists and their Patients.* London: Piatkus Publishers.

Zahavi, D. (2004). *Hidden Resources.* Exeter: Imprint Academic.

7

CBT APPROACHES

Angela Ioanna Loulopoulou

In this chapter you will read about the origins of the cognitive-behavioural therapeutic approach, its theory and modern-day development. The theory will be applied to practice with the provision of case examples and you will be given the opportunity to practice the main components of this approach. Furthermore, the evolution of cognitive-behavioural therapy (CBT) into 'third-wave' CBT approaches will be discussed. Holding more than one therapeutic approaches in mind and having a working knowledge of them is of the essence in the professional identity and work of a counselling psychologist; therefore the aim of this chapter is to introduce you to CBT as another applied approach in the toolkit you would have as a counselling psychologist.

Introduction

The British Association for Behavioural and Cognitive Psychotherapies (BABCP) was established in 1972 giving accredited and professional status to therapists practising CBT. Moreover, all training programmes in counselling psychology, accredited by the HCPC and the BPS, include teaching and practice of CBT within their curriculum, so that all BPS Chartered and HCPC Registered counselling psychologists can have a working knowledge of CBT. CBT has gained a lot of ground in the last fifteen years and has inadvertently become a known commodity in today's society. The fact that CBT is structured, with concrete concepts, has enabled it to be an approach that is measurable, using widely accessible scales. CBT has gained an evidence-based status amongst psychological therapies as a result of the volume of research conducted into its effectiveness. Due to this status, as well as its fairly rapid symptom reduction, CBT arguably appears as more financially viable than many other therapeutic approaches. Thus, CBT finds itself strongly founded within all sectors of mental health provision and has contributed to the formation of new systems of therapeutic provision, such as the Improved Access to Psychological Therapies (IAPT) services founded in 2007. Therefore, a working knowledge of CBT potentially increases one's employability in the current climate.

So far in this book, and in particular in the present section, you have read about two seemingly different approaches in therapeutic care; the essence of the difference is not only in how the person is viewed, but also how healing is expected to occur. CBT is not completely dissimilar to what you have read so far, but has a more logical and structured way of considering the individual and the path to positive change. 'Change' is a keyword in CBT, because through the therapy the aim is to alter one's way of thinking and behaviour. Change is discussed and practiced within CBT on several occurrences, at different levels and on various fronts until the new and positive thoughts and behaviours have been established. In CBT, words that represent polar opposites are often used: dysfunctional/negative thinking to positive thinking; unhelpful behaviours to helpful behaviours; negative vicious cycle to positive cycle of change and so on. In CBT the person seeking support needs to be an active participant in the process and must be motivated towards engaging in behaviours that will facilitate change. CBT involves doing homework in between sessions and actively pushing oneself to challenges that will promote change. CBT theorists consider it a very collaborative approach, because of the active involvement of the client in the improvement of well-being. Let us however take matters from the beginning and start with the origins of cognitive-behavioural theory so that its development into a therapeutic approach and practice can be better understood.

Cognitive-behavioural theory

In cognitive-behavioural theory it is argued that the cognitive developed as a response to the behavioural component. As you will have probably learnt in your degree so far, Skinner in the 1950s and 1960s was the pioneer of behavioural theory (considered the first wave of behavioural theory).The behavioural theory developed by Eysenck (1960) first discussed the notion that individuals learn certain conditions to live by and consequently develop the relevant behaviours and begin behaving in a certain way. For instance, a child can learn that his parent/carer shouts at him when he does not get a good grade of B or above at school. Therefore, according to the behavioural theory, a child would learn to be studious in order to avoid getting shouted at; i.e. learn this behaviour in order to maintain a positive emotional state. Such a theory nonetheless, was considered as lacking the cognitive element, of explaining why for instance a child experiencing similar parental responses might become a high academic achiever, whereas another one might become a low achiever.

Cognitive-behavioural theory (the second wave) was developed due to dissatisfaction with behavioural theory not being able to explain and account for mental processes such as thoughts, beliefs, interpretations, imagery and so on, which play an important role in the development and maintenance of behaviours (Beck, 2011). The forerunners of adding the 'cognitive' element to the behavioural were Aaron Beck (1976), a psychoanalyst, and Albert Ellis (1962). According to Beck, Rush, Shaw and Emery (1979), CBT is a type of psychological therapy in which the goal is to resolve psychological distress by altering dysfunctional cognitions, emotions and behaviours through a procedure that is systematic, goal-oriented and focused in the present. While underpinned by theories, which were rather different, these traditions were integrated on the common ground of alleviating symptoms of psychological distress (Beck, 2011). It was advocated that most emotional problems arise from errors in thinking and that therefore the change can occur when there is change both in thinking and behaviour. Consequently, in the above given example regarding being studious, cognitive theory would suggest that the beliefs of the child about himself and the interpretations of his environment would affect how he'd behave. For instance, if the child believes: 'I am capable and my parents only want the best for me and that is why they are strict' s/he is likely to study harder. If the child

TABLE 7.1 Cognitive principle versus behavioural principle

The Cognitive Principle	*The Behavioural Principle*
• People's emotional reactions and behaviours are strongly influenced by *cognition* (thoughts, images, beliefs, interpretations). • People act differently to similar events; i.e. the *meaning* they give to the event, themselves or others can differ from person to person.	• What we *do* is important in understanding how emotional states are maintained and can change.

however believes 'I am going to fail anyway and no matter what I do my parents will not be happy', s/he is likely to give up trying in her/his schoolwork.

In Table 7.1 you can see the two separate principles of the cognitive and the behavioural, which are then combined in cognitive-behavioural theory.

ACTIVITY BOX 7.1

(Allow 5–10 minutes)

1. Write down an event. It does not have to be a negative event necessarily, or something big, maybe even an interaction you had with someone. What happened and what were your thoughts? Your feelings?
2. What did you do (behaviour) in response to how you thought and felt?
3. Did others give the same meaning to this event when you discussed it with them?
4. Observe how easy or not it is to recognise such processes (thoughts, feelings, behaviours) within you.

Aaron Beck (1976) amalgamated the cognitive and behavioural. He constructed the backbone of CBT, in terms of the terminology and interventions used in therapeutic practice.

The theory and practice of cognitive-behavioural therapy

Beck (1976) advocated that while growing up, people form certain beliefs about themselves, others and the world based on the behaviours and thoughts of significant others in their environments. These were termed as the **core beliefs** or schemas of the individual and relate to her/him, others and/or the world. For instance 'I am unlovable'; 'I am worthless'; ' I am dull'. The core beliefs lead the person to make rules and assumptions of everyday living (Beck, 2011). Such rules can be 'Unless I do perfectly everyone will think I am useless', 'If I do not please others no one will like me'. Such rules and assumptions create negative thoughts about oneself and others in the situation at hand; they are called **negative automatic thoughts**, (NATs), because they have become automatic since the person lives by the rules and assumptions emanating from the core beliefs (Greenberger and Padesky, 2015). Such thoughts can be 'People are staring because I am ugly'; 'People laugh at me because I stutter'. The NATs can be triggered by various stimuli (triggers) that are particular to the situation, for example someone looking at the person. The NATs create feelings of anxiety and low mood and lead to behaviours the person perceives as helping her/him to cope (maladaptive coping mechanisms) (Beck, 2011). Therefore, for example a belief of 'I am not good enough', in a situation where the person has been asked to give a presentation at school may lead to the NATs of 'everyone will think I am talking rubbish, everyone will laugh at me', which can lead to feelings of increased anxiety. Such feelings can lead the person to finding an excuse not to appear at the presentation so that the fear (ridicule, negative impression on others) does not happen. The fact that the person resorts to this behaviour has the effect of relieving him of the anxiety in relation to the anticipated event (the presentation). Nonetheless, the core belief of 'I am not good enough' does not change and hence the NATs in relation to the event do not shift.

According to CBT, the catalyst in change is the challenging of the NATs, which can then have an effect in changing one's behaviour and eventually shifting the core belief(s) of the individual (Beck, 1976; Beck et al., 1979; Greenberger and Padesky, 2015). Once the NATs have been identified in everyday examples of the person's life, links can be made between their thoughts, emotions and behaviours; hence recognition comes that change can happen by changing aspects of these interlinked systems, which have been interfering with their life and goals (Beck, 2011).

As long as there is no challenging of the established pattern of unhelpful thoughts and behaviours, one feeds into the other, into the vicious cycle of maladaptive thinking and behaviour (see Figure 7.1).

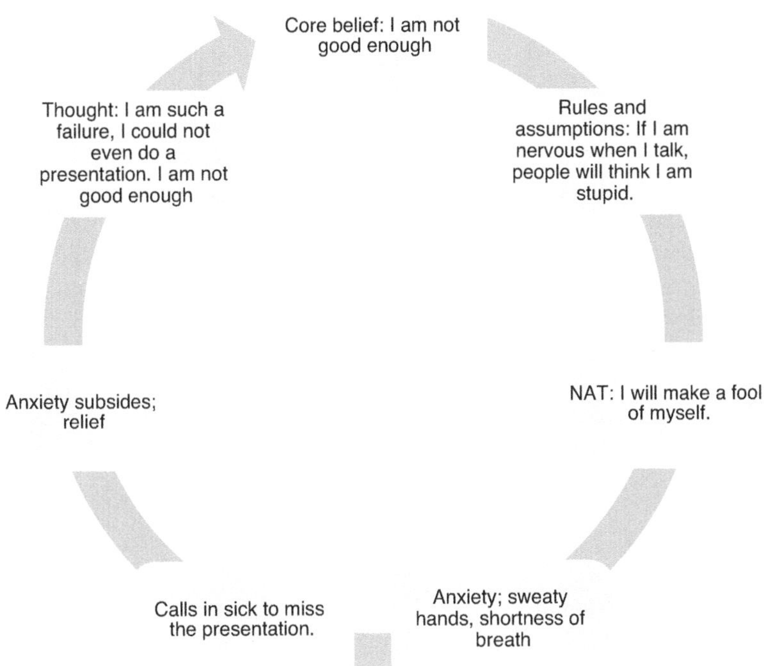

FIGURE 7.1 Vicious cycle in cognitive-behavioural therapy based on an individual being asked to give a presentation

TABLE 7.2 Examples of cognitive distortions

Cognitive Distortion	*Example*
Black-and-white thinking	*Everyone else gets it right; I never do anything worthy.* It is all or nothing, without a grey area in between.
Mind reading	*Everyone else must think I am boring.* Concluding that one knows what others are thinking or feeling.
Crystal ball gazing	It will not work, there is no point in trying. Making negative predictions about the future.
Overgeneralising/Catastrophising	*I will never get another job; I will probably lose my house and end up in the street.* Seeing one negative event as an indication of everything being negative.

According to Beck's model of CBT (1976), the core beliefs and the NATs represent different levels of cognition along a continuum (Westbrook et al., 2007 cited in Beck, 2011), from more specific and accessible to general and not as accessible. Along this continuum are the core beliefs and the cognitive distortions and the NATs. The cognitive distortions refer to the fact that the person can have distorted thinking about reality and the rules and assumptions are affected by the cognitive distortions. You can see examples of such distortions in Table 7.2.

Even though the core beliefs are harder to access, the cognitive distortions and NATs are fairly easily identified. The NATs are the first to be tackled in CBT because the effect that they have on one's emotional state is tangible. For instance going from 'I am useless', which is general, to 'Unless I do everything perfectly people will see I am useless' (rule and assumption), to 'My manager thinks all my work is rubbish', which is the NAT with the cognitive distortion, relevant to a particular situation. In a typical CBT session early on in therapy, the therapist and the client would discuss many instances of NATs and associated feelings and would then develop a formulation. The formulation is in itself a therapeutic intervention, and it is designed with the client, in the session. It is the tool to help the client and the therapist to understand where and when the problem originated, how its status has changed over time and what it is like at present and the factors that maintain it (Greenberger and Padesky, 2015). A formulation model in CBT (see Figure 7.2) is designed in a pictorial way so that the client and therapist can view it and add/amend information on it together.

ACTIVITY BOX 7.2

In pairs (Allow 15–20 minutes).

The theory of CBT will be put into practice in the following case example.

Take a few minutes to read it and locate how the information fits into the formulation model in Figure 7.2. Do you see any other information that could go in the formulation?

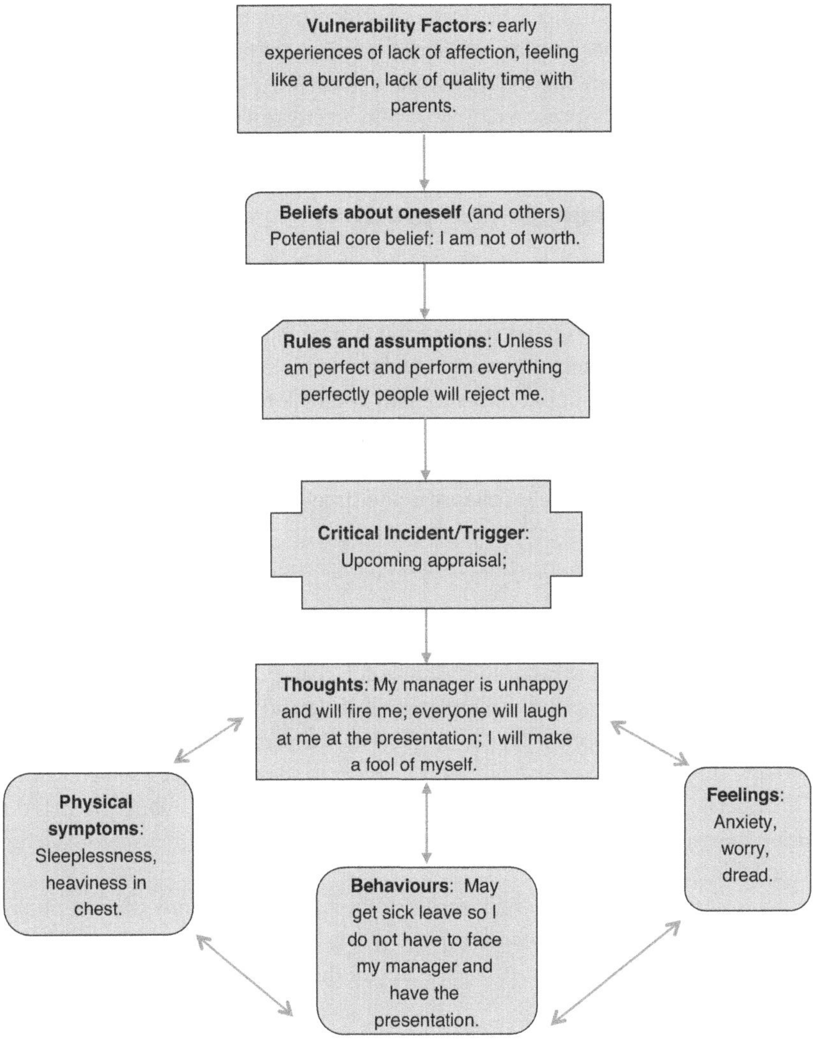

FIGURE 7.2 Formulation (Beckian model)
Jennifer's case formulation

Case example 1 – Jennifer

Jennifer (a pseudonym) has come to therapy because she is feeling really anxious. She thinks her manager does not like her, she catches him staring at her. She feels like her work is never good enough. She has her appraisal meeting soon and she is worried that he will fire her. Her anxiety has been intensified because she has to do a presentation in front of the whole department in a few weeks. Jennifer gets very nervous speaking in public. She worries that people will start sniggering as soon as she starts to talk. She cannot sleep very well and she is considering going to the GP to be signed off on long-term sick leave due to stress.

Jennifer also tells you that her parents had her when they were very young and would not pay much attention to her. She does not remember her parents being affectionate towards her and often her parents would argue in front of her about whose responsibility it was to look after her. She always felt like a burden.

Now read the following case example and try to create a case formulation, fitting the information for client Rameek, using the model in Figure 7.2.

Case example 2 – Rameek (self-practice)

Rameek (a pseudonym) really struggles to get out of the house and particularly to be in places with many people. Whenever he leaves the house, he starts getting sweaty hands and shortness of breath. His heart starts racing and he thinks he will have a heart attack. He thinks everyone is staring at him and laughing at him. Rameek just runs back home. His neighbour does big shopping trips for him and he feels very embarrassed about his inability to get out and worries his neighbour thinks he is just lazy. Yesterday he decided to push himself and take the bus to the big supermarket, but he was feeling so sick after getting out that he thought he'd collapse in the street and ran back home. Rameek feels useless and angry with himself.

The Thought Record Sheet is another vehicle for change, which is used to elicit NATs at the initial stages but also throughout the therapy, during and in-between the sessions. It is an essential part of the homework aspect of CBT. The Thought Record exists in a few forms, such as a basic three-column one (first three) in order to identify NATs, which can be useful in the initial session of therapy when an assessment of the client is taking place and there is formulation designed. The seven-column thought record however, goes into challenging the NATs (see Table 7.3).

The therapist usually asks the client to fill in the first few columns or even more if possible; then with the method of Socratic questioning as developed by Dennis Greenberger and Christine Padesky the therapist tries to access the client's core beliefs and furthermore

TABLE 7.3 Seven-column thought record using case example 1 – Jennifer

Situation	*Emotion % of intensity*	*NAT*	*Evidence supporting the NAT*	*Evidence contradicting/ not supporting the NAT*	*Alternative thought*	*Emotion or feeling and % of intensity*
At my desk, manager staring at me.	Anxiety 70%	He thinks I am rubbish at work and will fire me.	He commended my colleagues' work yesterday except mine.	Heard him telling the Head of Department how capable I am.	Just because he praised the others on one job, this does not mean he is unhappy with my work.	Anxiety 40%

to challenge the NATs, cognitive distortions and maladaptive behaviours by asking the client to find 'evidence' that contradict all of the above. Christine Padesky (1993),[1] defined Socratic questioning as a guided discovery. The term is rooted in the method of questioning used by the ancient Greek philosopher Socrates, in an effort to teach his disciples to reach conclusions using only arguments based on logical thinking. Socratic questioning is relevant to the philosophical underpinnings of cognitive-behavioural theory, which can be traced back to the philosophers of ancient Greece and to the movement of stoicism (Beck et al., 1979) that postulated that errors in judgement caused destructive emotions, and that a sage or an individual of "moral and intellectual perfection," was not to suffer these emotions. Padesky argues that Socratic Questioning involves:

> a) asking the client questions that he can answer; b) draw the attention of the client to information which is relevant to the issue being discussed but which may be outside of the client's current focus; c) generally move from the concrete to the more abstract so that d) the client can, in the end, apply the new information to either re-evaluate the previous conclusion or construct a new idea.
>
> *(Padesky, 1993, p. 4)*

In relation to point b in particular, Padesky clarifies that such information might be about the client's history or past. For example, in Jennifer's case above presented in the thought record sheet:

> Questioning what other thoughts were coming to her mind when her manager was staring at her might elicit answers such as her manager staring at her makes her feel worthless (NAT, Column 3).

This would be followed by a question asking whether she had experienced this with anyone else. The accessing of these worries might lead to a connection about the lack of affection and attention from her parents which she experienced as a child.

The therapist could then ask for exceptions to those experiences, when Jennifer would have felt loved by or valued by people around her.

Such information would then potentially guide Jennifer to re-evaluating the previous conclusions of never feeling appreciated, which could allow her to find evidence against the NAT and elicit an alternative thought.

The fact that she came up with an alternative thought herself and that this had an effect in decreasing her self-reported anxiety could eventually steer Jennifer towards avoiding the maladaptive coping mechanism of calling in sick and missing her appraisal meeting and presentation.

If then Jennifer succeeded in controlling her anxiety and cognitive distortions and conducted her meeting and/or presented to the department, she would have evidence that she is not worthless/useless.

This evidence would then be 'added in her toolkit of evidence' against further NATs, which would bring a further improvement in her mood and decrease her anxiety.

Greenberg and Padesky (2015), as well as Beck and other prominent CBT therapists and developers, such as Clark (2011) and Salkovkis (2002), emphasise that in CBT, as in person-centred therapy, there is a need for empathic listening and frequent summarising of what has been concluded so far. The point of the exploration in CBT is not to prove the client wrong but to be curious about the meaning they attribute to their experience.

Once the client is engaged with the cognitive aspects of her/his symptoms, the behavioural interventions can come into place. Such an intervention is behavioural activation; the therapist and the client agree together to activities the client can do in order to help her/him feel more positive and build up confidence. This activities need to be defined as pleasurable and/or meaningful by the client. For instance, one client may find pleasure in going for a walk, whereas another person may find pleasure in volunteering at a local charity. The importance is to keep revisiting the activities, evaluating them and building upon them to keep on challenging the NATs and core belief(s). Another intervention, useful when the maladaptive behaviour leads to complete avoidance of the anxiety-provoking situation, is behavioural experiments which permit exposure to the fearful stimulus. This exposure is gradual and controlled and in constant collaboration between client and therapist. The gradual exposure is referred to as 'experiments' because the exposure activities will be a 'testing' of the NATs. For instance, for an agoraphobic client, the gradual exposure would aim towards the client being able to go out to a busy place by himself.

ACTIVITY BOX 7.3

In pairs (Allow10 minutes per person.)

So far in this part of the chapter you have learned the key terms used in CBT and the main interventions. Explain to your peer, in your own words, the following terms, giving an example from one of the cases given above (Jennifer or Rameek) or using an example from your own experiences.

- Core Beliefs
- Rules and Assumptions of everyday life
- Cognitive Distortions: give examples of at least two types
- Negative Automatic Thoughts
- Socratic Questioning
- Thought Records: Try practicing doing one. How did you find it?
- Behavioural Activation
- Behavioural Experiments: Can you think of one?

CBT practice can be modified and applied to a wide variety of symptoms; its core is the identifying of a dysfunctional belief system, which leads to distorted thinking and maladaptive behaviours. Therefore, all symptoms are theorised and explained within this spectrum (Beck, 2011; Greenberger and Padesky, 2015). For instance, with panic disorder the person has panic attacks in response to her/his anxiety and thus, in order to avoid having panic attacks avoids stimuli associated with panic attacks (speaking in public, busy spaces etc.). In obsessive-compulsive disorder, the person engages in obsessive and compulsive thoughts and behaviours in an effort to control anxiety. In depression, the person is likely to believe s/he is unworthy and thus avoids doing anything that s/he perceives as a circumstance for further failure. The formulation and explanation of how the core belief(s) lead to NATs and maladaptive behaviour is in essence the same across many symptoms and diagnoses identified. However, in current applied CBT a therapist can find 'protocols of practice' which are diagnosis-specific, using the relevant language and behavioural techniques (Clark, 2011).

In the following section CBT will be discussed as an evidence-based therapy, within the contemporary field of mental health and counselling psychology practice.

CBT as evidenced-based: application and ethical considerations

One of the great strengths of cognitive-behavioural therapy has always been its practitioners' eagerness to strongly associate themselves with a scientific paradigm of psychological and psychopathological process (Athanasiadou-Lewis, 2014). Salkovkis (2002), as a leading CBT advocate, has pointed out that evidence-based therapies (EBTs) evolve partly because of the good linkage between theory, research studies and outcome research. Indeed, CBT has become so embedded in psychological science that Gilbert and Leahy (cited in Athanasiadou-Lewis, 2014) argue that it is basically evidence-based psychological therapy. Arguably, the pinnacle of this development is the fact that CBT is the most common therapeutic approach used within the NHS and in IAPT services. The National Institute for Clinical Excellence guidelines (NICE, 2009, 2011, 2013) include CBT amongst the preferable therapeutic approaches for the treatment of anxiety and depression. CBT is currently used widely for the treatment of anxiety disorders, depression, addictions, eating disorders, phobias and obsessive-compulsive disorders (Clark, 2011). Recent research suggests that CBT is most applicable to work in multicultural settings. It is argued that the collaborative and psycho-educational nature of CBT makes it more widely acceptable among different cultures. The NICE (2009, 2011, 2013) recommends individual-CBT as a treatment for all ethnic minority groups. In particular, in relation to British Ethnic Minority (BME) men, since CBT interventions are problem-focused and directive (Beck, 2011), men seem to find such interventions suitable. According to Mahalik (2001), BME men are more likely to avoid or to terminate therapy as the work starts to focus on their feelings. Moreover, Berger (2010) argues that CBT techniques can promote self-empowerment because they enhance the clients' ability to examine coping strategies.

CBT claims to be a therapeutic approach that is continuously evidence-based and ever developing. Its application acts as both a foundation and a platform for evolution. IAPT and other services produce research advocating that CBT works. Self-reporting measurements such as the Patient Health Questionnaire-9, the CORE-OM, and the Generalised Anxiety Disorder-7 amongst others, are routinely used to measure any shift in the client's mood and/or anxiety in response to the CBT received; thus they inadvertently measure the effectiveness of CBT. The wealth of research in the field show that clients observe improvements in their anhedonia and anxiety and a reduction in maladaptive behaviours fairly quickly. The general length of a course of CBT is between a minimum of six weeks to a maximum of twenty, for more chronic and complex symptoms (Beck, 2011).

The criticisms of CBT and its effectiveness have been numerous, however. One of the main arguments against its stronghold in psychological care is the fact that, although other psychological therapies (e.g. person-centred, existential and psychodynamic approaches) do not have as wide an evidence base, their value should not be undermined. In particular, in person-centred and existential psychotherapy, the person's concerns, worries and perceived inabilities are not considered as 'symptoms'. Consequently, the shift towards a better state of being may not be palpable in a similar way to how it is in CBT. Psychodynamic approaches have been trying recently to establish and strengthen their position in the therapy field, utilising evidence-based research on par with CBT (Athanasiadou-Lewis, 2014). A recent meta-analysis conducted by Fonagy, Roth and Higgitt (2005), and two reviews of psychodynamic psychotherapy (Leichsenring, Rabung and Leibing, 2004; Leichsenring and Leibing, 2007), presented twenty-four methodologically sufficient randomised controlled trials of psychodynamic psychotherapy for a range of psychiatric disorders. Both reviews yielded substantial evidence for the efficacy of brief psychodynamic treatments.

A further concern, relating to ethical considerations, is that because CBT is structured around collaboration, it may implicitly promote the coercion of clients to respond to the therapist in a way that indicates improvement, because they want to please the therapist and/or be liked by her/him. There is concern that even though CBT promotes itself as a therapeutic approach encouraging equality, it can actually set a relationship, which is perceived as didactic by the client and within which the client may feel the pressure to succeed. The genuineness of the effectiveness of CBT can hence be hard to measure because, as has been observed, clients can quickly become quite adept in answering in a mode that they believe will show them as achieving well (Gilmour, 2016). The sense of achievement and 'need to do well' appears as an alarm in relation to the reliability (not in statistical terms) of the tools used for measurement of improvement, such as the scales mentioned earlier. It has been noted that clients can fairly quickly become proficient in completing the scales, understanding how they need to answer in order to show improvement (or not). As an effect, the phenomenon of discrepancy between how the client presents in the session and what her/his self-report measures indicate is commonly notable.

Recent research has shown that the potential incongruence observed in CBT has a negative effect on the experience of CBT both in practitioners and in clients. Athanasiadou-Lewis (2014), in a study on the experiences of clinical and counselling psychologists working within IAPT services utilising CBT, found that one of the negative aspects of the therapists' experience was the continuous measurement of the clients' improvement. The measurements were perceived as (a) interfering with the therapeutic relationship and (b) as pressurising on the therapists, since they appeared to indicate the quality of the therapists' work. In light of the fact that IAPT services need to meet client contact and discharge targets in order to gain further funding, the therapists in the study argued that a lot rests on CBT appearing as an EBT because it has become a political tool. In relation to the clients' experience, it is worth noting that in numerous qualitative studies on the experience of CBT for enduring psychological problems, the clients seem to always identify the therapeutic relationship as the vehicle for change rather than specific CBT tools (Gilmour, 2016; Weston, 2016; Virdee, 2014). Within the counselling psychology practising framework, it is advocated that CBT should be practiced with some flexibility so that the practising counselling psychologist can adapt the therapeutic work and interventions to the personality and needs of the client; there is a strong relational value placed on the therapy as opposed to a strict adherence to a treatment protocol.

Irrelevantly of the critical and ethical considerations, however, the continuous research in the field of CBT and the debate it has elicited has sparked research in the field of psychological therapy; further ideas have been, and are, being developed. The following section will outline some of these more recent therapeutic approaches that loosely fall under the term of 'third-wave behavioural therapy'.

Third-wave behavioural therapy approaches

In the last fifteen to twenty years, especially with the introduction of positive psychology as a discipline in psychological science and practice (Seligman and Csikszentmihalyi, 2000), a shift has been noted within the wider circles of CBT. 'CBT subsidiaries' are becoming strength-focused, acknowledging resilience and growth as dynamic processes, and encouraging personal awareness and reflection. There are quite a few therapeutic approaches that fall under the third-wave CBT umbrella. In this chapter, three will be outlined.

1. Positive Psychotherapy (PP)

PP devised by Seligman, Rashid and Parks (2006) is structured along the same principles as CBT, in the sense that it is believed that dysfunctional thinking can lead to maladaptive cognitions and behaviours. However, in PP the focus becomes the positives in one's life and the strengths that a person has. Similarly to Rogers' concept of self-actualisation (1957), positive psychology advocates that all people have the potential for growth. Peterson and Seligman (2004), through devising the Character Strengths and Virtues Inventory Scale, identified that individuals possess numerous strengths and virtues. If these are tapped, then the person can lead a fulfilling life. PP employs interventions such as 'writing three good things that happened today' and 'the gratitude letter' as a way of assisting individuals in focusing on what is possible and good in one's life. PP strives to first of all maintain the positive(s) and then, improve upon it. Rashid indicates what the main philosophy of PP is: "By default, we remember and retrieve negative experiences and emotions more easily than the positives ones. Positive interventions essentially are re-education of attention and memory. The function of psychotherapy . . . is also to restore and nurture courage, kindness, modesty, perseverance, and emotional and social intelligence" (Rashid, 2009, p. 463). PP is still in its early days and research so far has been criticised as not being applicable to individuals with more enduring concerns (Loulopoulou, 2010). Nonetheless, positive psychology and the possibilities for clinical application are continuously being developed and are likely to become further established.

2. Acceptance and Commitment Therapy (ACT)

ACT was devised by Hayes, Strosahl and Wilson (1999) and is considered a transdiagnostic approach, in that the focus is on using the same treatment principles and applying them across mental health difficulties (Watson et al., 2010). ACT aims to increase psychological well-being by increasing 'psychological flexibility'. Psychological flexibility (Hayes, Luoma, Bond, Masuda and Lillis, 2006) is the ability to, on the one hand, be aware of personal experiences in the present moment and, on the other, respond to these without avoidance or struggling (Acceptance); furthermore it entails taking committed action towards directions to contribute to a rich and fulfilling life (Commitment). Acceptance is framed as the alternative to avoidance; by reducing the struggle in trying to avoid these experiences, individuals can more effectively use their energy into taking workable actions in line with the life they value. The commitment involves engaging in behaviours that lead individuals towards their values whilst being willing to experience any discomfort that may arise. ACT is utilised widely in group contexts, because the sharing and normalising qualities of the group context are particularly helpful in promoting self-acceptance (since acceptance is mirrored by a group) and commitment to change, since the commitment and the struggle is shared (Yalom,1995).

3. *Mindfulness-Based Cognitive Therapy (MBCT)*

MBCT was coined by Segal, Williams and Teasdale (2002) and it is another transdiagnostic approach, most often delivered in a group format. Mindfulness refers to intentionally and non-judgementally paying attention to the present moment. It was initially designed for people prone to recurring bouts of depression. It combines techniques like meditation and breathing exercises with cognitive interventions, aimed at breaking persistent negative thought patterns. MBCT teaches people to be present in the current moment and prevent rumination of negative events and thoughts that can perpetuate the depressive state. Moreover, by enabling people to have greater awareness of their own body, MBCT assists individuals in recognising earlier symptoms that can tip them over into depression. A recent study by Kim et al. (2009) compared the effectiveness of MBCT versus an anxiety education group for clients with anxiety. Clients in the MBCT group showed significant improvements in the anxiety measures. Additionally, two studies (Finucane and Mercer, 2006; Ree and Craigie, 2007), which explored the outcomes of MBCT in a heterogeneous group suffering from depression and/or anxiety, showed that MBCT was associated with significant reductions in both symptoms. Mindfulness is increasingly recognised as a tool for the maintenance of healthy mental equilibrium in individuals; because it draws from widely used and acceptable practices such as meditation and breathing exercises, it can further have the effect of de-pathologising people's symptoms.

So far in this chapter you have learnt about the origins of CBT, the main concepts of CBT and have been introduced to the skeleton of CBT interventions. Furthermore, CBT has been discussed within the current context of the mental health field, discussing potential limitations and ethical considerations. Finally, three contemporary therapeutic approaches were introduced, which, whilst maintaining certain cognitive and behavioural elements in their philosophy, appear to share a common feature: an emphasis on the elements that are good in one's life and their robust establishment in everyday living.

Conclusive thoughts

Already a counselling psychologist, I attended a symposium, named 'Life isn't Like That'[2] organised by Prof. Peter Fonagy on 17 November 2006 in London, UK. Therapists from different therapeutic approaches (CBT, systemic and psychodynamic) presented how they would work with given case examples. Each case was discussed within the three approaches. The therapists representing the various approaches became quite passionate supporting the effectiveness and pureness of their approach, which was surprising to me. During my training in counselling psychology (CoP) I had learnt to work within three different therapeutic approaches; and even though by the end I had a clear idea of which approach 'fitted me' more than another, I did not have any 'strong allegiance to a particular camp'. Fonagy, at the end of the symposium emphasised that the aim of therapists is not to compete on the effectiveness of therapeutic approaches, but to recognise how to best apply their therapeutic knowledge in order to support their client as well as possible. Even though my psychological thinking and practice have developed further since then, his words have stayed within me, because to me, they express the archetype of CoP: the client is put at the centre; and the approach is adapted along with the interaction in the therapy room. In CoP, it is not the CBT interventions that shape the client, but the clients' needs and personality that mould the interventions.

ACTIVITY BOX 7.4

In pairs discuss the following, taking turns. (Allow 20 minutes.)

- Explain, in your own words, CBT theory and how it works.
- Offer a challenge in relation to CBT's claim of being evidence-based practice, as opposed to the therapeutic approaches you have studied so far.
- Explain what you understand the main difference between traditional CBT and the third-wave approaches presented in this chapter to be.
- Discuss how you think CBT fits within counselling psychology philosophy and ethos and consider how key concepts of the other therapeutic approaches presented in this book are represented in the theory and practice of CBT.

These are points you can revisit again and again whilst going through this book and you may find that your perception and opinions change over time, as you learn about counselling psychology.

Learning outcomes

When you have completed this chapter, you should be able to:

- Describe the basic theory behind the CBT approach.
- Devise a CBT formulation.
- Have an understanding of the main therapeutic interventions.
- Have some familiarity with contemporary approaches that have evolved from CBT.

Key concepts

- Core Beliefs
- Negative Automatic Thoughts
- Socratic Questioning

Sample essay titles

1. 'Triggers', 'Rules and Assumptions', 'Core Beliefs' and 'Negative Automatic Thoughts', ' Cognitive Distortions' and 'Maladaptive-Behaviours'. Describe what each of these concepts mean within the theory of cognitive-behavioural therapy and discuss how they fit in with each other.
2. What is the purpose of the Thought Record Sheet in Cognitive-Behavioural Therapy? Discuss in particular its role in the formulation process and during the therapeutic work.
3. How is knowledge relevant to the client's issue(s) elicited in Cognitive-Behavioural Therapy? Discuss the relevant techniques and interventions, giving examples as well, if possible.

4. 'Cognitive-Behavioural Therapy is considered an evidence-based practice and is recommended by the NICE guidelines as the therapy of preference for the treatment of anxiety and depression'. Discuss your understanding of this statement and the implications in the provision of psychological care.
5. Describe one third-wave CBT approach and discuss it in relation to the traditional CBT approach.

Further reading

Hawton, K., Salkovskis, P. M., Kirk, J., & Clark, D. M. (Eds.). (1998). *Cognitive behaviour therapy for psychiatric problems: A practical guide.* Oxford: Oxford University Press.
Simmons, J., & Griffiths, R. (2009). *CBT for beginners.* Los Angeles: Sage.

Websites

All the websites below can provide you with useful information and resources to practice CBT (e.g. formulations, Thought Records)
http://psychology.tools
www.getselfhelp.co.uk
www.padesky.com and www.mindovermood.com

Notes

1 Padesky, C. (1993). Keynote Speech at the European Congress for Behavioural and Cognitive Therapies. Retrieved from http://padesky.com/newpad/wp-content/uploads/2012/11/socquest.pdf.
2 "Life isn't like that: the challenge of complex clinical work to our models of psychological therapy". The Tavistock and Portman NHS Trust, 17 November 2006, London, UK.

References

Athanasiadou-Lewis, C. (2014). Exploring the experience of protocol driven practice in counselling psychology through critical theory, reflective practice and doctoral research. Unpublished PsychD Thesis, City University, London.
Beck, A. T. (1976). *Cognitive therapy and the emotional disorders.* New York: Meridian.
Beck, A. T., Rush, A. J., Shaw, B. F., & Emery, G. (1979). *Cognitive therapy of depression.* New York: The Guilford Press.
Beck, J. S. (2011). *Cognitive behavior therapy: Basics and beyond.* New York: The Guilford Press.
Berger, R. (2010). Increasing clinical and contextual awareness when working with new fathers. In C. Z. Oren & D. C. Oren (Eds.), *Counselling fathers* (pp. 187–206). New York: Routledge Taylor & Francis.
Clark, D. (2011). Implementing NICE guidelines for the psychological treatment of depression and anxiety disorders: The IAPT experience. *International Review of Psychiatry*, 23, 375–384.
Ellis, A. (1962). *Reason and emotion in psychotherapy.* New York: Lyle Stuart.
Eysenck, H. (1960). *Behavior therapy and the neuroses.* Oxford: Pergamon Press.
Finucane, A., & Mercer, S. (2006). An exploratory mixed methods study of the acceptability and effectiveness of mindfulness-based cognitive therapy for patients with active depression and anxiety in primary care. *Biomed Central Psychiatry*, 6, 1–14. doi:10.1186/1471-244X-6-14
Fonagy, P., Roth, A., & Higgitt, A. (2005). The outcome of psychodynamic therapy for psychological disorders. *Clinical Neuroscience Research*, 4, 367–377.

Gilmour, A. (2016). Counselling psychology trainees' experiences of working with adult survivors of childhood sexual abuse: An Interpretative Phenomenological Analysis. Unpublished thesis, Professional Doctorate in counselling psychology, Metropolitan University, London.

Greenberger, D., & Padesky, C. (2015). *Mind over mood: Change how you feel by changing the way you think* (2nd ed.). New York: Guilford Press.

Hayes, S., Luoma, J., Bond, F., Masuda, A., & Lillis, J. (2006). Acceptance and commitment therapy: Model, processes and outcomes. *Behaviour Research and Therapy*, 44, 1–25. doi:10.1016/j.brat.2005.06.006

Hayes, S., Strosahl, K., & Wilson, K. (1999). *Acceptance and commitment therapy: An experiential approach to behavior change*. New York: The Guilford Press.

Kim, Y., Lee, S., Choi, T., Kim, B., Kim, C., & Yook, K. (2009). Effectiveness of mindfulness-based cognitive therapy as an adjuvant to pharmacotherapy in patients with panic disorder or generalized anxiety disorder. *Depression and Anxiety*, 26, 601–606.

Leichsenring, F., & Leibing, E. (2007). Psychodynamic psychotherapy: A systematic review of techniques, indications and empirical evidence. *Psychology and Psychotherapy: Theory, Research and Practice*, 80, 217–228.

Leichsenring, F., Rabung, S., & Leibing, E. (2004). The efficacy of short-term psychodynamic psychotherapy in specific psychiatric disorders: A meta-analysis. *Archives of General Psychiatry*, 61, (12), 1208–1216.

Loulopoulou, A. I. (2010). Positive psychology and the refugee experience: Shifting perceptions and attitudes towards refugees. Unpublished Ph.D. thesis, Essex University, Colchester, UK.

Mahalik, J. R. (2001). Cognitive therapy for men. In G. R. Brooks & G. E. Good (Eds.), *The new handbook of psychotherapy and counselling with men: A comprehensive guide to settings, problems, treatment approaches* (Vol 2, pp. 544–564). San Francisco: Jossey-Bass.

National Institute for Health & Clinical Excellence (NICE) (2009). *Depression: The treatment and management of depression in adults (update)*. London: National Institute for Health and Clinical Excellence.

National Institute for Health & Clinical Excellence (NICE) (2011). *Generalised anxiety disorder and panic disorder (with or without agoraphobia) in adults: Management in primary, secondary and community care*. London: National Institute for Health and Clinical Excellence.

National Institute for Health & Clinical Excellence (NICE) (2013). *Social anxiety: Recognition, assessment and treatment*. London: National Institute for Health and Clinical Excellence.

Padesky, C. (1993). Keynote Speech at the European Conference for Behaviuoural and Cognitive Therapies. Retrieved from http://padesky.com/newpad/wp-content/uploads/2012/11/socquest.pdf

Peterson, C., & Seligman, M. (2004). *Character strengths and virtues: A handbook and classification*. New York: Oxford University Press.

Rashid, T. (2009). Positive interventions in clinical practice. *Journal of Clinical Psychology*, 65, (5), 461–466.

Ree, M., & Craigie, M. (2007). Outcomes following mindfulness-based cognitive therapy in a heterogeneous sample of adult outpatients. *Behavior Change*, 24, 70–86.

Rogers, C. R. (1957). The necessary and sufficient conditions of therapeutic personality change. *Journal of Consulting Psychology*, 21, 95–103.

Salkovkis, P. M. (2002). Empirically grounded clinical interventions: Cognitive-behavioural therapy progresses through a multi-dimensional approach to clinical science. *Behavioural and Cognitive Psychotherapy*, 30, (1), 3–9. doi:http://dx.doi.org/10.1017/S1352465802001029

Segal, Z., Williams, J., & Teasdale, J. (2002). *Mindfulness-based cognitive therapy for depression: A new approach to preventing relapse*. New York: Guilford Press.

Seligman, M. E. P., & Csikszentmihalyi, M. (2000). Positive psychology: An introduction. *American Psychologist*, 55, 5–14.

Seligman, M. E. P., Rashid, T., & Parks, A. C. (2006). Positive psychotherapy. *American Psychologist*, 61, 774–788.

Virdee, S. (2014). It was quite helpful: An interpretative phenomenological analysis of Indian fathers' experience of family therapy. Unpublished thesis, Professional doctorate in counselling psychology, Metropolitan University, London.

Watson, H., McEvoy, P., Smith, L., Saulsman, L., Campbell, B., & Nathan, P. (2010). Affective disorders: Bridging the gap between efficacy and practice. In R. A. Carlstedt (Ed.), *Handbook of integrative clinical psychology, psychiatry, and behavioral medicine: Perspectives, practices, and research* (pp. 281–308). New York: Springer.

Weston, H. E. (2016). How do counselling psychologists make sense of their clients' psychiatric diagnoses: An IPA. Unpublished thesis, Professional doctorate in counselling psychology, Metropolitan University, London.

Yalom, I. (1995). *The theory and practice of group psychotherapy* (4th ed.). New York: Basic Books.

8

PSYCHODYNAMIC APPROACHES

Stelios Gkouskos

Chapter overview

The aim of this chapter is to provide you with a conceptual map that can serve as a starting point for becoming more familiar with psychodynamic approaches and understand how these approaches can inform the therapeutic practice of counselling psychologists. I will begin by pointing out that psychoanalysis has diversified and proliferated widely since its inception by Freud and that the term 'psychodynamic' is currently used to encompass the different schools of psychoanalytic thought. I will then offer a rudimentary synopsis of Freud's psychoanalytic model, since this is the reference point for all psychodynamic approaches and his theories dominated psychoanalysis for its first half-century. This synopsis will then serve as the basis for suggesting guidelines, along with a learning activity, that can help you navigate through some of the important ways that psychodynamic approaches have evolved and diversified since Freud. Next, I will focus on relational psychoanalysis, one of the contemporary developments in this field, since I consider it to be a good fit with the values and principles of counselling psychology and I will use a clinical example from my own practice to demonstrate how this theory can assist counselling psychologists in their therapeutic work with people who suffer from psychological distress. Moreover, since within counselling psychology we adopt the scientist-practitioner model and believe in the value of evidence-based practice, I will conclude the chapter by discussing research evidence that offers support to the tenets of relational psychoanalysis and the effectiveness of psychodynamic approaches.

'One nation, many tribes'

The expression 'One nation, many tribes', which has been used by Warner in an article where she discusses a number of diverse theoretical developments in person-centred psychotherapy (2000), could be applied equally aptly to psychoanalysis. Since its inception by Freud, psychoanalysis (both as a theoretical system and as a form of psychotherapeutic practice) has diversified and proliferated widely, as psychoanalysts have continuously tried to further develop, refine and sometimes change quite drastically Freud's original work in order to address unresolved theoretical questions and contradictions or clinical issues that had not been addressed by Freud himself. In fact, these changes have often generated great conflicts and disagreements amongst psychoanalysts, that have even led to expulsions from the psychoanalytic society, such as those of Jung, Rank, Adler and Ferenczi or to schisms such as those between proponents of Anna Freud and Melanie Klein and are documented in the 'Controversial Discussions' that took place between 1942 and 1944 in the British Psychoanalytical Society (Mitchell & Black, 1995). Regardless though of these debates and diversifications, all these 'tribes' of psychoanalytic thought share some common features (see Focus box 8.1) that unify them under the same 'nation' which has come to be represented by the umbrella term 'psychodynamic'.

FOCUS BOX 8.1

Some of the key common features of psychodynamic approaches

- The investigation and illumination of **unconscious** processes, since they are considered to play a determinant role in how we, humans, function; how we come to understand and interact with the world and others; as well as how we experience psychological distress.
- Psychological symptoms have meaning and can help us understand underlying psychological processes and what troubles us.
- We consciously and unconsciously use a number of **defence mechanisms** to help us keep out of our awareness unacceptable wishes, parts of ourselves, conflicts that, if they were to become conscious, would make us experience intense anxiety; these defences may be helpful or harmful.
- The central role of **transference** and **countertransference** in therapeutic work.
- The important role of early formative years in the development of personality and our ability to manage psychological distress in our adult lives and lead fulfilling lives.

The aforementioned diversification, the clashes and schisms within psychoanalysis make a fascinating read for those who are captivated by this framework. However, navigating through the world of psychodynamic approaches as a newcomer can prove to be quite a challenge for a number of reasons. First, as Mitchell and Black (1995) have noted, psychodynamic authors often use language which is dense, full of psychoanalytic 'jargon' and complex argumentation and, if one does not have a certain degree of familiarity with the nomenclature and an understanding of the meaning of basic concepts, it can be difficult to follow the presented arguments. Even when someone develops that understanding, the expansion of competing schools of thought can still make it difficult to comprehend what is being argued by different authors, since different psychodynamic theories may be based on very different philosophical premises and employ different languages, while at times the same concept may convey different meanings for different authors (Milton, Polmear, & Fabricius, 2004). Moreover, some theories may seem quite dated and for this reason difficult to grasp. For example, Freud's propositions about the pivotal role of sexual drive in the development of personality and its repression in the development of psychological distress can only be fully appreciated if they are examined within the scope of his era. That is, a historical period when sex was often associated with untreatable venereal diseases; while masturbation was considered to lead to, or be the result of, insanity (Decker, 1991) and often treated with painful restricting measures (e.g., wearing spiked metal rings on the penis at night) or even with mutilation (for a description of how sex was often associated with dread in Freud's era see Smith, 1999).

Evidently then, one important question for the newcomer to this field is: 'how can I navigate myself through the world of psychodynamic approaches?' This question though, cannot be addressed before one develops, at least, a basic understanding of Freud's theories. Hence, I will now attempt to provide a rudimentary synopsis of the basic propositions behind Freudian psychoanalysis.

Freudian psychoanalysis

Freud's intentions to establish and promote psychoanalysis not only as a clinical method but, primarily, as a well-respected scientific theory for the study of the mind led him to continuously evaluate, change and develop psychoanalysis throughout his lifetime. Each time that he identified incompatibilities between his clinical findings and his theoretical propositions he revised his theory. Essentially though, Freud offered us a physiological model of psychology. Giving primacy to our biology, he proposed that our sexual instincts (**Libido**) are the driving force for all our psychic life (i.e., mental life; our thoughts and feelings) and the main motivator behind our behaviour (Freud, 1905). More specifically, he proposed that as animals we are born with an intense need to gratify (**Pleasure Principle**) our innate sexual impulses (**Id**).[1] Quickly though we experience frustration of our needs due to constraints in external reality (**Reality Principle**) that leads to the emergence of a new structure of our personality (**Ego**). This is, according to Freud, the part of us that tries to mediate the demands between Id and external reality. Subsequently, we also learn that our instinctual wishes and needs may, at times, come in opposition to the rules and prohibitions of society, which we have grown to internalise in the form of our **Superego** (our conscience and sense of guilt). From that point on, the Ego has the difficult task of continuously mediating the needs and demands between the Id, the Superego and external reality (Freud, 1923). According to Freud, if we were conscious of these conflicts, we would experience intense and debilitating 'Angst' (feelings of anxiety) as well as guilt and shame. Thus, our Ego, in an effort to protect us, employs a number of psychological defences in order to keep these conflicts out of our awareness (i.e., in our unconscious). Nevertheless, psychological distress cannot be avoided as our defences cannot be effective in mitigating conflict all the time. It is at that point that we experience psychological distress in the form of different symptoms (e.g., depression, phobias, bulimia, etc.), which are the external expressions and symbolisations of our **intrapsychic** conflicts (i.e., conflicts that take place within our minds).

Following the above understanding about the origins and development of psychological distress, the aim of therapy in Freudian, also known as Classical or Orthodox, psychoanalysis is to help the patient become aware of these conflicts and their origins (i.e., making the unconscious conscious), work them through and come to a more satisfactory resolution. To accomplish this, the therapist needs to provide a therapeutic space that does not 'contaminate' the patient's psyche. This is primarily achieved by adopting the neutral stance of a detached observer who listens attentively to all aspects of the patient's narrative. By adopting such a style, the therapist also becomes a 'neutral screen' onto which the patient's conflictual wishes can be transferred. Change in therapy takes place primarily by the therapist interpreting the ways that the patient distorts his experience of the analyst by projecting onto the analyst wishes and experiences from the past (i.e., Transference Analysis), as well as interpreting the role of psychological defences and the meaning of psychological symptoms. By doing so, psychoanalysis patients are provided with insight about the meaning and origins of their intrapsychic conflicts and become aware of how these determine the ways they experience the world, relate to others and make choices in their lives. This then gives them the opportunity to find better ways of resolving these conflicts and not to be defined or limited by them.

In summary, Freud offered us a vision of an isolated mind consisting of different internal structures/agencies, derived from our efforts to gratify our instinctual needs and in constant conflict with each other (hence the term 'dynamic', which implies constant movement). In our everyday lives, these conflicts are beyond our awareness and control and motivate our behaviour. Accordingly, classical psychoanalysts were trained to objectively analyse the intrapsychic conflicts of their 'patients' and considered to be the 'experts' in essentially informing the 'patients' about what was happening inside their minds.

Navigating through the diversification

Having provided a precis of Freud's theory and its implications for therapeutic practice, I would now like to return to my earlier point that psychodynamic approaches have evolved and diversified in important ways since Freud. While it is beyond the scope of this chapter to present the progression and development of the different psychodynamic schools (see Young-Bruehl & Dunbar's (2009) *One Hundred Years of Psychoanalysis: A timeline, 1900–2000* for a comprehensive diagrammatic timeline), I would like to suggest two particular ways that I believe can serve as organising frameworks for helping newcomers understand some of the variations within this field, so that they can more effectively navigate themselves through this complex and diverse theoretical universe.

The first aspect that one needs to appreciate is that most of the developments within psychodynamic approaches have come out of debates around dichotomous concepts, such as "drive or relational; intrapsychic or interpersonal, biological or social, inner world or outer world, conflict or developmental arrest, oedipal or preoedipal, psychic reality or actuality, and so on" (Mitchell, 1988, p. 41). The efforts of different psychodynamic theorists to explicate their perspective and take a stance somewhere along the line between these various polarities have resulted in the development of diverse theoretical propositions about human nature and about what motivates our behaviour. To further explicate this point, I will try to particularly focus on the debate around 'drive or relational', since Gill (1983), in his seminal article 'The point of view in psychoanalysis: Energy discharge or person?', has persuasively proposed that this is the fundamental question that faces psychoanalysis and lies at the basis of all other debates. In short, the focal point of dispute about 'drive or relational' has been whether the forces that motivate our behaviour and constitute the very basis for the formation and development of our internal world and our personality are primarily the sexual and aggressive drives or our early experiences with our primary caregivers. In the continuum of these two polarities some have adopted and further developed Freud's Drive/Structural model (e.g., **Ego psychologists** such as Anna Freud, 1936; Hartmann, 1939; Mahler, 1968). Others have proposed modifications in some important respects to Freud's **Drive Theory** but still retained its major premise that the starting point of everything is the Id (e.g., Klein, 1975). Others have offered a creative synthesis of both drive-based and relational models (e.g., Winnicott, 1958). Finally, others have offered a radical reformulation of Freud's **metapsychology** as they have proposed that our relationships to other people ('Objects') are not secondary to our biological functions but constitute the very basis of our psychological existence and the motivating factor in the development of our personality. Typical examples of such theories are Fairbairn's (1952) and Bowlby's (1969) models from the **Object-Relations** School, Sullivan's (1953) **Interpersonal Psychoanalysis** and Kohut's (1971) **Self-Psychology**. However, it must be noted that although this group of theorists are all connected by their belief in the primacy of relationality, their theoretical propositions are not the same as they differ in "the manner in which they establish relational primacy within human experience" (Mitchell, 1988, p. 20). Overall, we see a vast array of proposed 'solutions' to this debate, which to the uninitiated may look like mere disagreements around terminology but in essence they become the basis for quite dissimilar visions about the development of personality and the origins and development of psychological distress. These differences have then important implications about therapeutic practice and about the role of therapist within the therapeutic endeavour.

ACTIVITY BOX 8.1 CLASS LEARNING

Separate into groups. Each group will read one of the first six chapters from Mitchell's and Black's book *Freud and Beyond: A History of Modern Psychoanalytic Thought* (1995) and then present in class the assigned theorist's vision about: (a) the development of our minds and personalities, (b) the reasons that we develop psychological distress, and (c) the basics of how psychoanalysis helps.

The other way which one can use to try to understand these diversifications, which is complementary and by no means exclusive to the above, is to understand the principal **epistemological** assumptions that have played a key role in shaping psychodynamic theory from its inception to this day. Psychoanalysis, as all forms of science, did not develop in a vacuum. It developed in an era that was dominated by **modernism** and quite naturally its views have evidently permeated early psychodynamic theories. Thus, for example, we predominantly see models, such as Freud's, that are very much based on concepts of a mind that more or less operates in isolation (as a closed system), an understanding of the patients' experience in therapy solely as a product of their intrapsychic processes, and a view of the therapist as a neutral and objective observer, whose only contribution to therapy is to interpret the real meaning that lies behind the patients' narratives. However, over the second half of the 20th century, when **post-modernist** assumptions started gaining momentum, we see the development of psychodynamic models that adopt the values of **pluralism** (i.e., all perspectives are equal in the pursuit of knowledge), subjectivity (i.e., there is no such thing as an objective reality, only subjective reality), intersubjectivity (i.e., meaning is co-created and negotiated between people), and contextualism (i.e., our knowledge and experience is relative to our context). Thus, we see a relational turn in many psychodynamic theories, where development is considered to be the product of our relationships to others. Moreover, the therapist becomes a co-participant in the therapeutic endeavour, who is no longer a distant expert that holds the key to the 'truth' but fully engages in a relationship with clients in order to help them explore the subjective meaning of their experience. In essence, we see a move from a psychology which was based on a "monadic theory of mind (a **one-person psychology**)" to a psychology which is based on "relational theory of mind (a **two-person psychology**)" (Aron, 1990, p. 475).

Having read the first two sections of this book, I expect you can easily identify that such models are very much congruent with the values and principles of counselling psychology, which, as Rizq notes, has itself been "the psychotherapeutic child of this post-modern turn" (2010, p. 90). Hence, I would now like to discuss one of these contemporary developments within psychodynamic approaches that is very much based on these values and as such can fittingly be applied by counselling psychologists in their therapeutic practice.

Relational psychoanalysis

Relational psychoanalysis is not a single theory. It encompasses a wide spectrum of psychoanalytic theories that are unified by a common set of central assumptions about human nature (Perlman & Frankel, 2009). Greenberg and Mitchell's ground-breaking book *Object Relations in Psychoanalytic Theory* (1983) is widely considered the first significant articulation of a relational school in psychoanalysis since they used the term 'relational' to bring together the traditions of Interpersonal Psychoanalysis, Object-relations, Self-Psychology and Intersubjective theory (Mitchell & Aron, 1999). More specifically, they identified that all these theories are united by an acceptance of the primacy of our relational nature over our instinctual impulses in understanding human motivation and personality and focus on how "people's embeddedness in a matrix of relationships, past and present, continually shape the development of personality" (Wachtel, 2008, p. viii). Thus, they maintained that a dialogue between these schools of thought and a cross-fertilisation of their ideas could provide us with a richer understanding of human nature and experience. As this school of thought embraces heterogeneous points of view from an array of psychoanalytic thinkers, it is not possible to provide a neat summary of the propositions that all relational psychoanalysts agree on. For the purposes though of this chapter, I will provide an outline of the basics that more or less are agreed by most within the school. Evidently, this summary, for purposes of enhancing comprehension and accessibility, will gloss over some of the important differences between relational theorists, such as for example, the different views about the degree to which contextual factors play a role in the development of our personalities and dynamics (Wachtel, 2008) (for comprehensive reviews on relational psychoanalysis see suggestions on Further reading).

Perlman and Frankel have eloquently summarised the starting point for all relational psychoanalysts. This is, "the premise that human beings are born with a primary need for relatedness and communication with other human beings. This need is seen as fundamental to the human organism, and its satisfaction is held to be necessary for normal development and survival. In the relational perspective, then, social experience is primary as a motivation and as an organizer of mental life" (2009, p. 106). Thus, all relational theorists agree that our early relationships in life become the building blocks of our minds and personality. These relationships come to be represented in our minds as '**relational configurations**', which then serve as guiding principles, models, for our relationships in adult lives. These configurations, according to Mitchell (1988), include three dimensions: the 'self', 'object' and the psychological 'space' between them. They are based on actual early relationships but are not what one would say 'true and accurate' representations of them; they have been imbued by our own perceptions and fantasies as children. Once developed, they come to shape our perceptions and expectations of others and ourselves, and our behaviour and choices in relationships. Still, although they are fairly stable, they are not 'fixed'. New relational experiences throughout our lives have the potential of 'reshaping' these configurations.

The above understanding of human nature and experience points to a conceptualisation of psychological distress that is characterised "by relational configurations that are conducive to painful relationships, constrictions in our capacity for authenticity, mutual intimacy and love, and impairments in the quality of self-experience" (Perlman & Frankel, 2009, p. 110). Moreover, psychological distress is seen as a result of rigid relational configurations that are resistant to change, with different relational theorists though offering a variety of explanations about the reasons for the rigidity and resistance. Change takes place in therapy by helping clients become aware of persistent maladaptive relational configurations and assisting them to develop more flexible and adaptive ones. This change is promoted by insight but also by the novel, reparative, experience with the therapist. It must be noted here that when we refer to insight in relational psychoanalysis we don't presume that the therapist can ever be in a position of interpreting what is happening in the client's mind or ever discovering an objective reality. Insight is the outcome of an intersubjective process, where the client's own understanding about their experience comes in contact with the subjective meaning of the therapist about the client's predicament, evidently influenced by his own theories and personal and clinical experience. It is this meeting of minds (Aron, 1996) that creates new meanings, relational experience and eventually change. The relationality of this process has been best encapsulated by Mitchell and Aron (1999), who following Winnicott's (1960) famous statement "there is no such thing as an infant" "the infant and the maternal care form together a unit" (p. 587), have proclaimed that "there is no such thing as either the patient or the analyst – only the patient-analyst unit" (p. xv). I hope the following vignette from my clinical work will help illustrate some of what I have been describing.

CASE STUDY LINKING THEORY WITH PRACTICE

Mary, a young woman in her early 20s, came to personal therapy hoping to alleviate long-standing symptoms of depression and putting an end to frequent and severe episodes of self-harm (primarily cutting and burning herself). This was the first time that Mary had come to therapy. She came regularly to our weekly sessions and made active use of the time that we had at our availability.

Our work initially focused on providing her the space to describe her life-story and the regular incidents of self-harm. At the beginning of therapy, her narrative was mainly focused on berating herself for not being able to stop hurting herself and for not being as happy and successful as other people at her age, which in her view was entirely her fault as she was "pathetic" and somehow "defective". Gradually though, she began unfolding a long history of physical abuse by her mother and neglect by her father, which was followed by an array of abusive and neglectful partners in her intimate relationships, with the exception of a few caring partners with whom she had split up very quickly. This recounting was done in almost a detached and unemotional manner, where Mary would talk as if she was describing the life of someone else. From my end, during our sessions, I often felt overwhelmed by the intensity of my emotions, which predominantly oscillated between intense anger and sadness about the abuse and neglect she had suffered and, at times, a need to withdraw and disconnect from her. I also felt stuck, as for the better part of the first year of our five-year-long therapy my efforts to empathise with her pain and feelings were often met with outright rejection and condemnation. For instance, she would often rebuff my interventions by telling me that I was only listening to her because she was paying me and I was nice to her because it was my job to be so. While, a couple of times she had even got up from her chair and started shouting at me.

Through our work, I began trying to make sense of what was happening in her life and in our therapeutic relationship. More specifically, I hypothesised that through her relationships with her parents she had internalised a relational configuration where others were seen as uncaring, critical, frightening and abusive, while she saw herself as someone who was unworthy of love, care and happiness. This configuration served then as an unconscious template for choosing partners and shaping her current relationships. It was also resistant to change as any experiences that contradicted her expectations about herself and others were outrightly dismissed. As, for example, had happened with my attempts to empathise with her or the couple of relationships that she had quickly terminated, when boyfriends had shown her signs of affection and respect. This understanding gave me the space to also reflect on my feelings of disengagement and disconnection, which evidently could affect our therapeutic work. Aside from understanding my feelings as an expected reaction to being constantly rebuffed and rejected by Mary, I realised through my supervision that these feelings were also attributed to my own intense, but unacknowledged, anxiety about being a 'good' therapist, as I had only just started my own private practice. This understanding steadily dissipated my feelings of disengagement, helped me withstand Mary's rejections and stay attuned to her underlying pain. I was then able to tentatively share with Mary my hypothesis about the ways that her past experiences might be guiding her expectations about me, which then helped us begin exploring the ways that her main relational configuration was shaping and limiting her current experience and life choices.

By providing Mary with a sustained and consistent experience of someone who cared for her and did not retaliate or abandon her when she 'pushed back', she gradually came to trust me. Her rejections weakened and, for the first time in her life, she began expressing her sadness and rage about the abuse and neglect she had endured. As this process evolved, she was able to recount the very first time that she self-harmed, which according to her she had completely forgotten. She recalled that, about the age of 11, she had broken a mirror in her house and her mother beat her and then, by pushing her head to the floor, forced her to collect all the broken pieces. Once her mother let her go, she went straight to the bathroom and started cutting herself with one of the broken pieces of glass that she had kept.

Following that point, we began working on her anger/rage towards her parents and at the same time hypothesising about the meaning of the self-harm. We noticed that the incidents of self-harm were almost always preceded either by an altercation with her mother, which sometimes would become physical, or ruminations about past arguments and abusive incidents with her mother. Hence, we ended up hypothesising that her self-harm might be connected to her underlying, and previously unacknowledged, rage towards her parents, which she felt terrified to express as she was worried that she would end up physically harming them. In other words, her self-harm seemed to be an unconscious compromise between being in touch with her intense pain and rage without though having to worry about her wishes to hurt her parents, as these were kept out of her consciousness since her anger was thus far displaced towards herself. This hypothesis, which admittedly was very much influenced by my own inclination in psychodynamic theory, proved to be a useful way for helping Mary create meaning to an experience (i.e., self-harm), which more or less up to that point seemed nonsensical to her.

In the safe and contained space of therapy we continued working through her rage towards her parents and exploring the ways that her main relational configuration was influencing her everyday life and relationships. Mary also began grieving for the pain she had endured, started learning to externalise and express her anger and eventually stopped self-harming.

Before leaving this vignette, it is important to note that I have only selected a few key points from my therapeutic work with this client for the purposes of this illustration, which I hope has shown how relational psychoanalysis informed my therapeutic work with this client. In particular, how this work involved an examination of both unconscious intrapsychic (i.e., the client's relational configurations) and interpersonal processes (i.e., past and current relational experiences) and how change was the product of both insight (i.e., bringing my own theories and experience to help the client create new ways of understanding and organising her experience) and novel relational experience (i.e., a new experience with someone who was consistently caring, did not retaliate to her anger or rejections and allowed her to express her feelings). I do not of course pertain that this is the only or the best way of understanding the client's experience or what happened between us. Evidently, due to the brevity of the illustration it has also not been possible to communicate the highly emotional and very deep experience between the client and myself and the far more slow and 'messy' progression of therapy, which was markedly different from the above 'clean' and linear-presented account.

Evidence-based practice

As counselling psychologists espouse the scientist-practitioner model, which places great value on therapeutic practice that is based on research evidence, I would now like to turn to current research that provides support for the foundational tenets of relational psychoanalysis and to research that discusses the effectiveness of psychodynamic approaches in alleviating psychological distress. Starting with the basic premises of relational psychoanalysis (i.e., our relational nature; and the pivotal role of intersubjectivity and relational configurations in our psychological functioning and well-being), I would put forward the claim that these are well grounded in research as we now have evidence from a wide range of disciplines, such as research on infants, attachment and neuroscience that provide substantial support for them. For example, numerous research studies (e.g., Beebe & Lachmann, 1988; Meltzoff, 1985; Trevarthen, 1998; Stern, 1985) that have examined the early interactions of infants with their mothers have persuasively demonstrated that humans come prepared from birth with an ability, albeit rudimentary, to perceive their primary caregivers' mental states and a tendency to actively seek and participate in communications that promote caregiving and the development of emotional bonds. As soon as they are born, infants enter into dyadic interactions with their primary caregivers, which are mutually regulated and co-created, naturally though with parental interactions having more weight in shaping and regulating these communications. Through these intersubjective interactions infants come to build expectations about themselves, others and relationships which gradually become mental representations that implicitly guide the ways they feel and think about themselves and relate to others. As demonstrated by research from the field of attachment in adolescence and adulthood (Pietromonaco & Barrett, 2000), these internal representations[2] have been found to be fairly stable through our lives.

The claims from infant researchers about our innate ability to interact with others seem to be further supported by recent research from neuroscience. Particularly, Gallese's (2009) current work on 'mirror neurons' indicates that we seem to have an innate embodied ability to empathise with others. That is, in our brain structure there are neurons that get activated when we observe someone doing something. What is interesting about this finding is that if we were to engage in the same activity as the one we observed, the same neurons would be activated. In essence, it is hypothesised that these neurons provide us with the ability to understand other people's actions and intentions 'as if' they were our own. In fact, researchers such as Iacoboni (2008) have even proposed a connection between autism and a lack of sufficient mirror neurons. Although, this research is admittedly still in its infancy, it seems to suggest that the structure and physiology of our brain is organised in a way that orients us to the interpersonal world from the very beginning of our lives. Therefore, it corroborates the assertions from infant researchers that we come to life with, what Trevarthen (1979) has called, a 'primary intersubjectivity' and thus we are 'programmed' to be social (Mitchell, 1988). Finally, the fundamental importance of our social nature in our psychological development is further supported by the work of Schore (2015). A neuropsychologist, who for the past 30 years, has provided compelling evidence about the ways that early socio-emotional experiences influence the maturation of the brain and shape our ability to self-regulate our emotions and manage psychological distress as adults. More specifically, Schore has demonstrated that the interplay of the subjectivities of the primary caregiver and the infant create an affective co-regulatory system, which helps the infant regulate their affect. Through these interactions, the infant gradually develops more complex affect regulatory capacities, which over time lead to the emergence of an ability to self-regulate and manage distress. In essence, we are provided with a framework that describes the emotional development of a person through a two-person psychology. Thus, as Seligman and Harrison point, there "is now consensus among development researchers that the relationship between infant and parent is the fundamental unit in which development takes place, and that the creation and maintenance of ties to other people are central motivations for infants" (2012, p. 339).

The substantial support that we see for the theoretical foundations of relational psychoanalysis does not seem though to be matched with an equally convincing case for the effectiveness of psychodynamic approaches in clinical work. In fact, one of the steady criticisms towards psychodynamic approaches is that their effectiveness is not backed up as extensively as CBT. The reasons for this shortage of evidence are multiple and well beyond the remit of this chapter (see Fonagy, Roth, & Higgitt, 2005; Levy & Ablon, 2009 for recent extensive reviews of these matters) but I would like to refer here to some recent reviews that show promising results for the effectiveness of psychodynamic approaches for various clinical conditions. In particular, in a recent meta-analytic study, that included 11 randomised-control trials (RCTs) and 12 observational studies that had examined the effectiveness of long-term psychodynamic psychotherapy (LTPP) on various mental disorders, Leichsenring and Rabung (2008) concluded that LTPP (defined as at least 50 sessions or one-year weekly therapy) has been shown to be effective for "personality disorders, chronic mental disorders (defined as lasting at least a year), multiple mental disorders, or complex depression and anxiety disorders" (p. 1522). While, a previous meta-analytic study of 17 RCTs, that had focused on the efficacy of short-term psychodynamic psychotherapy (STPP) on various mental disorders, showed that STPP was equally efficacious to CBT and significantly superior to no treatment and 'treatment as usual' (Leichsenring, Rabung, & Leibing, 2004). Of course, as the authors of both these meta-analytic studies have noted, the number of RCTs were not enough to conduct separate meta-analyses for specific disorders and have pointed to the need for further research of both LTPP and STPP in specific psychiatric disorders. Finally, Fonagy, Roth, and Higgitt (2005) conducted an exhaustive review of research on psychodynamic approaches that has been carried out in various countries and on various mental disorders. Their 58-page-long review, concluded with mixed messages. On one hand, they argued that overall we now have considerable evidence for the effectiveness of psychodynamic approaches for a range of psychiatric disorders. On the other hand, in no area the evidence seems to be that compelling. Moreover, in some areas, such as major depression or anxiety disorders, there is little evidence supporting the approach and more research is needed to be able to draw conclusions. Nevertheless, in areas where systematic investigations have been carried out the evidence indicates that psychodynamic approaches perform equally well to other therapeutic methods (e.g., personality disorders and anorexia nervosa) and sometimes even outperform them (e.g., borderline personality disorder). As previous researchers though, they end their article by emphasising the critical need for further outcome research. Thus, overall, one could say that, although as Holmes (2002) has noted that absence of evidence should not be confused with lack of effectiveness of an approach, the jury is still out regarding the effectiveness of psychodynamic approaches for a number of clinical conditions.

Summary

This chapter has provided you with an overview of Freud's theory and organisational frameworks for understanding the ways that psychodynamic approaches have evolved and diversified since their inception. The main focus has been on relational psychoanalysis, one of the contemporary psychodynamic approaches, as its theory and application to practice fit well with the discipline of counselling psychology. A clinical illustration has also demonstrated the application of this theory to practice, while the chapter ends with an overview of research that supports the effectiveness of psychodynamic approaches and the theoretical premises of relational psychoanalysis. Admittedly, it has not been possible within the space of a single chapter to do justice to the sheer volume, richness, nuances and complexities of all the different theories within the psychodynamic framework. Nevertheless, I hope that the above brief account of psychodynamic approaches has introduced you to one of the core psychotherapeutic approaches that is utilised in the clinical work of counselling psychologists and has sparked your curiosity and desire to learn more about this exciting field.

Learning outcomes

When you have completed this chapter you should be able to:

- Describe the core elements of Freud's Drive/Structural Theory.

- Understand the various ways that psychodynamic approaches have evolved and diversified.
- Understand the foundational tenets of relational psychoanalysis and how it can inform the therapeutic practice of counselling psychologists.
- Have an understanding of the research that supports relational psychoanalysis and the status of research regarding the effectiveness of psychodynamic approaches.

Key concepts and terms

- Countertransference
- Ego Psychology
- Defence Mechanisms
- Drive Theory
- Epistemology
- Id-Ego-Superego
- Interpersonal Psychoanalysis
- Intrapsychic
- Libido
- Metapsychology
- Modernism
- Object Relations
- One- and Two-Person Psychologies
- Pleasure Principle
- Pluralism
- Postmodernist
- Reality Principle
- Relational Configurations
- Relational Psychoanalysis
- Self-Psychology
- Transference
- Unconscious

Sample essay titles

1. Describe the basic premises of Freud's Drive/Structural theory and then discuss its propositions about the development of psychological distress and the ways it can be alleviated by psychoanalysis.
2. Choose two psychodynamic approaches that fall on different ends of the continuum 'drive vs relational' and compare and contrast their propositions about the motivational basis of our behaviour, the reasons that we develop psychological distress and the aims of psychotherapy.
3. Describe the foundational tenets of relational psychoanalysis and critically evaluate them by referring to current research.
4. Critically evaluate the statement "relational psychoanalysis fits closely with the values and principles of counselling psychology".

Note

The name and any identifying details of the client in the vignette have been changed in order to protect their anonymity and preserve the confidential nature of our work.

1 In his later theorising, in 1920, he also added aggressive impulses to the Id.

2 It must be noted that although researchers from the above disciplines have used a number of names to refer to these internal representations (e.g., 'Representations of Interactions that have been Generalised' (RIGs) (Stern, 1985); 'Internal Working models' (Bowlby, 1973)), essentially these are the same as the 'relational configurations' described by relational psychoanalysts.

Further reading

Curtis, R. C. & Hirsch, I. (2011). Relational psychoanalytic psychotherapy. In S. B. Messer & A. S. Gurman (Eds.), *Essential psychotherapies: Theory and practice* (3rd ed.) (pp. 72–104). New York: The Guilford Press.

Mitchell, S. A. & Black, M. J. (1995). *Freud and beyond: A history of modern psychoanalytic thought.* New York: Basic Books.

Perlman, F. & Frankel, J. (2009). Relational psychoanalysis: A review. *Psychoanalytic Social Work, 16*, 105–125.

References

Aron, L. (1990). One person and two person psychologies and the method of psychoanalysis. *Psychoanalytic Psychology*, 7(4), 475–485.

Aron, L. (1996). *A meeting of minds: Mutuality in psychoanalysis.* Hillsdale, NJ: The Analytic Press.

Beebe, B. & Lachmann, F. M. (1988). Mother-infant mutual influence and precursors of psychic structure. In A. Goldberg (Ed.), *Progress in self psychology*, Volume 3 (pp. 3–25). Hillsdale, NJ: Analytic Press.

Bowlby, J. (1969). *Attachment and loss: Volume 1. Attachment.* New York: Basic Books.

Bowlby, J. (1973). *Attachment and loss: Volume 2. Separation: Anxiety and anger.* New York: Basic Books.

Decker, H. (1991). *Freud, Dora, and Vienna 1900.* New York: Macmillan.

Fairbairn, W. D. (1952). *Psychoanalytic studies of the personality.* London: Tavistock.

Fonagy, P., Roth, A., & Higgitt, A. (2005). Psychodynamic psychotherapies: Evidence-based practice and clinical wisdom. *Bulletin of the Menninger Clinic, 69*(1), 1–58.

Freud, A. (1936). *The ego and the mechanisms of defense.* London: Hogarth Press.

Freud, S. (1905). Three essays on the theory of sexuality. In J. Starchey (Ed.), *The standard edition of the complete psychological works of Sigmund Freud*, Volume 7 (pp. 123–246). London: Hogarth Press.

Freud, S. (1920). Beyond the pleasure principle. In J. Starchey (Ed.), *The standard edition of the complete psychological works of Sigmund Freud*, Volume 18 (pp. 1–64). London: Hogarth Press.

Freud, S. (1923). The ego and the id: Volume 11. In J. Starchey (Ed.), *The standard edition of the complete psychological works of Sigmund Freud*, Volume 19 (pp. 1–66). London: Hogarth Press.

Gallese, V. (2009). Mirror neurons, embodied simulation, and the neural basis of social identification. *Psychoanalytic Dialogues, 19*(5), 519–536.

Gill, M. M. (1983). The point of view in psychoanalysis: Energy discharge or person? *Psychoanalytic Contemporary Thought, 6*, 523–552.

Greenberg, J. R. & Mitchell, S. A. (1983). *Object relations in psychoanalytic theory.* Cambridge, MA: Harvard University Press.

Hartmann, H. (1939). *Ego psychology and the problem of adaptation.* New York: International Universities Press.

Holmes, J. (2002). All you need is cognitive-behavioral therapy? *British Medical Journal, 324*(7332), 288–294.

Iacoboni, M. (2008). *Mirroring people: The new science of how we connect with others.* New York: Farrar, Strauss and Giroux.

Klein, M. (1975). *Love, guilt and reparation and other works: 1921–1945.* New York: The Free Press.
Kohut, H. (1971). *The analysis of self.* New York: International Universities Press.
Leichsenring, F. & Rabung, S. (2008). Effectiveness of long-term psychodynamic psychotherapy: A meta-analysis. *JAMA, 300*(13), 1555–1565.
Leichsenring, F., Rabung, S., & Leibing, E. (2004). The efficacy of short-term psychodynamic psychotherapy in specific psychiatric disorders: A meta-analysis. *Archives of General Psychiatry, 61*(12), 1208–1216.
Levy, R. A. & Ablon, J. S. (Eds.) (2009). *Handbook of evidence-based psychodynamic psychotherapy: Bridging the gap between science and practice.* New York: Humana Press.
Mahler, M. (1968). *On human symbiosis and the vicissitudes of individuation.* New York: International Universities Press.
Meltzoff, A. (1985). The roots of social and cognitive development: Models of man's original nature. In T. Field & N. Fox (Eds.), *Social perception in infants* (pp. 1–30). Norwood, NJ: Ablex.
Milton, J., Polmear, C., & Fabricius, J. (2004). *A short introduction to psychoanalysis.* London: Sage.
Mitchell, S. A. (1988). *Relational concepts in psychoanalysis: An integration.* Cambridge, MA: Harvard University Press.
Mitchell, S. A. & Aron, L. (Eds.) (1999). *Relational psychoanalysis: The emergence of a tradition.* New York: Routledge.
Mitchell, S. A. & Black, M. J. (1995). *Freud and beyond: A history of modern psychoanalytic thought.* New York: Basic Books.
Perlman, F. & Frankel, J. (2009). Relational psychoanalysis: A review. *Psychoanalytic Social Work, 16*, 105–125.
Pietromonaco, P. R. & Barrett, L. F. (2000). The internal working models concept: What do we really know about the self in relation to others? *Review of General Psychology, 4*(2), 155–175.
Rizq, R. (2010). Psychodynamic approaches. In R. Woolfe, S. Strawbridge, B. Douglas, & W. Dryden (Eds.), *Handbook of counselling psychology* (3rd ed.) (pp. 85–104). London: Sage.
Schore, A. N. (2015). *Affect regulation and the origin of the self: The neurobiology of emotional development.* New York: Routledge.
Seligman, S. & Harrison, A. (2012). Infancy research, infant mental health, and adult psychotherapy: Mutual influences. *Infant Mental Health Journal, 33*(4), 339–349.
Smith, D. L. (1999). *Approaching psychoanalysis: An introductory course.* London: Karnac Books.
Stern, D. (1985). *The interpersonal world of the infant.* New York: Basic Books.
Sullivan, H. S. (1953). *The interpersonal theory of psychiatry.* New York: Norton.
Trevarthen, C. (1979). Communication and cooperation in early infancy: A description of primary intersubjectivity. In M. Bullowa (Ed.), *Before speech: The beginnings of human communication* (pp. 321–347). London: Cambridge University Press.
Trevarthen, C. (1998). The concept and foundations of infant intersubjectivity. In S. Braten (Ed.), *Intersubjective communication and emotion in early ontogeny* (pp. 15–46). Cambridge, UK: Cambridge University Press.
Wachtel, P. L. (2008). *Relational theory and the practice of psychotherapy.* New York: The Guilford Press.
Warner, M. S. (2000). Person-centered psychotherapy: One nation, many tribes. *The Person-Centered Journal*, 7(1), 28–39.
Winnicott, D. W. (1958). *Through paediatrics to psychoanalysis.* London: Hogarth Press.
Winnicott, D. W. (1960). The theory of the parent-infant relationship. *International Journal of Psycho-analysis, 41*, 585–595.
Young-Bruehl, E. & Dunbar, C. (2009). *One hundred years of psychoanalysis: A timeline: 1900–2000.* Toronto, ON: Caversham Productions.

SECTION 4

Personal and professional issues in counselling psychology

9

ETHICAL AND PROFESSIONAL PRACTICE, AND WORKING RESPECTFULLY WITH DIVERSE CLIENTS

Lewis J. Blair

Introduction

This chapter discusses the ethical and professional practice guidelines for the profession of counselling psychology in order to introduce the standards and competencies required by practitioners, and sign-posts readers to the relevant guidelines for more detail. These standards and competencies are briefly contextualised in terms of the history and current political climate of the helping professions as well as linked to key values and philosophical underpinnings of counselling psychology. The chapter then discusses specific issues such as ethical decision-making, professional boundaries, **competence**, **confidentiality** and **supervision**. Finally, the chapter focuses more specifically on being mindful of **diversity** and the required considerations and competencies when working with diverse clients.

Counselling psychology values as basis for ethical and professional practice

Some key features of counselling psychology in the UK which are especially pertinent to this chapter are summarised below, drawing from Woolfe (2016), Strawbridge (2016), and Cooper (2009), and which are elaborated in Chapters 1 and 3 of this volume:

- an appreciation of subjectivity and inter-subjectivity
- a sense of the importance of the **therapeutic relationship**
- a humanistic ethos which welcomes and deeply respects the 'other'.

In particular, the humanistic ethos of valuing and respecting the other in all aspects of counselling psychology practice provides a meaningful basis for ethical attitudes and practice. In this respect, **ethical practice** goes beyond simply the avoidance of harm (***non-maleficence***) to a more proactive doing good (***beneficence***), which respects and thrives on difference, rather than simply tolerating difference and trying to avoid discrimination. Counselling psychology also places considerable emphasis on the belief that the client is a unique and meaning-making human being, and is therefore an autonomous and respected partner in the therapeutic relationship (Cooper, 2009).

Furthermore, the doctoral level of training and the standing of the profession in society ought to be, and usually is, matched by an aspiration towards high standards of ethical and professional practice. Qualifying as a counselling psychologist implies not just a doctoral level of competence but also a deep reflective capacity, a profound commitment to the welfare of others, and an ongoing effort towards growth in our skills and knowledge. Therefore, ethical and professional practice is not simply about avoiding complaints. Whilst this incentive is important, high standards of practice also ought to be positive aspirations.

The social and historical context of professional regulation

Counselling psychology sits within and contributes to a very long history of helping professions and psychological study (Woolfe, 2016; Strawbridge, 2016; chapter 1, this volume). Throughout much of this history, the practice of therapy was largely private and took place with relatively little oversight by state bodies, though voluntary professional organisations have long held some responsibility for the practice of their members. However, counselling psychology practice in the 21st century takes place within the context of state regulation, a well-informed consumer society, greater technological complexity, and a wide variety of demands on the practitioner's time, energy, and skill (Carroll & Shaw, 2016).

The helping professions have done and continue to do a great deal of good, in part due to the commitment, skill, and good motives of individual therapists. Unfortunately, the history of the helping professions is also replete with examples of the misuse of the power of the helper. The intimacy and relative privacy of therapeutic relationships, and the power inherent in the therapist role, can make it easier for therapists to take advantage of their positions of power and the vulnerabilities of clients, whether deliberately or otherwise. For many years, therapy professions have, in effect, regulated themselves through bodies such as the **British Psychological Society** (BPS), United Kingdom Council for Psychotherapy (UKCP), and the British Association for Counselling and Psychotherapy (BACP). Since 2009, practitioner psychologists in the UK have been regulated by the **Health and Care Professions Council (HCPC)**. Psychologists not offering services to the public (such as those who work solely in teaching or research) do not need to be registered with the HCPC.

Professional practice guidelines (BPS and HCPC)

To practice as an applied psychologist in the UK, one must be registered with the HCPC as a Practitioner Psychologist. The seven Practitioner Psychologist 'domains' regulated by the HCPC are clinical, counselling, educational, forensic, health, occupational, and sports and exercise. As such, these are legally protected titles, and can only be used by practitioners who are registered with the HCPC. This arrangement is intended to maintain the integrity of the profession, and to ensure that the public can trust that anyone using these titles is competent to practice to the appropriate standards. It is no longer strictly necessary to be chartered with the British Psychological Society, given that registration of psychologists was taken on by the HCPC in 2009. However, the BPS and its Division of Counselling Psychology continue to work on behalf of counselling psychologists and thus membership of the BPS can mean further support to develop and thrive throughout one's career (Blair, 2016; and see chapter 13 within this volume).

The Health and Care Professions Council (HCPC) publishes Standards of Conduct, Performance and Ethics, which applies to all professionals registered with the HCPC (HCPC, 2016). It also publishes Standards of Proficiency for Practitioner Psychologists (HCPC, 2015), which are the benchmark for qualified psychologists. It is worth reading the Standards of Proficiency in full, but broadly speaking they highlight the importance of the following factors.

FOCUS BOX 9.1

- practicing safely and effectively within your scope of practice and within the legal and ethical boundaries of the profession
- maintaining fitness to practice as an autonomous professional
- being aware of the impact of culture, equality, and diversity and practising in a non-discriminatory manner
- maintaining confidentiality, maintaining records appropriately, and working appropriately and collaboratively with others
- being able to reflect on and review practice
- understanding the key concepts of the knowledge base of the profession and drawing on appropriate knowledge and skills to inform practice

On this last point, the Standards of Proficiency detail knowledge and skills to span all domains (clinical, counselling, etc.) but also detail knowledge and skills *particular* to each domain. As well as publishing and promoting the Standards of Proficiency, the HCPC holds the power to hear and investigate complaints about applied psychologists, as well as to impose measures to try to improve the conduct of psychologists and to protect the public from poor or abusive practice.

In parallel with the HCPC, the British Psychological Society publishes Professional Practice Guidelines for all psychologists (BPS, 2008) *and* guidelines more specific to each specialty including counselling psychology (BPS DCoP, 2005).

The BPS Generic Professional Practice Guidelines summarise professional practice as being underpinned by four key ethical values:

- Respect
- Competence
- Responsibility
- Integrity

and five core competencies:

- Assessment
- Formulation
- Intervention or implementation
- Evaluation and research
- Communication.

(BPS, 2008: p. ii)

The BPS Division of Counselling Psychology Professional Practice Guidelines (2005) flesh out some of these themes with particular reference to the philosophy and values of counselling psychology, and these have been further updated in the Standards for the Accreditation of Doctoral Programmes in Counselling Psychology (BPS DCoP, 2015). As we examine various aspects of ethical and professional practice, key points from the BPS and HCPC guidelines will be highlighted and elaborated.

Ethical principles

Before we turn to the **ethical guidelines** that shape our ethical decisions, it is worth recognising the *ethical principles* that underpin such guidelines. Perhaps the most established ethical principles of any profession are the Principles of Biomedical Ethics (Beauchamp & Childress, 2013).

FOCUS BOX 9.2 BEAUCHAMP AND CHILDRESS (2013) – PRINCIPLES OF BIOMEDICAL ETHICS

- Respect for autonomy
- Beneficence ("do good")
- Non-maleficence ("do no harm")
- Justice

These principles derive from a long tradition in moral philosophy as well as medical practice, and have in turn profoundly influenced ethics in other professions such as counselling psychology.

In addition to these four principles, Thompson (1990) suggests the addition of two further principles, namely Fidelity and Self-Interest. In this context, fidelity refers to honouring the promises and trust between client and therapist. Self-interest refers to the therapist's entitlement to the other five principles. Thompson suggests the explicit inclusion of self-interest because self-interest *inevitably* influences our ethical decision-making, and thus we ought to 'own' this factor, rather than delude ourselves that our judgements and actions are entirely altruistic. Self-interest is more dangerous in ethical decision-making if we deny its influence (Bond, 2015). Alternatively, if we acknowledge self-interest as a factor, through reflection and discussion with others we can recognise how self-interest may be influencing our thinking. Ethical perspectives are therefore subjective, and change over time.

Ethical guidelines

Ethical guidelines (also sometimes called ethical codes, ethical frameworks, ethical statements, etc.) are intended to offer guidance to practitioners in their ethical discernment and decision-making, and are based partly on the principles discussed earlier. The main such guideline for counselling psychologists in the UK is the BPS Code of Ethics and Conduct, which summarises neatly in its introduction the role and limitations of ethical guidelines:

> Psychologists are likely to need to make decisions in difficult, changing and unclear situations. The Society expects that the code will be used to form a basis for consideration of ethical questions, with the principles in this code being taken into account in the process of making decisions, together with the needs of the client and the individual circumstances of the case. However, no code can replace the need for psychologists to use their professional and ethical judgement.
>
> *(BPS 2009: p. 4)*

Working as a counselling psychologist can present a number of ethical dilemmas. In some cases, the correct course of action is reasonably clear to the practitioner. In some cases, considerable reflection and consultation of the relevant ethical guidance and with colleagues may be necessary to select the most ethical decision. Where the dilemma is extremely complex and/or unusual, we may never know whether we have made the best decision, and may have to live with that uncertainty (Carroll & Shaw, 2016). Ethical guidance such as the BPS Code of Ethics and Conduct (2009) is therefore a valuable resource, but has to be considered alongside one's professional judgement, and the specific context of the dilemma. Carroll and Shaw (2016) offer a discerning exploration of the different aspects of mature, ethical decision-making. They describe six components of ethical maturity, which are not necessarily sequential stages but conditions that make for good ethical decision-making.

FOCUS BOX 9.3

1. *Ethical sensitivity.* Alertness and watchfulness for ethical issues.
2. *Ethical discernment.* Making ethical decisions maturely.
3. *Ethical implementation.* Implementing the decisions made.
4. *Ethical accountability.* Defending our ethical decisions.
5. *Ethical peace.* Living with the ethical decisions made.
6. *Learning from the experience of the ethical process.*

(Carroll & Shaw, 2016: p. 254)

Similarly to the Generic Professional Practice Guidelines (BPS, 2008), the BPS Code of Ethics and Conduct outlines four ethical principles or domains of responsibility:

- Respect
- Competence
- Responsibility
- Integrity

The BPS Code of Ethics and Conduct further highlights that the following aspects of work produce the majority of ethical concerns:

- Multiple relationships
- Personal relationships (with clients)
- Unclear or inadequate standards of practice

- Breaches of confidentiality
- Competence
- Research issues

These ethical principles and areas of work are explored in more detail throughout this chapter (with the exception of research issues, which are discussed in Chapter 12). These are complex and broad ideas, and what follows is, by necessity, a brief introduction. Professional training and qualified practice in counselling psychology allow for much deeper exploration of these matters, but this chapter aims to generate some working knowledge of the concepts and their place in practice.

Professional relationships, boundaries, and contracts

The practice of counselling psychology is rooted in relationships (see Chapter 4). This includes relationships with clients, others in the client's life, colleagues, and other professionals. These relationships with clients, in particular, are powerful and are known to be an important element of therapeutic change, potentially accounting for about 30% of therapy outcome (Hubble, Duncan & Miller, 1999). The intimacy and privacy of therapeutic relationships adds to their power, but this power contains the potential for damage to be done by such relationships. Therefore, "inevitably, ethical decisions in counselling psychology will have a relational dimension" (Carroll & Shaw, 2016: p. 252).

Ethical and effective counselling psychology practice demands the ability to establish and maintain appropriate boundaries in these multiple relationships (HCPC, 2015: standard 2). The concept of boundaries has become commonly used in the therapeutic milieu but is not often defined, partly because it can have a multitude of meanings (Hermannson, 1997). At a basic level, boundaries are the distinctions between selves, the edges of the individual. In this respect, a boundary violation involves stepping over the line, infringing on the other's protected or private space. We can also speak of boundaries between different types of relationship, such as the difference between a therapeutic relationship and a friendship. In this respect, a boundary violation occurs when we move from an appropriate relationship to a relationship which is deemed inappropriate from our own perspective and/or the perspective of the wider profession.

Appropriate boundaries for the therapeutic relationship include:

- Working within your competence (e.g. referring them elsewhere if you do not have the skills and knowledge to work effectively with them)
- Maintaining appropriate confidentiality
- Staying within a professional relationship (e.g. not beginning friendships, relationships, or business dealings with clients)
- Being clear with the client about therapy arrangements (e.g. what type of therapy, how many sessions, what type of contact is appropriate outside of sessions, etc.)
- Being clear with the client about confidentiality and the limits thereof (*this is discussed more fully later in the chapter*)

Often, these types of details can be included in a ***contract***, which details in writing, what the client can and should expect from therapy.

ACTIVITY BOX 9.1

This exercise can be done individually, in pairs, or in small groups. Having read the preceding section on contracts, and using your own ideas, write a contract for individual therapy in a setting of your choice (e.g. NHS, independent practice, drug and alcohol service, voluntary sector counselling service, etc.). This contract should be written in such a way that it is understandable for clients with a variety of reading abilities. It should cover all the points about which you think clients should know when they start a period of therapy in your chosen setting.

PSYCHOLOGICAL THERAPY INFORMATION AND CONTRACT

A psychologist or therapist is someone who has training in and experience of working with people in distress or who want to change something about themselves or their lives. Psychological therapy cannot 'cure' problems, but it is an effective way of tackling problems and challenges 'as a team'.

I may draw on a number of different theories of psychology and therapy, trying to 'fit' these to you and the nature of your aims in therapy, informed by research evidence and national guidelines. I am happy to discuss this further with you if you wish.

I may also discuss and reflect on our work with my supervisor, who is another psychologist or therapist. All therapists use this type of supervision to monitor and improve their own practice.

I will only work with you if I am competent to do so. I would refer you to another service elsewhere if I felt I did not have the skills, knowledge, time or resources to work effectively with you.

Other than in exceptional circumstances, I will only see you at our sessions, and any telephone or written contact outside of our sessions will relate to our therapy work together.

Contract for Psychological Therapy

In order for psychological therapy to be useful to you and taking into account the high demand for this service, it will be helpful for us to agree to the following conditions for the duration of our work together.

1. As therapist, I will respect your privacy and confidentiality as fully as I can. This means:
    - I will maintain written records about you securely and professionally.
    - I will only discuss details about you with other professionals where necessary (e.g. GP, psychiatrist, Community Psychiatric Nurse, etc.) and will be open with you about this.
    - I will not discuss any details about you or your attendance at therapy with anyone else in your life, unless you explicitly ask me to do so.

- I will break confidentiality only if I perceive that you or someone else is at risk of harm and I feel I have a duty to intervene to prevent harm occurring. In such a case, I would make every effort to discuss this with you first, and my communication would most likely be with your GP or other health professionals.

2. On the rare occasions when I am not able to see you due to ill health or unforeseen circumstances, I will do my best to make sure you are informed as early as possible.
3. As far as possible, I will try to arrange appointments with you that suit your schedule.
4. I ask you to:
   - Attend scheduled sessions as agreed. We will meet weekly/fortnightly/ monthly (delete as appropriate). We will review our work after every 6 sessions, to discuss whether you feel you are making progress, and for us to together identify any changes we want to make to your goals, or to how we are working together.
   - Inform me as soon as possible if you have to cancel or re-arrange a session – if you fail to attend without contacting me beforehand, I will assume that you may no longer wish to be seen. If you cancel a significant proportion of agreed appointments, I will discuss with you whether it is realistic for you to attend regular sessions and discuss any factors that might be getting in the way of you attending (such as ill health, other commitments, low motivation, etc.).
   - Inform me if your address or phone number changes.
   - Discuss with me what your aims and expectations are for therapy.
   - Take an active role in your therapy. This might involve:
     - Thinking through difficult issues together in session;
     - Continuing this process between sessions;
     - Using our sessions to start to question or change some of the ways in which you think and act; and
     - Trying out different ways of doing things outside of therapy.

If you have any questions or concerns about any aspect of therapy, please feel free to discuss these with me. That way I can help address any difficulties to help you feel confident and safe about therapy.

Competence and fitness to practice

The BPS DCoP Professional Practice Guidelines summarise neatly the importance of competence by stating, "practitioners will offer their best practice while recognising their current limitations in terms of training and ability and not practise beyond them" (DCoP, 2005). Competence should develop considerably throughout the training period (see Chapter 14, this volume). However, qualifying as a counselling psychologist is "a good start, rather than the whole race" (Blair, 2016: p. 557). Therefore, the practice of counselling psychology demands and encourages a strong commitment to ongoing learning and development. Indeed therapists in general tend to be highly committed to continual improvement (Ronnestad & Skovholt, 2012; Orlinsky & Ronnestad, 2005).

Maintenance and development of competency can be achieved through:

- reading and implementing of theory and research
- attending training courses, conferences, and workshops
- broadening professional and personal experience (e.g. working with unfamiliar presenting problems, discussion/consultation with a variety of colleagues, supervising trainees and colleagues, carrying out research, etc.)
- review of our own strengths, needs, and performance
- eliciting and noticing implicit and explicit feedback from clients and colleagues.

As well as developing our abilities, it is sometimes necessary to non-defensively recognise the current limits of our abilities. Furthermore, counselling psychologists are not immune from the vicissitudes of life, and will sometimes be temporarily unable to work effectively due to physical or psychological ill health, or circumstances in their personal or professional lives. It is the duty of the practitioner to recognise temporary impairments to their professional functioning and to take appropriate measures such as time off therapeutic practice, or improve their self-care (see Chapter 10 of this volume). It is also the duty of practitioners to recognise such difficulties in colleagues and take action for the sake of clients and the profession (BPS DCoP, 2005), challenging though this may be.

Confidentiality

Confidentiality is one of the key elements that make therapy different from most other forms of human interaction, and which enable clients to establish a trusting therapeutic relationship. Most clients come to therapy with some awareness and expectations about confidentiality, keen for the privacy this entails, and ready to share of themselves deeply as long as the therapeutic container is 'safe'. Furthermore, Bond (2015) points out that, "confidentiality acts as a shield to protect client autonomy by putting them in control of how they use their counselling in everyday life. Confidentiality protects against unwelcome intrusions from the counselling room into other areas of a client's life" (Bond, 2015: p. 169).

It is therefore crucial, ethical, and respectful towards the client, that counselling psychologists hold clients' information in confidence. It is also crucial, ethical, and respectful that clients are made aware of confidentiality standards and practice at the point of first contact (BPS DCoP, 2005). This includes an explicit explanation of the *limits* to confidentiality. Generally speaking, disclosure of confidential information may be deemed appropriate when such information shows a clear risk of harm to the client or others, where there is a legal obligation to disclose, where the client consents to disclosure, or in the balance of public interest (see Bond, 2015 for an excellent overview of exceptions to the duty of confidentiality). It is usually ideal to try to obtain valid consent from the client for the disclosure of their information, but there are legitimate exceptions, such as where the safety or welfare of the client or someone else would be put at risk by informing the client of the disclosure in advance. Risk of harm and public interest are exceedingly subjective matters. For example, the probability of harm and type of harm required to justify breaking confidentiality will depend on law, government policy, political climate, organisational policies, the mental state of the client, and the judgement of the psychologist.

In short, confidentiality is an increasingly complex ethical and professional tightrope. Whilst there is a presumption towards confidentiality in therapeutic work, counselling psychologists need to be very aware of the exceptions (HCPC, 2015: standard 7), and of the often subtle pressures to breach confidentiality, as the following case example illustrates.

CASE STUDY 1

Colin, a counselling psychologist, is working in therapy with Anna, a 19-year-old woman, who has difficulties with low self-worth, self-harm, and loneliness. Whilst discussing Anna in supervision, Colin's supervisor Maria realises that Anna's mother is one of her own clients, and Maria therefore knows some of the family history from her work with Anna's mother. Colin is unsure whether he should be discussing Anna with Maria. Maria acknowledges that it is a complicated situation, but concludes that she can 'bracket' or 'lay aside' her knowledge of the family, in order to offer unbiased supervision to Colin regarding his therapeutic work with Anna. Colin is concerned that Anna's confidentiality may be threatened, and doesn't agree that his supervisor can fully 'bracket' her knowledge of the family.

Supervision

Supervision in the therapy professions has a meaning and set of purposes quite different from what is usually meant by 'supervision'. Supervision support can be defined as:

> A contractually negotiated relationship between practitioners for the purpose of supporting, evaluating and developing professional practice . . . in an atmosphere of integrity and openness for the purpose of enhancing reflective skills, maximising the effectiveness of therapeutic interventions, informing ethical decisions and facilitating an understanding of the use of self.
>
> *(BPS DCoP 2005: p. 5)*

In most cases, and ideally, the practitioner's supervisor is not their line manager, so that the supervisee feels free in supervision sessions to discuss difficulties in their work or to discuss frankly how the organisational context may be influencing their work and morale. Instead, the supervisor is a fellow practitioner (perhaps with more experience but not necessarily so) who can *facilitate* the practitioner's ongoing development of skills and knowledge, whilst also offering an alternative perspective, for example, on therapeutic challenges being faced by the supervisee. The profession of counselling psychology in the UK has, from its beginnings, affirmed the value of and necessity for appropriate supervision for all counselling psychologists, regardless of their level of expertise.

The supervisor also has a responsibility to monitor the appropriateness of the supervisee's actions, particularly in regard to clients. On occasion, the supervisor has to raise with the supervisee their concerns about the supervisee's competence or decisions. More broadly, regular supervision is an important resource for the skills, use of self, and choices which are examined in this chapter.

Working with difference and diversity

Now that some of the key dimensions of ethical and professional practice have been introduced, we turn to what it means to work ethically and professionally with 'difference' and 'diversity'. Diversity is often considered in terms of differences of race, culture, religion, gender, sexuality, and (dis)ability. Other aspects of difference which are perhaps under-examined in the current literature include class, socio-economic status, and mental health diagnosis/difficulty. It is worth noting that difference is inherently relative – there needs to be a privileged, majority, or hegemonic group, compared with which other groups are 'different'. Therefore difference is in the eye of the beholder (Lago, 2006).

Why might it be important to recognise these diversities and understand some of their implications? The work of therapy requires a process of *empathic understanding*, a good-faith effort to imaginatively see the world as the client sees it (Rogers, 1957). The professional practice guidelines of the **BPS** Division of Counselling state that, "practitioners will make themselves knowledgeable about the diverse life experiences of the clients they work with" (BPS DCoP, 2005: p. 7). To use the dimension only of culture/ethnicity, we may miss a great deal when working with Eastern European immigrants, refugees from Syria, or Chinese students, if we fail to explore the cultural milieu that has shaped them, or ignore the complexities of coming to a different culture where they exist as 'minorities'.

Counselling psychology claims to be committed to social **justice** and counselling psychologists are expected to have a critical awareness of power structures (e.g. Cutts, 2013). This is especially true in the United States where such principles have a more prominent place in the profession and its training courses (Goodman et al., 2004). Counselling psychology (including therapy) can have an empowering function, encouraging minority or marginalised peoples to articulate their experiences, challenging discrimination, and working for social change (Vera & Speight, 2003). Practitioners ought to "challenge the views of people who pathologise on the basis of such aspects as sexual orientation, disability, class origin or racial identity and religious and spiritual views" (BPS DCoP, 2005: p. 7). There are, however, important questions asked regarding the actual fulfilment of these ideals by counselling psychologists (Moller, 2011). It is also possible that positive ideas such as 'empowerment' and 'giving voice to' can seem patronising to those we deem to need our empowerment.

A commitment to **anti-discriminatory practice** and a developing awareness of diversity are also advantageous if we wish to discern the values and assumptions which underlie our psychological and psychotherapeutic theories and models. It has been argued that these theories and models tend to be quite rooted in Western, individualistic, and patriarchal cultural norms (Parritt, 2016, Moodley, 2009; Tindall, Robinson & Kagan, 2010). To use myself as an example, as a white, British man, these underlying assumptions can be almost invisible to me, but may be much more obvious to those outside of my hegemonic in-group. Perspectives from 'outsiders' can therefore highlight our blind spots. For example, a colleague was developing a questionnaire of psychological wellbeing and had it translated for use in other countries. In some other countries, even within Europe, she found that participants experienced the constant use of "I" as jarring and difficult to relate to fully. For some cultures, identity and wellbeing are less an individual matter and more a collective one (Triandis, 2001). For those of us raised in the highly individualistic modern West, it is very hard to think in a different way, and it may be a surprise to realise that there are more collectivist ways of thinking about self, wellbeing, distress, decision-making, and so forth.

There has been effort to develop models for understanding the experiences of people of any minority status, focussed on what it is like to be 'outside of' the hegemonic, majority, or privileged groups. As Parritt states, "although oppressed and minority groups are, by their very nature, distinct and uniquely different, they share much in relation to their experience of the dominant culture and ideology and the underlying issues that confront them" (Parritt, 2016: p. 198). For example, Meyer (2003) articulates the Minority Stress Model, which identifies the stress caused by mismatch between oneself and one's society, and the discrimination and prejudice that can take place. It is also worth remembering that those qualities which make us 'different' may not be static throughout the course of one's life (such as illness/disability).

Competencies and values for working with diverse clients

Having recognised the phenomenon of diversity and some of its implications, we now consider how we can best work with those who are 'different' to ourselves in some way. Indeed, the HCPC Standards of Proficiency require counselling psychologists to, "be aware of the impact of culture, equality and diversity on practice," and, "be able to practice in a non-discriminatory manner" (HCPC, 2015: standards 5 & 6). There is a breadth of literature on working competently with each dimension of difference we have discussed, some of which is sign-posted at the end of the chapter. Furthermore, counselling psychology doctoral training provides opportunities (through therapeutic practice, teaching, supervision, personal therapy, etc.) to further develop the competencies required to effectively work with diverse clients.

Therefore, it is neither possible nor necessary to provide here a comprehensive guide to the knowledge and skills required for such work. Instead, the following are broad competencies which can give some direction to learning and development, and which apply to working therapeutically with people across a wide range of diversities. These guidelines are partly based on cross-cultural therapeutic goals detailed by Eleftheriadou (2010) but broadened to working with diverse clients more generally. Included here are dimensions of difference commonly discussed in the literature (race, culture, religion, gender, sexuality, and disability), but the same principles could apply to other dimensions of difference encountered in counselling psychology practice. For the sake of brevity, I have chosen here to focus primarily on therapeutic factors, but there are numerous other factors which can influence our work with diverse clients (e.g. language barriers, organisational behaviours, research, training, and supervision).

1. *To take into account the role of race/culture/religion/gender/sexuality/disability in the client's life.* In this process we ought to make no assumptions but can hold in mind some possibilities, whilst paying keen attention to the client's unique experience and their view of this role. For example, I may hold in mind the possibility that a Muslim man may have experienced some form of prejudice, particularly in the present political climate. It is wise to sensitively ask about the role of these factors, rather than ignore them out of politeness or fear of a difficult conversation (Lago, 2006).
2. *To sensitively explore the client's relationship to, understanding of, and feelings towards their race/culture/religion/gender/sexuality/disability.* The client may experience a mixture of feelings – belonging, pride, alienation, shame, confusion, fear, resentment, and so forth. Sensitive exploration requires that the counselling psychologist recognises and 'brackets' their assumptions and prejudices, in order to be very open to hearing the client's unique perspective. It

may be helpful to relate this to theoretical models on minority experience, such as the R/CID model discussed below.

3. *To understand any significance in the client's choice of therapist, and to reflect on potential and actual effects of similarity or difference between client and therapist in terms of race/culture/religion/gender/sexuality/disability.* Research suggests that whilst some clients desire a therapist of the same gender, race, the actual outcomes of therapy are unaffected by this matching (Cabral & Smith, 2011; Cottone, Drucker & Javier, 2002). It may be important, though, for the therapist to enquire with the client about their choice (if they made a choice) and about how they feel about working with someone who is similar or different in terms of gender, race, and so forth.
4. *To have clear awareness of and challenge one's own attitudes and stereotypes relating to differences in race/culture/religion/gender/sexuality/disability.* This is a significant and ongoing challenge, and requires a deep openness to learning from others about ourselves and our blind spots. It may be helpful for us to explicitly ask clients whether they are experiencing discriminatory attitudes in their therapeutic work with us, and to use supervision and personal therapy to bring these matters to conscious awareness where they can be understood and perhaps changed.
5. *To explore the client's conscious and unconscious relationship to the majority group.* Minority clients' experience of the majority group (or culture, in the broadest sense) may be very important to know about, and may influence their difficulties, their outlook on life, their relationships, work-life, and so forth. It is possible for people to have a wide variety of feelings towards and beliefs about the majority group, based on their experience of that group but possibly based also on their own stereotypes. These may act as barriers in therapy that need to be explicitly addressed, particular if the counselling psychologist belongs to the majority group.
6. *To actively explore how the client understands and presents their 'difference' rather than the societal or media portrayals of that 'difference'.* Again, it is important that we do not extrapolate from the group to the member of the group based on generalisations or prejudices. Research in social psychology shows, for example, that we are prone to the 'out-group homogeneity bias', believing members of the out-group to be less varied than our own in-group (Simon, 1989). It is possible for people to have a wide variety of feelings towards and beliefs about their minority even including unconscious internalised prejudice against their own minority group (e.g. internalised homophobia in a gay man, internalised racist stereotypes in a Pakistani woman).
7. *To have some understanding of what it may be like for the client to have this race/culture/religion/gender/sexuality/disability status, and the journey on which they may be in this regard.* This idea of journey or process is perhaps best researched in relation to culture, where there are many variations on the Racial/Cultural Identity Development Model (Sue & Sue, 2013; Lee, 2006). Sue and Sue (2013) state that, "The R/CID model defines 5 stages of development that minority individuals experience as they struggle to understand themselves in terms of their own culture, and the oppressive relationship between the two cultures" (p. 296). These stages are paraphrased below.

Stage 1: Conformity. The individual is relatively naive about his cultural position, and is more aligned to the dominant group.

Stage 2: Dissonance. A developing awareness of cultural issues and his own minority cultural identity creates dissonance and conflict.
Stage 3: Resistance and immersion. The individual more fully embraces his minority cultural identity, and may reject the realities of the dominant group.
Stage 4: Introspection. The individual questions and reflects on his mixed cultural situation, questioning the complete acceptance of the minority identity and questioning the rejection of the dominant identity.
Stage 5: Integrative awareness. The individual gains an internalised self-awareness as a cultural being and can appreciate both his minority group and selectively appreciate the dominant group.

Lee (2006) also details a converse process for individuals in dominant groups becoming more aware of their cultural identity, e.g. recognising the 'invisibility of whiteness' (Kincheloe et al., 1998).

8. *To develop some understanding of how the client's view of therapy and help-seeking may be influenced by their race/culture/religion/gender/sexuality/disability status.* Some cultures or religious groups may believe that therapy conflicts with their beliefs, or a lesbian woman may fear that her sexuality will be assumed by the therapist to be a source of conflict and tension. The following case example illustrates something of this issue.

CASE STUDY 2

Ahmed had fled his home country during the upheaval following the 'Arab Spring'. After arriving and settling in the UK, he had been referred to psychology by his GP because he seemed traumatised by the events of war he had experienced before coming to the UK. When the psychologist met with him to assess the potential value of therapy, Ahmed did not describe himself as traumatised, indeed he did not seem familiar with the concept. Nor did he seem particularly focussed on therapeutic help for himself. He continued to receive reports of the atrocities in his home country, and was passionately involved in efforts to achieve a political solution. From this perspective, it was inevitable and natural that he was exposed to traumatic events and reports. He did not seem focussed on his individual plight, but was more concerned for his community and his country. He was torn between returning home to help, but knew that his life would be in danger there. The psychologist thought that therapy might help Ahmed work through this decision. However, in the end, Ahmed and the psychologist amicably agreed that therapy would not 'fit' Ahmed and his situation, and the psychologist expressed **respect** for Ahmed's commitment to the wellbeing of his country.

9. *For the therapist to be aware of and take into account the role of race/culture/religion/ gender/sexuality/disability in their own life.* This requires an ongoing deepening of self-awareness, which can be aided by personal therapy, supervision, training activities, and so forth. This process is also made easier by open-mindedness, lateral thinking, perspective-taking, and engagement with literature that can reveal more about our relationship to race, gender,

and other issues. For example, practising a personal Christian spirituality in a relatively secular culture, and knowing the predominant (negative) stereotypes of Christians, I notice feeling 'different', feeling implicated in the failings of religious people in general, feeling concerned about divulging my faith to others, and noticing the implicit atheistic assumptions in some models of psychology. Yet conversely, in other aspects of my identity as a white, heterosexual male in a respected profession, I experience hidden privilege, relative power, and freedom to be who I am without fear of prejudice. Therefore, most of us can reflect on our own experiences of being part of majorities *and* minorities. Such reflection is likely to help us empathise a little more easily with others in their experience.

ACTIVITY BOX 9.2

Identifying and 'owning' your own cultural perspective. Take some time to write down on your own, or discuss in pairs/groups, your answers to the following questions:

Which culture and sub-cultures do you inhabit? (e.g. British culture, working class sub-culture, Jewish subculture)
In what ways have you experienced *privilege/inclusion/majority status* in society?
What does this feel like?
How might this experience influence your ability to work psychologically and to empathise with others who are culturally different from you?
In what ways have you experienced *disadvantage/exclusion/minority status* in society?
What does this feel like?
How might this experience influence your ability to work psychologically and to empathise with others who are culturally different from you?

Summary

This chapter has introduced the key guidelines and principles for ethical and professional counselling psychology practice. Areas of application have been explored, such as confidentiality, competence, and relationship boundaries, and we have considered some of the factors that support good practice, such as supervision and personal reflection. The chapter has also highlighted some key dimensions of difference between individuals, and considered the competencies and attitudes in working with difference, which are most helpful and respectful to clients, thus reflecting counselling psychology values.

Learning outcomes

When you have completed this chapter you should:

- Be familiar with professional practice guidelines relevant to counselling psychology in the UK.
- Understand the importance of ethical principles and guidelines in professional practice.
- Be aware of the areas of practice where ethical dilemmas can arise.

- Understand multiple areas of difference between people, and how these can influence their wellbeing and their engagement with counselling psychologists.
- Understand the desirable competencies for working with diverse clients.
- Be able to reflect openly on one's own assumptions and attitudes relating to diversity (e.g. in terms of race, culture, religion, etc.).

Key concepts and terms

- Anti-discriminatory practice
- Beneficence
- British Psychological Society (BPS)
- Competence
- Confidentiality
- Contracts
- Diversity
- Ethical guidelines
- Ethical practice
- Fitness to practice
- Health and Care Professions Council (HCPC)
- Justice
- Non-maleficence
- Respect
- Supervision
- Therapeutic relationship

Sample essay titles

1. How can counselling psychologists integrate ethical principles into their practice?
2. Describe the key features of Sue and Sue's (2013) Racial/Cultural Identity Development Model and critically evaluate its implications for counselling psychology practice.
3. Produce an up-to-date literature review on desirable competencies for working therapeutically with one of the following:
    - Spiritual/religious difference
    - Diversity of sexualities
    - Diversity of abilities/disabilities

Further reading

Books and guidelines

British Psychological Society. (2008). *Generic professional practice guidelines*. Leicester: BPS.

British Psychological Society. (2009). *Code of ethics and conduct: Guidance published by the ethics committee of the British Psychological Society*. Leicester: BPS.

British Psychological Society: Division of Counselling Psychology. (2005). *Professional practice guidelines for counselling psychology*. Leicester: BPS.

Douglas, B., Woolfe, R., Strawbridge, S., Kasket, E., & Galbraith, V. (Eds.). (2016). *The handbook of counselling psychology* (4th ed.). London: Sage.

Health & Care Professions Council. (2015). *Standards of proficiency for practitioner psychologists.* London: HCPC.

Journal article

Cooper, M. (2009). Welcoming the other: Actualising the humanistic ethic at the core of counselling psychology practice. *Counselling Psychology Review, 24*(3), 119–129.

References

Beauchamp, T. L., & Childress, J. F. (2013). *Principles of biomedical ethics* (7th ed.). New York: Oxford University Press.

Blair, L. J. (2016). The transition from trainee to qualified counselling psychologist. In B. Douglas, R. Woolfe, S. Strawbridge, E. Kasket & V. Galbraith (Eds.), *The handbook of counselling psychology* (4th ed., pp. 549–566). London: Sage.

Bond, T. (2015). *Standards and ethics for counselling in action.* London: Sage.

British Psychological Society. (2008). *Generic professional practice guidelines.* Leicester: BPS.

British Psychological Society. (2009). *Code of ethics and conduct: Guidance published by the ethics committee of the British Psychological Society.* Leicester: BPS.

British Psychological Society: Division of Counselling Psychology. (2005). *Professional practice guidelines for counselling psychology.* Leicester: BPS.

British Psychological Society: Division of Counselling Psychology. (2015). *Standards for the accreditation of doctoral programmes in counselling psychology.* Leicester: BPS.

Cabral, R. R., & Smith, T. B. (2011). Racial/ethnic matching of clients and therapists in mental health services: A meta-analytic review of preferences, perceptions, and outcomes. *Journal of Counseling Psychology, 58*(4), 537–554.

Carroll, M., & Shaw, C. (2016). Towards ethical maturity in counselling psychology. In B. Douglas, R. Woolfe, S. Strawbridge, E. Kasket & V. Galbraith (Eds.), *Handbook of counselling psychology* (4th ed., pp. 244–258). London: Sage.

Cooper, M. (2009). Welcoming the other: Actualising the humanistic ethic at the core of counselling psychology practice. *Counselling Psychology Review, 24*(3), 119–129.

Cottone, J. G., Drucker, P., & Javier, R. A. (2002). Gender differences in psychotherapy dyads: Changes in psychological symptoms and responsiveness to treatment during 3 months of therapy. *Psychotherapy Theory, Research, Practice, Training, 39*, 297–308.

Cutts, L. A. (2013). Considering a social justice agenda for counselling psychology in the UK. *Counselling Psychology Review, 28*(2), 8–16.

Eleftheriadou, Z. (2010). Cross-cultural counselling psychology. In R. Woolfe, S. Strawbridge, B. Douglas & W. Dryden (Eds.), *Handbook of counselling psychology* (3rd ed., pp. 195–212). London: Sage.

Goodman, L. A., Liang, B., Helms, J. E., Latta, R. E., Sparks, E., & Weintraub, S. R. (2004). Training counseling psychologists as social justice agents: Feminist and multicultural principles in action. *The Counseling Psychologist, 32*(6), 793–836.

Health & Care Professions Council. (2015). *Standards of proficiency for practitioner psychologists.* London: HCPC.

Health & Care Professions Council. (2016). *Standards of conduct, performance and ethics.* London: HCPC.

Hermannson, G. (1997). Boundaries and boundary management in counselling: The never-ending story. *British Journal of Guidance and Counselling, 25*(2), 133–146.

Hubble, M. A., Duncan, B. L., & Miller, S. D. (Eds.). (1999). *The heart and soul of change: What works in therapy.* New York: American Psychological Association.

Kincheloe, J. L., Steinberg, S. R., Rodriguez, N. M., & Chennault, R. E. (Eds.). (1998). *White reign: Deploying whiteness in America.* New York: St. Martin's Press.

Lago, C. (2006). *Race, culture and counselling* (2nd ed.). Maidenhead: Open University Press.

Lee, C. C. (2006). Updating the models of identity development. In C. Lago (Ed.), *Race, culture and counselling: The ongoing challenge* (2nd ed., pp. 179–186). Maidenhead: Open University Press.

Meyer, I. H. (2003). Prejudice, social stress, and mental health in lesbian, gay, and bisexual populations: Conceptual issues and research evidence. *Psychological Bulletin, 129*(5), 674–697.

Moller, N. (2011). The identity of counselling psychology in Britain is parochial, rigid and irrelevant but diversity offers a solution. *Counselling Psychology Review, 26*(2), 8–16.

Moodley, R. (2009). Multi(ple) cultural voices speaking 'outside the sentence' of counselling and psychotherapy. *Counselling Psychology Quarterly, 22*(3), 297–307.

Orlinsky, D. E., & Ronnestad, M. H. (2005). *How psychotherapists develop: A study of therapeutic work and professional growth.* Washington: APA.

Parritt, S. (2016). Working with difference and diversity. In B. Douglas, R. Woolfe, S. Strawbridge, E. Kasket & V. Galbraith (Eds.), *Handbook of counselling psychology* (4th ed., pp. 198–212). London: Sage.

Rogers, C. R. (1957). The necessary and sufficient conditions of therapeutic personality change. *Journal of Consulting Psychology, 21*, 95–103.

Ronnestad, M. H., & Skovholt, T. (2012). *The developing practitioner: Growth and stagnation of therapists and counselors.* New York: Routledge.

Simon, B. (1989). Perceptions of ingroup and outgroup variability: A meta-analytic integration. *Basic and Applied Social Psychology, 10*(3), 233–252.

Strawbridge, S. (2016). Science, craft and professional values. In B. Douglas, R. Woolfe, S. Strawbridge, E. Kasket & V. Galbraith (Eds.), *The handbook of counselling psychology* (4th ed., pp. 20–37). London: Sage.

Sue, D. W., & Sue, D. (2013). *Counseling the culturally diverse: Theory and practice* (6th ed.). Hoboken, NJ: John Wiley & Sons.

Thompson, A. (1990). *A guide to ethical practice in psychotherapy.* New York: John Wiley and Sons.

Tindall, C., Robinson, J., & Kagan, C. (2010). Feminist perspectives. In R. Woolfe, S. Strawbridge, B. Douglas & W. Dryden (Eds.), *Handbook of counselling psychology* (3rd ed., pp. 213–234). London: Sage.

Triandis, H. C. (2001). Individualism-collectivism and personality. *Journal of Personality, 69*(6), 907–924.

Vera, E. M., & Speight, S. L. (2003). Multicultural competence, social justice, and counseling psychology: Expanding our roles. *The Counseling Psychologist, 31*(3), 253–272.

Woolfe, R. (2016). Mapping the world of helping: The place of counselling psychology. In B. Douglas, R. Woolfe, S. Strawbridge, E. Kasket & V. Galbraith (Eds.), *The handbook of counselling psychology* (4th ed., pp. 5–19). London: Sage.

10

THE VALUE OF PERSONAL DEVELOPMENT IN COUNSELLING PSYCHOLOGY

Victoria Galbraith

The chapter will introduce **personal development** and **self-awareness** as integral to the practice and profession of counselling psychology. The importance of **self-care** and developing resilience will be discussed and research presented. The chapter will conclude with suggestions for self-care including the use of **mindfulness**-based techniques.

By this point in the text, you will be familiar with the philosophical underpinnings of the profession of counselling psychology and the way in which, as counselling psychologists, we always consider values and ethics in the work that we undertake. Therefore you may not be surprised to hear that we think of our clients first and foremost as individuals rather than as a potential diagnosis (e.g. "a person who experiences depression, rather than a *depressive*"; "a person who has a diagnosis of schizophrenia, rather than a *schizophrenic*"); that we use our psychological knowledge in a collaborative way in order that we are working *with* our clients, as opposed to *doing to* them; and that we generally do not have a view of ourselves as experts. After all, no one else can be the expert on another person's life until they have lived it and stood in their shoes. We recognise that language has a huge part to play here in the way that difficulties are understood and in how individuals narrate their existence, therefore we pay close attention to what is said, both verbally and non-verbally. Ultimately, we attempt to create a relationship of trust and equality with our clients.

Given that these understandings are inherent within the profession of counselling psychology, it may also not come as a surprise to hear that personal **self-reflection** is something that counselling psychologists themselves engage with. As psychologists who espouse the humanistic ethos, we are trained in the use of the self, the ways in which we use our own being as a vehicle to facilitate change in others. In order therefore to be in a position to do this effectively, there is a need to understand oneself in the first instance before we can dedicate ourselves to the understanding of others. Our philosophical underpinnings are built on the premise of striving for growth and development with the work of Maslow and Rogers being central to our professional identity. Therefore, given the equality that we attempt to promote, on both a therapeutic, professional and more global scale, we recognise that the first step in doing so is to become agents of our own personal development; and in order to do so, there is a need to engage, at various levels, with personal self-reflection.

The wounded healer

On beginning the journey into the profession of counselling psychology, it is important to consider the reasons for this choice. When asking a less reflective person "why do you want to be a counselling psychologist?", their thoughts may include "I want to help and care for people". There are so many different careers or vocations that would assist others, from support work to nursing, from emergency service personnel to teaching. So what is it that attracts people to the profession of counselling psychology? Each person's story will be unique and there could be a whole host of different reasons, perhaps academic, professional or personal. It is always worth considering the question in detail through self-reflection (an activity in Chapter 15 allows for some initial reflections on this question). Perhaps one has had their own experience of being supported by a psychologist; perhaps another has witnessed the change in someone close to them as a result of a psychologist; or yet another is perhaps intrigued by people, wondering what factors may influence one person to suffer when another does not. There is an argument within academic literature that some counselling psychologists (and according to DiCaccavo (2002) other helping professions) are motivated towards their choice of career due to their own difficult life experiences (Barnett, 2007; Farber, Manevich, Metzger & Saypol, 2005; Guggenbuhl-Craig, 1999; Martin, 2011; Sedgwick, 1994; Sussman, 2007; Zerubavel & O'Dougherty Wright, 2012). This understanding has come to be known by the term '**wounded healer**'. However, according to Rice (2011) and Zerubavel and O'Dougherty Wright (2012), the personal experience of difficulty may not be the primary catalyst for this chosen profession but rather that the development or recovery process enables a level of self-reflection and understanding, which in turn enables the facilitation of others' on their quest towards **growth** or change. And according to Jung and Jaffe (1962: 134), "the doctor is effective only when he himself is affected. Only the wounded physician heals". It is therefore essential for a person to feel emotionally fit and stable enough to work in this capacity, due to the responsibility of working clinically with people who are oftentimes considered to be vulnerable.

Introspection

Wilhelm Wundt (1832–1920), who formed the first psychology laboratory in Leipzig, Germany, coined the term 'introspection' with his self-observation experiment. This involved researchers analysing their own inner thoughts and feelings (Galbraith, 2016a). Introspection has since become commonplace within the profession of counselling psychology with self-awareness, self-reflection and personal development being supported. Indeed, self-analysis, originating at the time of Freud, has come to be seen as integral to therapeutic efficacy, particularly within the psychoanalytic tradition. Furthermore, Wilkins (1997: 63) states that therapists must address their own conditions of worth, irrational beliefs and suppressed early experiences in order to become "fit" to accompany others on their "sometimes fearful and painful journey of personal growth". However, in order to do so, they must engage in reflection and self-analysis. One method of beginning the process of self-reflection is to use a concept known as Johari's Window (Figure 10.1), which was developed by psychologists Joe Luft and Harry Ingham in 1955. They believed that there are certain things we know about ourselves and also things we do not know; that there are certain things that other people know about us and certain things they do not know. Through self-reflection and personal therapy,

1. **Known Self** Things we know about ourselves and others know about us.	2. **Hidden Self** Things we know about ourselves that others do not know about us.
3. **Blind Self** Things others know about us that we do not know about ourselves.	4. **Unknown Self** Things neither we nor others know about us.

FIGURE 10.1 Johari's Window

we become more aware of our 'blind self window' and perhaps even our 'unknown self' window; and we may feel more trusting and confident about allowing others to see those hidden parts of ourselves in the 'hidden self window'.

Personal therapy

> *Trainee counsellors [counselling psychologists] are . . . qualitatively like their clients, even if they differ quantitatively in the degree to which their perception of the world is distorted. In other words, although they may be in less need of counselling than the clients they intend to help, they can still benefit from it.*
>
> *(Donati & Legg, 2016: 50)*

Inevitably through the study of psychological theory, we consider our own lives in relation to psychotherapeutic models, however within counselling psychology, we go a step further with **personal therapy** being a specific mandatory requirement of counselling psychology training. Indeed, how would it be possible to understand someone else and their life narrative if we fail to understand our own? This does not mean that we become infallible in the way that some believe (Callahan & Ditloff, 2007). On the contrary, there are many instances of psychologists who experience mental health difficulties, relationship difficulties, life difficulties, in the same way as any other person. Through engaging in personal therapy, however, we recognise that, regardless of theory, we are all victims (or, should I say, survivors!) of the human condition. "None of us are invincible or superhuman; we experience the vicissitudes of life in the same way as every other mortal" (Galbraith, 2016a: 214).

In order to ensure that a counselling psychologist is **self-aware** and reflective, a minimum of 40 hours (usually more) of personal therapy is a mandatory requirement of training, with many counselling psychologists continuing to fund this as a personal resource well beyond training; and/or in instances whereby difficult life experiences take place. Indeed, the BPS Standards for Doctoral Programmes in Counselling Psychology (2014: 13) require that trainees will continually evaluate their practice in the light of the following principles and, by the end of the programme, will (8.3) understand the experience of therapy through active and systematic engagement in personal therapy, which will enable them to:

i) Demonstrate an understanding and experience of therapy from the perspective of the client, which will be utilised to guide their own practice;
ii) Demonstrate an understanding through therapy of their own life experience, and understand the impact of that experience upon practice;
iii) Demonstrate ability for critical self-reflection on the use of self in the therapeutic process.

It is essential that a counselling psychologist can look after themselves first in order that they are then in a position to work with the complexities that clients may present with. It is highly likely that we will become faced with stories which resonate with us, perhaps we have been through similar or perhaps we are familiar with the theme being presented. In these instances, we must ensure that we do not cloud the work with our own subjective view of the difficulty. Although we may have experienced similar issues, this does not mean that we will feel the same, cope the same or react the same. We therefore need to be in a position to bracket off our own prior assumptions in order to remain with the client and within their frame of reference.

Self-reflection and personal therapy can also assist us in deciphering our own assumptions, judgements and stereotypes. It would be idealistic to assume that counselling psychologists do not hold values or beliefs of our own which may, at times, conflict with those of our clients. It is therefore through personal (and professional) development work that we may recognise our own limitations and vulnerabilities and consider ways of managing these in the therapeutic encounter, should they arise. Engaging in personal development and self-reflection can assist us in ensuring that we are in a position to work with individuals regardless of this possible conflict. Self-reflection can teach us that as long as we respect the person that we are working with, regardless of their behaviour, values or beliefs, that we have a chance of developing a therapeutic relationship with them. And it may be that we realise, through personal development work, that there are certain client groups that we would just not be able to work with, for whatever reason. This then provides us with an informed choice as to how to proceed in such a situation. Essentially, personal therapy allows us the opportunity to invest in ourselves as a person but also as a professional. In a therapeutic relationship, I use myself as a tool, so personal therapy ensures that I have worked through my own issues to a level that would enable me to sit comfortably in a room with a client. It is also a form of self-care, an investment in me. For an exercise on seeking the right personal therapist for you, please see Chapter 11 of this text.

Various pieces of research (e.g. Grimmer & Tribe, 2010; Williams, Coyle & Lyons, 1999) have been conducted to assess how counselling psychologists view this mandatory requirement of training. Williams, Coyle and Lyons (1999) found that 88 per cent of participants were in favour of personal therapy as a mandatory requirement with most reporting positive personal therapy outcomes. Grimmer and Tribe (2010) performed a qualitative study and found that mandatory personal therapy can lead to

> perceived positive outcomes in terms of professional development including: a sense of the self as a professional through developing reflexivity as a result of being in the role of

> client; socialization into a professional role through validational and normative experiences such as the therapist modelling good and poor practice; support during times of personal difficulty; and, personal development that leads to a perceived improved ability for the participant to distinguish between personal issues and those of the client. An important effect for participants who did not have a previous substantial experience of personal therapy appeared to be the validation of therapy as an effective psychological intervention.
>
> *(p. 287)*

So far, we have focused on personal therapy but counselling psychology training programmes encourage personal and professional development by a variety of means, including personal development exercises, **reflexive journals** and the sharing of oneself within a group situation (Galbraith, 2016b). These groups are usually referred to as personal development groups, which are often considered to be somewhat of a mystery. They are formed of a cohort of trainees and an external facilitator, which provides trainees the opportunity to engage in, observe and be part of a group process.

FOCUS BOX 10.1

Each individual trainee will have a different experience of the group process but this quote from Keys (2004) captures her self-reflection and growth as a result of the experience.

> *At the beginning of the course I spent a lot of time feeling isolated because I did not feel 'heard': I imagined that no-one could understand or respond to me adequately, and perversely I pushed away any attempts to do so. Gradually, with help, I began to recognise that this was a self-destructive pattern that alienated me from what I most desperately wanted. . . Much of our work on the course took place in a group in which there was nowhere to hide and where an awareness and acceptance of difference was paramount. I was challenged to accept myself; my uniqueness, my right to a voice, my inevitable weaknesses and strengths. It was hard to show myself unconditional positive regard and accept, for example, that I had prejudices. It did not fit with my view of myself as open-minded and non-judgemental.*
>
> (Keys, 2004: 75)

She continues "*I am slowly, however, learning to chastise myself less*" (2004: 75).

Personal and professional challenges

However, the personal development work undertaken will not immunise us from the impact of the stories we hear on a daily basis. Whilst we may attempt to leave our clients' stories at the clinic door when we return home after a day's work, it is likely that certain narratives will resonate with us or may be particularly harrowing so that it becomes more difficult than usual to switch off. In some instances the experiences of our clients can impact on our home lives, in both positive and negative ways. This can, on occasion, create a perspective such as "I'm so fortunate to be living the life that I do", whereas at other times, it may bring back memories of our own experiences or we could find ourselves ruminating over the stories we hear. Dryden and Thorne (1991) discuss the periods of distress and bewilderment that can occur during the counselling psychology training period which can lead trainees to struggle with anxiety, depression and/or relationship difficulties. It is probable that qualified professionals will also find themselves in a position where they feel affected by their clients stories from time to time. This can be due to several factors, such as "over-identification with the client or their difficulty, a countertransference reaction, advanced empathic attunement, vicarious trauma and compassion fatigue (Baker, 2003), secondary trauma, feeling de-skilled with particular client(s), discomfort with the characteristics or behaviours that clients engage in, or through something else entirely" (Galbraith, 2016a: 219). Working with traumatised individuals can also impact on counselling psychologists, as discussed by Jenkins and Baird (2002) and Trippany, Kress and Wilcoxon (2004). When we find ourselves struggling, it is important to be able to take the necessary steps to ensure we take care of ourselves in order that we are able to continue providing a quality service for our clients. In these less positive moments, gaining a sense of equilibrium rather than being suffocated by the affect would be the aim (Galbraith, 2016a).

Self-care contract

It is inevitable that we will encounter situations which overwhelm us and that we will be emotionally touched by our clients, potentially having an impact on the professional service we are able to provide. Therefore entering into a self-care contract can be invaluable. Becoming aware of our own emotional thermometer can be a good starting point, in other words developing an understanding of how we react or respond in certain situations, and being aware of what our own personal needs are and how to meet them.

ACTIVITY BOX 10.1 'KEEP A REFLEXIVE JOURNAL' – IN-CLASS ACTIVITY

Consider the following questions by firstly spending some time considering the following questions and writing a journal entry reflecting your answers. Secondly, if it feels comfortable, share your responses with a trusted and supportive small group.

1. When you are feeling overwhelmed within your personal life, academic studies or work life, what do you notice? How do you feel, behave, think? What do you notice physiologically?

   (Some examples might be that you may overeat, undereat or experience insomnia, migraine, anxiety, panic, stress, you may shut people out, become angry, experience negative thinking with themes of overgeneralisation or catastrophising; or that you may cry a lot).

2. In what way do you know that you are struggling? What are the alarm bells that you might look out for?
3. Do you normally recognise these signals? If not, how might you come to recognise them? What type of support do you feel that you need when you encounter such situations?
4. List a variety of support strategies which you may find useful.

Keeping a reflexive journal can help with monitoring our emotional state and with a variety of other personal development needs.

FOCUS BOX 10.2

Bolton (2014) states that we write in order to:

- Communicate with and advise the self: about overcoming personal prejudices perhaps
- Clarify beliefs and goals: how current thinking is partly formed by family of origin and past history, perhaps
- Make and evaluate decisions
- Be self-indulgent
- Reflect upon dreams and disappointment
- Rehearse future behaviour
- Reflect on current events, situations and people
- Work towards clarity and order where appropriate
- Exercise self-responsibility, and reinforce self-trust, -respect and -confidence
- Reflect upon and reinforce value of occasions when things went right
- Be expressive and creative
- Examine areas hard to voice with others
- Respond to, and reflect on how to apply, professional theory.

(adapted from Wright and Bolton, 2012: 7–8)

There are many other ways of engaging with self-care and personal development, including the practice of mindfulness. Jon Kabat-Zinn, who developed the Mindfulness-Based Stress Reduction model at the University of Massachusetts defines it in the following way, "Mindfulness means paying attention in a particular way; on purpose, in the present moment, and nonjudgmentally" (1994: 4). Mindfulness aims to facilitate awareness of internal and external experiences that take place in the present moment, which can then lead to a change in ways of behaving, for example moving away from reacting to a situation towards a more measured way of responding, and stepping away from habitual ways of behaving or thinking (Segal, Williams & Teasdale, 2001). According to Kabat-Zinn, "the simple act of recognizing your thoughts as thoughts can free you from the distorted reality they often create and allow for more clear-sightedness and a greater sense of manageability in your life" (pp. 69–70). Many believe that mindfulness involves clearing one's mind of clutter and thought but this is, in fact, not the case. We are human beings who have this incredible gift of consciousness and thought. We therefore cannot expect to rid our mind of thought, but rather it allows us the opportunity to observe thoughts rather than to live our lives as though being stuck in them. Furthermore, the benefit of mindfulness is that it isn't purely about meditative activities (although practicing meditation daily is recommended). It also involves informal practices that can be incorporated into daily life, so rather than rushing around from one job to the next, mindfulness assists in slowing down the pace and allows us to reframe the way we experience everyday activities or habits.

It has been argued that mindfulness training would be useful if incorporated into counselling psychology training programmes due to its positive effects. Christopher and Maris (2010) conducted a study of counselling and psychotherapy trainees' experiences of a 15-week "Mind-Body Medicine and the Art of Self-Care" class which incorporated mindfulness techniques. Their qualitative summary of a variety of studies conducted over several years demonstrated that trainees became more emotionally aware, with some recognising development within their interpersonal relationships too. Research also concluded that trainees noticed a positive change in their therapeutic work from a range of different dimensions, for example, feeling more present in the relationship rather than thinking about the next intervention, and thus feeling better able to contain their clients. Williams and Penman (2010) report that mindfulness practice not only significantly impacts on wellbeing after a short 8-week period but that parts of the brain associated with happiness, empathy and compassion become stronger and more active too. Consequently, by learning the act of presence, we may also be in a better position to provide this invaluable gift to our clients.

Aside from mindfulness, there are of course additional self-care strategies available and each person will have their own way of taking care of themselves. These may include clinical supervision, networking and gaining support from other professionals, managing time effectively, learning the art of saying no, taking time off when feeling unwell, doing the work out of choice rather than compulsion, gaining support from friends and family and taking time out for hobbies (Galbraith, 2016a). Keeping a reflexive journal (Bolton, 2014), engaging in physical activity and spending time in nature can also assist (Gatersleben, 2008; Wheeler, White, Stahl-Timmins & Depledge, 2012; Nichols, 2014). Ultimately, ensuring a healthy work-life balance is imperative to self-care and in reducing stress-related difficulties.

Conclusion

Personal development is not a one-off event but rather a life-long process (Johns, 1996), which counselling psychologists are required to commit to. "To be able to stand compassionately in someone else's shoes and dethrone ourselves for a time from the centre of our world demands an enormous, principled, ethical and imaginative effort – and considerable self-knowledge: hence the need for personal development as a core focus in counselling [psychology] training" (Johns, 2012: 26).

Learning outcomes

When you have completed this chapter you should be able to:

- Describe the reasons for personal development being integral to the profession of counselling psychology.

- Understand the concept of the wounded healer.
- Understand the functions of personal therapy, reflexive journaling and mindfulness.
- Demonstrate awareness of various ways of engaging in self-care and developing resilience.

Key concepts

- Growth
- Mindfulness
- Personal development
- Personal therapy
- Reflexive journal
- Self-aware
- Self-care
- Self-reflection
- Wounded healer

Sample essay titles

1. Discuss the differences between self-reflection, self-awareness and personal development and the ways in which they are interlinked.
2. Describe the reasons for personal therapy being included as a mandatory requirement on counselling psychology training programmes.
3. Discuss the ways in which reflexive journaling and mindfulness can be useful for self-care and in developing resilience.

Further reading

Bolton, G. (2014). *Reflective Practice: Writing and Professional Development* (4th ed.). London: Sage.

Douglas, B., Woolfe, R., Strawbridge, S., Kasket, E., & Galbraith, V. (2016). *Handbook of Counselling Psychology* (4th ed.). London: Sage (see Chapters 5 and 13).

Donati, M. & Legg, C. (2016). *The Trainee Handbook: A Guide for Counselling and Psychotherapy Trainees* (4th ed.). London: Sage.

Useful journal article

Martin, P. (2011). 'Celebrating the wounded healer', *Counselling Psychology Review*, 26 (1), 10–19.

Web resources

Division of Counselling Psychology – British Psychological Society: dcop.bps.org.uk/
Health and Care Professions Council: www.hcpc-uk.co.uk

References

Baker, E. (2003). *Caring for Ourselves: A Therapist's Guide to Personal and Professional Wellbeing*. Washington, DC: American Psychological Association.

Barnett, M. (2007). 'What brings you here? An exploration of the unconscious motivations of those who choose to train and work as psychotherapists and counselors', *Psychodynamic Practice*, 13, 257–274.

Bolton, G. (2014). *Reflective Practice: Writing and Professional Development* (4th ed.). London: Sage.

BPS (2014). *Standards for Doctoral Programmes in Counselling Psychology.* Leicester: BPS.

Callahan, J. L. & Ditloff, M. (2007). 'Through a glass darkly: Reflections on therapist transformations', *Professional Psychology: Research and Practice*, 38, 547–553.

Christopher, J. C. & Marris, J. A. (2010). 'Integrating mindfulness as self-care into counselling and psychotherapy training', *Counselling & Psychotherapy Research*, 10 (2), 114–125.

DiCaccavo, A. (2002). 'Investigating individuals' motivations to become counselling psychologists: The influence of early caretaker roles within the family', *Psychology and Psychotherapy: Theory, Research and Practice*, 75, 463–472.

Donati, M. & Legg, C. (2016). *The Trainee Handbook: A Guide for Counselling and Psychotherapy Trainees* (4th ed.). London: Sage (pp. 49–65).

Dryden, W. & Thorne, B. (eds) (1991). *Training and Supervision for Counselling in Action.* London: Sage.

Farber, B. A., Manevich, I., Metzger, J., & Saypol, E. (2005). 'Choosing psychotherapy as a career: Why did we cross that road?', *Journal of Clinical Psychology: In Session*, 61, 1009–1031.

Galbraith, V. (2016a). Developing self-care and resilience. In Douglas, B., Woolfe, R., Strawbridge, S., Kasket, E., & Galbraith, V. (eds.) (2016). *Handbook of Counselling Psychology* (4th ed.). London: Sage (pp. 212–227).

Galbraith, V. (2016b). Engaging with training and academia. In Douglas, B., Woolfe, R., Strawbridge, S., Kasket, E., & Galbraith, V. (eds.) (2016). *Handbook of Counselling Psychology* (4th ed.). London: Sage (pp. 75–92).

Gatersleben, B. (2008). 'Humans and nature: 10 useful findings from environmental psychology research', *Counselling Psychology Review*, 23 (2), 24–23.

Grimmer, A. & Tribe, R. (2010). 'Counselling psychologists' perceptions of the impact of mandatory personal therapy on professional development – an exploratory study', *Counselling Psychology Quarterly*, 14 (4), 287–301.

Guggenbuhl-Craig, A. (1999). *Power in the Helping Professions.* Putnam, CT: Spring Publications.

Jenkins, S. R. & Baird, S. (2002). 'Secondary traumatic stress and vicarious trauma: A validational study', *Journal of Traumatic Stress*, 15 (2): 423–432.

Johns, H. (1996). *Personal Development in Counsellor Training.* London: Sage.

Johns, H. (2012). *Personal Development in Counsellor Training* (2nd ed). London: Sage.

Jung, C. G. & Jaffe A. (1962). Memories, Dreams, Reflections. London: Collins.

Kabat-Zinn, J. (1994). *Wherever You Go, There You Are: Mindfulness Meditation in Everyday Life.* New York: Hyperion (p. 4).

Keys, S. (2004). Singing out. In Harding Davies, V., Alred, G., Hunt, K., & Davies, G. (eds.). *Experiences of Counsellor Training: Challenges, Surprise and Change.* London: Palgrave (pp. 71–79).

Martin, P. (2011). 'Celebrating the wounded healer', *Counselling Psychology Review*, 26 (1), 10–19.

Nichols, W. J. (2014). *Blue Mind: The Surprising Science That Shows How Being Near, In, On, or Under Water Can Make You Happier, Healthier, More Connected and Better at What You Do.* New York: Little Brown and Company.

Rice, C. A. (2011). 'The psychotherapist as "wounded healer": A modern expression of an ancient tradition' in R. H. Klein, H. S. Bernard, and V. L. Schermer (eds.). *On Becoming a Psychotherapist: The Personal and Professional Journey.* New York: Oxford University Press (pp. 165–189).

Sedgwick, D. (1994). *The Wounded Healer: Countertransference from a Jungian Perspective.* East Sussex: Routledge.

Segal, Z. V., Williams, J. M. G., & Teasdale, J. D. (2001). *Mindfulness-Based Cognitive Therapy for Depression: A New Approach to Preventing Relapse.* New York: Guilford Press.

Sussman, M. B. (2007). *A Curious Calling: Unconscious Motivations for Practicing Psychotherapy* (2nd ed.). New York: Jason Aronson.

Trippany, R. L., Kress, V. E., & Wilcoxon, S. A. (2004). 'Preventing vicarious trauma: What counsellors should know when working with trauma survivors', *Journal of Counselling & Development*, 82, 31–37.

Wheeler, B. W., White, M., Stahl-Timmins, W., & Depledge, M. H. (2012). 'Does living by the coast improve health and wellbeing? *Health & Place*, 18 (5), 1198–1201.Available online 30 June 2012. ISSN 1353–8292. doi: 10.1016/j.healthplace.2012.06.015.

Wilkins, P. (1997). *Personal and Professional Development for Counsellors*. London: Sage.
Williams, F., Coyle, A., & Lyons, E. (1999). 'How counselling psychologists view their personal therapy', *British Journal of Medical Psychology*, 72 (4), 545–555.
Williams, M. & Penman, D. (2010). *Mindfulness: A Practical Guide to Finding Peace in a Frantic World*. London: Piatkus.
Wright, J. & Bolton, G. (2012). *Reflective Writing in Counselling and Psychotherapy*. London: Sage.
Zerubavel, N. & O'Dougherty Wright, M. (2012). 'The dilemma of the wounded healer', *Psychotherapy*, 40 (4), 482–491.

SECTION 5

Evidence-based practice and practice-based evidence

11

THE SCIENTIST-PRACTITIONER AND THE REFLECTIVE-PRACTITIONER

Terry Hanley and India Amos

This chapter explores two models that have been identified as appropriate for the training and ongoing practice and professional development of counselling psychology practitioners and researchers. These are the **scientist-practitioner** model and the **reflective-practitioner** models. An overview of both models is presented, as well as an exploration of the potential problems that arise out of their development. Finally, the chapter aims to discuss and consider how these two models might be integrated in order for them both to complement the training and ongoing practice of counselling psychologists.

The development of counselling psychology

Established within the humanistic movement, the emergence of counselling psychology was influenced by conceptualisations of counselling psychology as it is practiced in the United States (US), European psychotherapy, as well as mainstream psychology. In the US, the profession of counselling psychology has had a much longer history; it being established in 1946 at a time when numerous individuals returned from the Second World War needing additional psychological support. In the UK however, the inception of counselling psychology did not begin until the 1980s when an increasing number of individuals who had studied psychology were interested in applying their knowledge within the helping professions. A working party was set up, within the British Psychological Society, to consider the relationship between psychology and counselling (BPS, 1980). In 1994 counselling psychology achieved divisional status, according it equivalent status to other applied psychological disciplines and a corresponding outline of the defined area of theory and practice relevant to the profession. At the time of writing, counselling psychology is now the third-largest division in the BPS, after clinical and occupational psychology.

There exists a diversity of influence on the development of counselling psychology which some suggest has created a tension for the profession. The emphasis of counselling psychology on engagement with notions of subjectivity, inter-subjectivity, values, and beliefs is often considered to be at odds with the empirical-positivistic approach to 'science' which underlies scientific psychology, as it is traditionally defined. Ideas about 'science', especially within western psychology may not appear compatible with the concept of 'the person'. Counselling psychology developed distinct from its fellow forms of applied psychology because of its philosophical underpinning. With an explicit focus on a humanistic value base, counselling psychology is built on the understanding of people as 'relational beings', and it is this conception of the human which informs the way in which counselling psychologists practise, adopting a strongly relational stance (Cooper, 2008). On this basis, practitioners seek to cultivate democratic, non-hierarchical client-therapist relationships, preferring to take a collaborative position alongside their client rather than positioning themselves as the expert over the client.

Counselling psychologists are required to negotiate diverse, and at times competing, ideologies which inform both their research activity and clinical practice. As a result, practitioners and researchers within the field of counselling psychology are tasked to *hold* this tension, and to form a professional identity which seeks to coherently integrate the thinking of the varied influences which have shaped its development. One key debate within the field of counselling psychology refers to the way in which counselling psychologists conceptualise their practice in relation to research. Strawbridge and Woolfe (2010), when considering this relationship, assert that counselling psychologists are scientist-practitioners, and suggest that there should be an increasing recognition of what constitutes the scientific aspects of the counselling psychology identity. The next section aims to explore the implications of this label for counselling psychology practitioners and researchers, and to speculate whether the scientist-practitioner model is the only model suitable to guide the practice of counselling psychologists.

The scientist-practitioner model

The concept of the scientist-practitioner was originally conceived within the clinical psychology field. It was first introduced at the Boulder Conference on Graduate Education in 1949 in which it was proposed that clinical psychology training should provide an equal emphasis on both the research (science) and applied (practice) aspects of the discipline. This prompted a significant shift in the training of clinical psychologists, and later for those training as counselling psychologists. In 1951 the scientist-practitioner model was also endorsed by 'The Division of Counseling and Guidance' as a central model to inform counselling psychology training and practice, and has become the most popular model underpinning the development of the profession. More recently the BPS guidelines for the professional practice of counselling psychology state that the aim of the profession is to develop models of practice and research which 'marry the scientific demand for rigorous empirical enquiry with a firm value base grounded in the primacy of the counselling or psychotherapeutic relationship' (BPS, 2005, p. 1). A research attitude and commitment to conduct research is a key feature of the professional knowledge base of counselling psychology, and this professional practice guideline refers directly to the important requirement of 'bridging' the gap between practice and research. It is precisely this aim which the scientist-practitioner model fundamentally encapsulates. Corrie and Callahan (2000) suggest that those trained as scientist-practitioners should be equally capable of producing theoretical and research knowledge as they are at using it to inform their clinical practice. Research and practice should therefore be integrated into a coherent way of working, and expressed with a scientific attitude. In summary, counselling psychologists should have a 'research-orientation in their practice, and a practice relevance in their research' (Belar & Perry, 1992, p. 72).

In seeking to extend the potential of research to inform clinical practice, the question surfaces of *what research* should be conducted and applied within the profession. The professional practice guideline for counselling psychologists, provided by the BPS, uses the terminology 'rigorous empirical enquiry'. So, what constitutes rigorous research, and how is the quality of research into therapy assessed? Policy initiatives in the area explicitly stress the importance of basing therapeutic practice on 'evidence', a viewpoint that has become commonly known as '**evidence-based practice**' (EBP).

FOCUS BOX 11.1 EVIDENCE-BASED PRACTICE AND PRACTICE-BASED EVIDENCE

In an effort to enhance the effectiveness of psychological therapy, two different, and sometimes considered competing, paradigms have developed which adhere to different models of research. ***Evidence-based practice*** refers to the use of current best evidence when making decisions about the care of individual clients. The best evidence is often considered to be that which develop psychological interventions via the testing of their efficacy in well-controlled and randomised trials; known as randomised controlled trials (RCTs). The comparison of the experimental condition versus the control group takes place under tightly controlled conditions in order to extrapolate a generalisable conclusion from the study. Outcomes of these research studies are then sought to be disseminated and applied in practice.

In contrast, ***practice-based evidence*** (PBE) seeks to study the effects of psychological therapy as they are delivered in routine clinical practice. In these studies, allowance is made for variation in the client's presentation, therapist competence and different therapy contexts. Unlike the controlled conditions which are sought within RCTs, in PBE real world practice is documented and measured, just as it occurs. It could be said that this type of research does not readily accept the 'cause and effect' model of science. Instead, research is understood to flow out from practice.

Since the advent of the EBP movement in the 1990s, and adoption of EBP as a key paradigm within the National Health Service (NHS) in the UK, professionals working in the field of counselling psychology have been confronted by the growing demand that they produce and utilise research which has a high level of scientific rigour; thus, they seek to employ exclusively those therapeutic practices that have empirical support (Barkham & Mellor-Clark, 2003). In the UK, clinical guideline groups, such as the National Institute for Health and Care Excellence (NICE), have an increasingly influential role in the commissioning and delivery of psychological therapies. NICE offer guidance on conducting good quality research that can be used in the NHS, viewing the quality of research evidence in a hierarchical manner. Quantitative research approaches are favoured. Systematic reviews and RCTs are considered to be at the top of this hierarchy of evidence, as research participants are allocated to different interventions, including a control group, in a randomised fashion. Qualitative research, on the other hand, is considered much lower down in the levels of evidence deemed suitable to inform therapeutic practice.

FOCUS BOX 11.2 RESEARCH METHODS

A well-known RCT conducted by King et al. (2000) set out to compare the efficacy of up to 12 weeks of non-directive counselling with usual general practitioner (GP) care for adults experiencing depression. A total of 467 individuals took part in the research. They asked participants to complete the Beck Depression Inventory (BDI; a common measure of depression, in which a higher score means a higher number of depressive symptoms) at the assessment and then again after 4 and 12 months. The results showed psychological therapy was a more effective treatment for depression than usual general practitioner care in the short term. However after 12 months there was no difference in outcome.

As a discipline, counselling psychology adopts a critically minded position when considering the validity and utility of evidence produced by RCTs. The limitations of RCTs on methodological and ethical grounds have been explored (Cartwright, 2007).

FOCUS BOX 11.3 ETHICAL ISSUES

Counselling psychologist Alexandra works in an acute inpatient setting. She is keen to carry out an evaluation of the mindfulness group she runs weekly on the ward. As a result she decides to conduct a service evaluation. Before members begin the group, and at each mindfulness session for the next nine weeks, she invites group members to complete a batch of questionnaires relating to their wellbeing and understanding of mindfulness. She also asks individuals to complete a feedback form asking questions about what they found most/least helpful about the session. At the end of each group Alexandra collects the questionnaire and feedback forms from group members, scores them and inputs the data into statistical software which she will later use to analyse the results.

What ethical problems might arise when considering conducting an evaluation of this sort?

Consider the following:

- The dual role of researcher and practitioner
- Conflicts of interest
- The storage of questionnaire and feedback forms

As well as examining the relevance of outcomes of RCTs for their practice, counselling psychologists have also questioned the assertion that the scientist-practitioner model is the only model capable of relating practice to evidence. The reflective-practitioner model provides an alternative framework for counselling psychologists to consider, and it is that which we turn to now.

The reflective-practitioner model

In the previous section, the vast professional knowledge base of counselling psychology began to be explored. Among the areas of knowledge which counselling psychologists are expected to grasp, including knowledge pertaining to psychological and philosophical dimensions, and awareness of ethical and professional issues, is reflexive knowledge. Reflexivity is a key characteristic of the counselling psychology profession, and has been referred to as one of the defining features distinguishing it from other applied psychology professions. Emergence of the reflective-practitioner model has provided counselling psychologists with an alternative model to the scientist-practitioner model, within which to establish their professional identity. Being a reflective-practitioner requires the individual to consider, and analyse, how they were impacted by the interaction within the therapeutic relationship, and how it may have been experienced by the client. Engaging in reflective practice therefore requires practitioners to assume the perspective of an external observer of their own assumptions and feelings which underlie their behaviour. It is then the responsibility of the reflective-practitioner to consider how these assumptions and feelings may have affected their practice. Where a lack of self-awareness may cause practitioners to be more likely to use their own values and assumptions to make judgements about the presenting problems of their clients, a practitioner's increased awareness of their subjectivity and the way their personal lenses may impact their decision-making indicates an increase in successful interpersonal understanding.

The term 'reflective practice' was initially developed by Schön (1983), who identified two types of reflection; reflection-in-action and reflection-on-action. The first, reflection-in-action, refers to the reflection of the practitioner on their behaviour as it occurs (e.g. within a therapy session); the reflexive process informs their immediate action. Reflection-on-action occurs after the situation has taken place (e.g. sometime after the therapy session), in which the practitioner may review, describe, analyse and/or evaluate the event in order to gain insights for the future. It is considered very important that practitioners understand why their practice was either productive or unproductive within the therapeutic context. It enables the promotion of effective, competent and ethical practice (Furr & Carroll, 2003), and permits an 'anticipatory reflection' process (Conway, 2001), which refers to the way in which the reflexive activities of the practitioner act to inform their subsequent practice.

FOCUS BOX 11.4 APPLYING THE SCIENCE: REFLECTION-IN-ACTION AND REFLECTION-ON-ACTION

Reflection-in-action

During a family therapy session counselling psychologist Aisha was facilitating with daughter Elise, and her parents James and Joanne, Elise's father James began to cry. Aisha felt unsure why James had become emotional at that moment, as there appeared to be no immediate and obvious cause. She wondered how best to manage the situation, and noticed that Elise had turned her gaze away from her parents. Aisha noticed her urge to acknowledge James' expression of emotion, however also recognised a felt-sense that the family may benefit from sitting with this experience before it was explored further. Aisha facilitated silence for another minute, and as a result witnessed Joanne take the hands of both her daughter and husband in what appeared to be a comforting gesture.

Reflection-on-action

Emma is reflecting on a role-play which she participated in earlier in the day, as part of a training course. The role-play involved various professionals, including the role of a psychiatrist and social worker. Upon reflection she recalled the events and processes which took place during the role play, including the way she responded to the other participants, particularly the psychiatrist, whose opinions she did not entirely agree with. Emma decided to take notes of the specific interaction, including how it made her feel, and how it could have been done differently.

If reflective practice requires the practitioner to include themselves within the frame in which they view their work, then in order for counselling psychologists to engage with subjectivity, intersubjectivity and the values and beliefs of the clients they work with, they too must be open to explore their own value base and implicit dimensions of their thinking and practice. With that in mind, learning the skills required to become a reflective-practitioner is often understood as stemming from participation in personal therapy and experiences in clinical supervision. The requirement to undertake personal therapy during training is one component that sets counselling psychology apart from other applied psychologies within the BPS. It is also an element that helps to demonstrate the discipline's commitment to viewing reflexivity as an essential skill for the work of psychologists. Please refer to Chapter 10 for further exploration of the personal development component of the profession.

FOCUS BOX 11.5 SUPERVISION TO SUPPORT REFLECTIVE PRACTICE

The supervision of clinical work is a requirement for counselling psychologists in training and after qualification, and is part of the ethical framework for practice. Clinical supervision offers a space to reflect upon our therapeutic practice, and as a result to support the development of skills essential to a reflective-practitioner. What factors make supervision effective? Driscoll (2007) considers the use of experiential learning to develop further knowledge as one function of supervision. In addition they suggest that the exploration of personal feelings that can surface as a result of client work also serves an important feature. These appear to be particularly appropriate to the reflective-practitioner.

There is a recognition that counselling psychology sits within a more creative realm than other psychologies, emphasising the importance of reflexivity and self-awareness. Perhaps this is why Woolfe (2012) considers the reflective-practitioner model to offer counselling psychology a 'narrative arc' which differentiates the discipline from the rest of the applied psychology family. However, insight from Joyce Scaife (2010), a clinical psychologist, about her understanding of reflexivity demonstrates the extent to which the reflective-practitioner model has successfully developed as a supplementary model to the scientist-practitioner across other areas of applied psychology too:

> My personal reactions are important and useful. I need to engage with the issues with energy and resourcefulness. In this context my feelings and thoughts are information

> and my task is to monitor these and generate ideas from among which I choose in deciding what next to do and say. I might jot down some of my ideas and return to these later if the direction of the work does not seem optimally useful. Successful analytical reflection on practice should lead to learning and skill development because it involves maintaining a stance of curiosity and questioning automatic responses. Instead of doing things in the way that they have habitually been done or according to a manual or technical prescription, the worker feels, thinks and modifies what he or she is doing responsively to the ongoing process. No wonder Schön referred to this as professional artistry. The creative element is forefront.
>
> *(p. 5)*

Conceptualisation of reflective practice, such as the one offered here by Scaife (2010) does not aim to deny the importance of theory and technique in conducting adept therapeutic practice. Instead, it encourages processes of reflection as a way in which to improve the practitioner's ability to adapt and improvise in accordance with what the therapeutic situation may demand, all the while working from a consolidated theoretical and practical knowledge base.

FOCUS BOX 11.6 CASE EXAMPLE: RESPONDING TO THE CLIENT'S CHANGING NEEDS

Kasimir has been working with his client, Gerard, for seven weeks. Gerard initially sought psychological therapy as he had been experiencing what he called 'unbearable performance anxiety' in relation to his work life. Gerard works as a manager of a restaurant and is often called upon to deliver series of training sessions for staff. When he came to see Kasimir, he was clear that his life on the whole was fine, all except his recurring anxiety in the weeks leading up to his training sessions. Gerard made it clear to Kasimir that what he wanted from counselling was to achieve his goal of 'being able to stand in front of staff without feeling so panicked'. Kasimir introduced Gerard to a cognitive model of panic and over the course of the first five sessions, after devising a formulation, they began to focus on how Gerard might be able to begin challenging some of his unhelpful thoughts and beliefs in order for him to gradually begin to make changes in his behaviour. During the sixth session Kasimir invited feedback from Gerard on how he thought the therapy was progressing. Gerard reported feeling more able to challenge his negative thoughts, since being able to apply the 'fact or opinion' skill that he and Kasimir had discussed in session. However, Gerard also expressed that he had recently started to wonder where his negative thought patterns first originated. As the session continued, Kasimir acknowledged that Gerard may also benefit from developing an understanding of the problem and how it developed, and that this may go some way in preventing it from reoccurring in the future. Following the session Kasimir reflected on the benefit of therapists requesting feedback from clients to ensure that they are working collaboratively with them to decide on how the therapeutic work should proceed. In the seventh session, Kasimir and Gerard begun to talk in more depth about his early life experience, beginning to make links between the past and present, including these insights into the formulation as they went.

Exploring the tensions

The consumption and production of research has been identified as an important component in the formation of the identity of counselling psychologists. In addition to this, the notion of reflexivity has also been recognised as a central process to inform the good practice of counselling psychologists. The next section explores some of the tensions which exist as a result of our commitment to being both scientist- and reflective-practitioners.

What is evidence?

Practice-led enquiry has been strongly endorsed by counselling psychology, despite it posing a number of challenges to the positivistic methodological framework which currently dominates. At the root of scientific enquiry is the underlying assumption that only objectively observable phenomena can be considered as evidence. Therefore, evidence-based practice and **practice-based evidence** are often viewed as opposing one another. However, there are ongoing debates between practitioners and academic researchers about what kind of knowledge counts as evidence, and counselling psychologists have been active in this discussion. While the notion of 'good' research is valued within counselling psychology regardless of which research method is used, practitioners have challenged the way in which more value is placed on particular research approaches over others (Hanley, Cutts, Gordon & Scott, 2013). For instance, one argument is that the use of quantitative methods in evidence-based practice has been developed entirely independently of practice in the caring professions. Such work commonly prizes the concept of *statistical significance*, where the change reported during a period of therapy is greater than that expected by chance, despite this potentially having little explicit relationship to peoples' lives. The *relevance* of such research findings for practice can therefore be open to question. In response, researchers have adapted quantitative methodologies to consider more practically applicable concepts. For example the concept of *clinical significance*, where the change reported during therapy reduces symptoms of distress below a pre-set threshold. This might be viewed as more meaningful to the therapeutic process.

FOCUS BOX 11.7 THE GENERALISABILITY OF RANDOMISED CONTROLLED TRIALS

The central goal of conducting an RCT is to test whether an intervention works by comparing it to a control condition, which means either no intervention is received by participants or an alternative one. In this kind of research, participants are randomly allocated to either treatment or control conditions. Procedures are sought to be controlled to ensure that all participants in all conditions are treated the same except for the factor that is unique to their group. However, how generalisable are the results to routine clinical practice? In order to operationally define the independent variable (the therapy) in RCTs, treatment manuals for therapists to follow are produced as an attempt to ensure that participants receive the same therapeutic treatment. However in clinical practice, the way psychological interventions are provided may (appropriately) vary between clients and between therapists. Furthermore, client characteristics such as capacity to form an alliance with the therapist and initial functioning have also proved to be important in predicting treatment outcome, and may not be easily accounted for within an RCT (Krupnick et al., 1996).

The scientist is considered to be concerned with knowledge that is rigorous, objective and generalisable. It could be said that the priority of the scientist is on the *product*. In contrast, the practitioner emphasises knowledge that is subjective, holistic and relevant to the individual. Therefore, it could be said that the emphasis for the practitioner is on the *person*. For this reason, some would argue that the scientist-practitioner model is an unsustainable model for counselling psychologists as it is unable to capture the essence of the therapeutic relationship. Barkham and Mellor-Clark (2003) recommend more research is needed that truly examines the applied clinical issues which psychologists come across daily in their practice. However, this need exists within a context of an increasing demand for evidence-based practice. Therefore, from this position, it is argued that practice must be grounded in the evidence which is available, even if this evidence appears less sensitive to diverse populations and unique contexts of delivery.

What influences therapeutic practice?

Before we think further about this question, have a go at completing the activity in Activity box 11.1.

ACTIVITY BOX 11.1 SEEKING THE THERAPIST FOR YOU

Imagine you are just beginning your professional training in counselling psychology and as a result are required to undertake a minimum of 40 hours of personal therapy. What expectations would you have of your therapist? What would be the most important factors for you? Rate the following therapist characteristics in order of importance (1 being unimportant and 5 being essential).

	An ability to develop a warm and responsive therapeutic relationship
	Over 20 years' experience as a therapeutic practitioner
	A non-judgemental attitude
	A knowledge of the most up-to-date research findings
	Experience of conducting research on the effectiveness of therapy
	A thorough knowledge of CBT techniques
	The knowledge that the therapist reflects upon their practice in clinical supervision

Consider your ratings in relation to what you now know about the scientist-practitioner and reflective-practitioner model. Which of the models do the elements you chose resonate most with?

Meier and Davis (1997) claimed that 'in no other profession does the personality and behaviour of the profession make such a difference as it does in counselling' (p. 61). Therefore there is an ongoing debate about the utilisation of knowledge counselling psychologists acquire throughout their training and ongoing professional development, and their subsequent behaviour within their clinical practice. What does influence the decision-making of therapists? Whilst evidence-based practice encourages the implementation of those therapies with the greater evidence base, the practice of counselling psychologists may be informed by a broader range of aspects than just research. Activity box 10.1 invited you to reflect on what elements would be most important to you when seeking out a therapist. Perhaps a clear knowledge of the most up-to-date evidence was considered most important to you, or maybe you felt it was more important that your therapist had a significant number of years' experience in therapeutic practice? It might be interesting to consider a piece of research conducted by Lucock, Hall and Noble (2006) which aimed to find out what is considered as most influential on the practice of psychotherapists and trainee clinical psychologists in the UK. What do you think the results demonstrated? The survey showed that professional training, clinical supervision and three related factors, client characteristics, client feedback and psychological formulation, were rated as the most influential factors for both the qualified psychotherapists and trainee clinical psychologists. Cognitive-behaviour therapists rated evidence-based guidelines, research-based journal articles and electronic journals higher than the other groups in the study; however on the whole, evidence-based factors including treatment manuals and evidence-based guidelines were rated less highly overall. Perhaps this is particularly surprising for clinical psychologists in training, who are primarily supported by the scientist-practitioner training model. Do you think this result would be the same for qualified and trainee counselling psychologists?

What makes therapy effective?

FOCUS BOX 11.8 *EFFICACY AND EFFECTIVENESS*

Roth and Fonagy (2005) draw attention to the important distinction between **efficacy studies** and the effectiveness of routine therapeutic practice, and the different purposes of each. **Efficacy studies** demonstrate outcomes achieved in the context of highly controlled research trials, where the aim is to discover the benefits or harm of an intervention. Effectiveness, on the other hand, refers to the performance of an intervention under real world conditions, with more heterogeneous populations and less standardised protocols of therapy.

With the above in mind, efficacy and **effectiveness studies** might be viewed as existing at opposite ends of a continuum of decision-making in research. Therefore, a focus on either efficacy or effectiveness will affect the research study design. How might the terms 'efficacy' and 'effectiveness' relate to those researchers/practitioners engaged in working within the paradigms of evidence-based practice, or **practice-based evidence**?

Systematic reviews have shown that, when compared, different mainstream therapies are actually as effective as each other (Cooper, 2008). This has given rise to phrase 'the dodo bird verdict', which references a story in Lewis Carroll 's *Alice in Wonderland*. In the story, a group of animals run a chaotic race, which is brought to an end when the Dodo bird declares '*everybody* has won, and all must have prizes'. In the context of psychological therapy, this result suggests that there must be effective components of practice that are common to all therapeutic approaches. To reflect upon what these active ingredients of therapy might be the American Psychological Association assembled a task force to review the empirical research.

They discovered that the specific techniques associated with certain types of therapy are less important than non-specific factors such as positive qualities of the therapeutic relationship. Focus box 11.9 provides more detail on the findings of this seminal work.

FOCUS BOX 11.9 RESEARCH METHODS: COMMON THERAPEUTIC FACTORS

In a book entitled *Psychotherapeutic Relationships that Work* by Norcross (2011), the elements of the therapeutic relationship that work were investigated. The common therapeutic factors considered as demonstrably effective in individual therapy were highlighted as follows:

- Alliance in individual psychotherapy
- Alliance in youth psychotherapy
- Empathy – communication of the therapists understanding of the client's emotional experience
- Collecting client feedback – asking for the client's views on their experience of therapy

It is important to note that the term *alliance* is often understood as consisting of a shared agreement between the therapist and client on the goals and tasks of therapy, as well as referring to the emotional bond between the therapist and client (Bordin, 1994).

Exploring the opportunities

Expanding the notion of evidence

We have identified that the creation of research that can be translated into practice is not a simple matter. The question of what type of knowledge and created by whom, in what context should be considered legitimate, still remains. The concept of '**methodological pluralism**' (Kasket, 2013) offers one way in which to reconcile the tension between assumptions underlying more positivist approaches with the humanistic and intersubjective concerns of counselling psychology. The concepts of methodological pluralism suggests that there are numerous research methods that can be useful in addressing a research question. The position is therefore opposed to the idea that there is only one valid way to approach the inquiry of any given question. By expanding the notion of what constitutes 'science' and 'valid evidence', an increasing inclusion of diverse methodological perspectives with different epistemological underpinnings can be appreciated and valued. Key concepts within counselling psychology such as meaning, values and insight are less amenable to be tested via strictly quantitative methods. Instead, they may be better explored via qualitative research approaches which provide rich and detailed pictures of human experience. A pluralistic approach to evidence enables more inclusive methods for the synthesis of evidence and highlights the useful contribution to counselling psychology practice from a diverse array of research approaches (Hanley & Winter, 2016). In the case of evidence-based practice versus practice-based evidence, seeing the two paradigms as complementary rather than competing may be the most appropriate way forward for counselling psychologists. Barkham, Stiles, Lambert and Mellor-Clark (2010) suggest that both are needed in order to build a relevant and rigorous science of the psychological therapies. Barkham and Mellor-Clark (2003) suggest that 'no single research paradigm can deliver all the requirements of rigorous and relevant research' (p. 320). Therefore it is suggested that practitioners and researchers should seek to value diverse research approaches which in combination enable a richer foundation of knowledge on both the process and outcomes of psychological therapy.

Forming a relationship with research

The findings from the Lucock et al. study (2006), which was mentioned earlier, showed the high ratings for client-centred factors and notions of intuition and judgement on the influence of practice. This would appear to support the idea that effective practice might be best seen as a combination of evidence-based practice guidelines with reflective practice elements such as clinical judgement and flexibility, in order to adjust the therapy to the individual. A conclusion from the Lucock study suggested that practitioners using predominantly CBT were more inclined to view the importance of evidence-based practice. However within CBT there have been developments of integrative training strategies which aim to enable practitioners an experiential learning process to facilitate the acquisition of therapeutic skill in a number of cognitive-behavioural therapy (CBT) competencies (Bennett-Levy, Lee, Travers, Pohlman & Hamernik, 2003). The self-practice component of the process involves the practitioner's engagement in a structured experience of using CBT on themselves, either in the form of self-guided completion of a manualised workbook of typical CBT tasks or the initiation of limited co-therapy with a colleague (Bennett-Levy & Lee, 2014). The therapists' self-reflection is encouraged on both the experience of the process of self-practice and the perceived implications of their experience on their subsequent understanding of CBT theory and practice. Within this paradigm, reflexivity is considered to play an essential role in therapist skill development, as it acts to mediate how knowledge is used in practice, and vice versa. Furthermore, reflection on clinical practice is also understood as having potential to consolidate or modify current declarative knowledge and, hence, contribute to new learning. Perhaps this particular approach provides one way in which to combine technical knowledge informed by research evidence, and reflective knowledge informed by the experience of its application.

FOCUS BOX 11.10 BEYOND THE FRONTIER: A RESEARCH-INFORMED APPROACH

As has been discussed counselling psychologists commonly advocate the use of the **scientist-practitioner** model to inform how practice relates to evidence. As a result, taking account of current research findings is considered important and useful for their practice. We have also discussed some of the potential tensions that may exist between the discipline's philosophical basis and what is currently considered appropriate research evidence to inform practice. A research-informed approach, as opposed to research-directed one, may be one way in which counselling psychologists can acknowledge the many things, including research, which can impact on the decision we make for each individual client we meet in therapy.

Conclusion

> *[A counselling psychologist must] be able to use professional and research skills in work with clients based on a* ***scientist-practitioner*** *and* ***reflective-practitioner*** *model that incorporates a cycle of assessment, formulation, intervention and evaluation.*
>
> (HCPC, 2015, p. 22)

The identity of the counselling psychology profession could be defined as one which seeks to hold tensions, rather than necessarily resolve them. The same could be said for the potential tension which exists between the two models presented in this chapter. The diverse forms of knowledge which constitute the counselling psychology profession may make it difficult to conform solely to the principles of evidence-based practice. However it is our continued engagement with the tensions which this debate generates that has the most potential to enable the formation of a distinct professional identity.

At present, evidence-based practices, primarily developed through the amalgamation of randomised control trials, dominate guidelines instructing what therapeutic approach should be utilised for whom. In contrast, counselling psychologists commonly advocate a broader understanding of how evidence is used to inform practice. From this perspective, the relationship between research and practice appears best seen as bi-directional, where research has a role in informing practice, as does practice in informing areas where further research is required to be conducted. In order for practitioners to respond to client needs, therapists will always be in a position whereby they are required to devise innovative methods. As practitioners gain experience, and more important reflect on that experience, they become better equipped to combine theoretical concepts and techniques with their clinical wisdom in order to serve the needs of their clients. Counselling psychology seems able to form a dual alliance with both the scientist-practitioner model and the reflective-practitioner model. As scientist-practitioners we can seek to both consume and produce research, and as reflective-practitioners we seek to always remain alert to the uniqueness of each practice situation as it develops.

This chapter has highlighted that the articulation of what constitutes practice knowledge appears hard to define. Training, and continued professional development models which support the experiential learning and reflexivity skills of counselling psychologists, as well as their suitable use of psychological research to inform their practice, offers one way in which to achieve a coherent integration of theory, research and practice. As a result, the models are seen as increasingly complementary rather than opposing forces. Counselling psychologists can therefore locate themselves in a position whereby they remain as both scientist- and reflective-practitioners (HCPC, 2015).

Learning outcomes

When you have completed this chapter, you should be able:

- To outline the key elements of the scientist-practitioner model and its relationship to the discipline of counselling psychology.
- To outline the key elements of the reflective-practitioner model and its relationship to the discipline of counselling psychology.
- To highlight the differences between EBP and PBE and their relevant contribution to counselling psychology practice.

- To critically engage with the debate on what constitutes as suitable research evidence to inform therapeutic practice.

Key concepts

- Effectiveness studies
- Efficacy studies
- Evidence-based practice
- Methodological pluralism
- Practice-based evidence
- Reflective-practitioner
- Scientist-practitioner

Sample essay titles

1. Critically discuss the reflective-practitioner model.
2. What challenges and opportunities do randomised control trials pose for counselling psychologists?
3. Describe and discuss a situation when it is appropriate for a psychologist not to use a recommended evidence-based practice.

Further reading

Barkham, M., Hardy, S. E., & Mellor-Clark, J. (2010). *Developing and delivering practice-based evidence: A guide for the psychological therapies*. London: John Wiley & Sons.

Hanley, T., Cutts, L., Gordon, R., & Scott, A. (2013). A research informed approach to counselling psychology. In G. Davey (Ed). *Applied psychology* (pp. 1–23 supplementary material). London: BPS Wiley Blackwell.

Kasket, E. (2013). The counselling psychology researcher. In G. Davey (Ed). *Applied psychology* (pp. 1–19 supplementary material). London: BPS Wiley Blackwell.

Wessley, S. (2001). Randomised controlled trails: The gold standard? In C. Mace, S. Moorey, & B. Robert (Eds). *Evidence in the psychological therapies: A critical guide for practitioners* (pp. 46–59). Hove: Brunner-Routledge.

Lane, D., & Corrie, S. (2006). *The modern scientist-practitioner: A guide to practice in psychology*. Sussex: Routledge.

Scaife, J. (2010). *Supervising the reflective practitioner: An essential guide to theory and practice*. Sussex: Routledge.

Useful journal articles

Blair, L. (2010). A critical review of the scientist-practitioner model for counselling psychology. *Counselling Psychology Review, 25*(4), 19–30.

Cartwright, N. (2007). Are RCTs the gold standard? *BioSocieties, 2*(1), 11–20.

Jones, J. L., & Mehr, S. L. (2007). Foundations and assumptions of the scientist-practitioner model. *American Behavioral Scientist, 50*(6), 766–771.

Myers, D. (2007). Implication of the scientist-practitioner model in counselling psychology training and practice. *American Behavioural Scientist, 50*(6), 789–796.

Rennie, D. L. (2004). Reflexivity and person-centered counseling. *Journal of Humanistic Psychology, 44*, 182–203.

Web resources

The NICE website provides an overview of the recommended evidence-based guidance for recognised mental health issues – www.nice.org.uk

References

Barkham, M., & Mellor-Clark, J. (2003). Bridging evidence-based practice and practice-based evidence: Developing a rigorous and relevant knowledge for the psychological therapies. *Clinical Psychology & Psychotherapy, 10*(6), 319–327.

Barkham, M., Stiles, W. B., Lambert, M. J., & Mellor-Clark, J. (2010). Building a rigorous and relevant knowledge-base for the psychological therapies. In M. Barkham, G. Hardy & J. Mellor-Clark (Eds). *Developing and delivering practice-based evidence: A guide for the psychological therapies* (pp. 21–61). London: Wiley & Sons.

Belar, C. D., & Perry, N. W. (1992). The national conference on scientist-practitioner education and training for the professional practice of psychology. *American Psychologist, 47*(1), 71.

Bennett-Levy, J., & Lee, N. K. (2014). Self-practice and self-reflection in cognitive behaviour therapy training: What factors influence trainees' engagement and experience of benefit? *Behavioural and Cognitive Psychotherapy, 42*(1), 48–64.

Bennett-Levy, J., Lee, N. K., Travers, K., Pohlman, S., & Hamernik, E. (2003). Cognitive therapy from the inside: Enhancing therapist skills through practising what we preach. *Behavioural and Cognitive Psychotherapy, 31*(2), 143–158.

Bordin, E. S. (1994). Theory and research on the therapeutic working alliance: New directions. In A. Horvath & L. Greenberg (Eds). *The Working Alliance: Theory, Research, and Practice* (pp. 13–37). New York: Wiley & Sons.

British Psychological Society (1980). *Counselling: The report of a working party*. Leicester: BPS.

British Psychological Society Division of Counselling Psychology (2005). *Professional practice guidelines*. Leicester: BPS.

Cartwright, N. (2007). Are RCTs the gold standard? *BioSocieties, 2*(1), 11–20.

Conway, P.F. (2001). Anticipatory reflection while learning to teach: From a temporally truncated to a temporally distributed model of reflection in teacher education. *Teaching and Teacher Education, 17*(1), 89–106.

Cooper, M. (2008). *Essential research findings in counselling and psychotherapy: The facts are friendly*. London: Sage.

Corrie, S., & Callahan, M. M. (2000). A review of the scientist – practitioner model: Reflections on its potential contribution to counselling psychology within the context of current health care trends. *Psychology and Psychotherapy, 73*, 413.

Driscoll, J. (2007). *Practising clinical supervision: A reflective approach for healthcare professionals*. (2nd edition). Philadelphia, PA: Elsevier.

Furr, S. R., & Carroll, J. J. (2003). Critical incidents in student counselor development. *Journal of Counseling & Development, 81*(4), 483–489.

Hanley, T., Cutts, L., Gordon, R., & Scott, A. (2013). A research informed approach to counselling psychology. In G. Davey (Ed). *Applied psychology* (pp. 1–23 supplementary material). London: BPS Wiley Blackwell.

Hanley, T., & Winter, L. (2016). Research and pluralism. In M. Cooper & W. Dryden (Eds). *The handbook of pluralistic counselling and psychotherapy* (pp. 337–349). London: Sage.

Health and Care Professions Council (2015). *Standards of proficiency – practitioner psychologists*. London: HCPC.

Kasket, E. (2013). The counselling psychology researcher. In G. Davey (Ed). *Applied psychology* (pp. 1–19 supplementary material). London: BPS Wiley Blackwell.

King, M., Sibbald, B., Ward, E., Bower, P., Lloyd, M., Gabbay, M., & Byford, S. (2000). Randomised controlled trial of non-directive counselling, cognitive-behaviour therapy and usual general practitioner care in the management of depression as well as mixed anxiety and depression in primary care. *Health Technology Assessment*, *4*, 1–83.

Krupnick, J. L., Sotsky, S. M., Simmens, S., Moyer, J., Elkin, I., Watkins, J., & Pilkonis, P. A. (1996). The role of the therapeutic alliance in psychotherapy and pharmacotherapy outcome: Findings in the National Institute of Mental Health Treatment of Depression Collaborative Research Program. *Journal of Consulting and Clinical Psychology*, *64*(3), 532.

Lucock, M. P., Hall, P., & Noble, R. (2006). A survey of influences on the practice of psychotherapists and clinical psychologists in training in the UK. *Clinical Psychology & Psychotherapy*, *13*(2), 123–130.

Meier, S., & Davis, S. (1997). *The elements of counseling*. (2nd edition). Pacific Grove, CA: Brooks/Cole.

Norcross, J. C. (Ed) (2011). *Psychotherapy relationships that work: Evidence-based responsiveness*. (2nd edition). Oxford: Oxford University Press.

Roth, A. & Fonagy, P. (2005). *What works for whom? A critical review of psychotherapy research*. (2nd edition). New York: Guilford Press.

Scaife, J. (2010). *Supervising the reflective practitioner: An essential guide to theory and practice*. London: Routledge.

Schön, D. A. (1983). *The reflective practitioner: How professionals think in action*. New York: Basic Books.

Strawbridge, S., & Woolfe, R. (2010). Counselling psychology: Origins, developments and challenges. In R. Woolfe, S. Strawbridge, B. Douglas & W. Dryden (Eds). *Handbook of counselling psychology* (3rd edition, pp. 3–22). London: Sage.

Woolfe, W. (2012). Risorgimento: A history of Counselling Psychology in Britain. *Counselling Psychology Review*, *27*(4), 72–78.

12

RESEARCH IN COUNSELLING PSYCHOLOGY

Isabel Henton and Elaine Kasket

Chapter overview

If we were to apply the 'relationship status' label that most accurately describes the historical connection between counselling psychology and research, it would probably be "it's complicated". There has been considerable discussion, even argument, about the centrality of research within the profession, with some counselling psychologists enthusiastically embracing research, and others questioning its relevance and usefulness to our day-to-day working lives. Whatever our relationship with research has been in the past, however, contemporary developments – such as the 'doctoralisation' of the profession, and the wider emphasis on evidence-based practice – are forcing us all to think more deeply about our attitudes towards research, and towards our own research activity. We argue that these developments offer opportunities to innovate, to renegotiate apparent tensions, and to foster a richer and more meaningful relationship between counselling psychology and research.

In this chapter, we examine the role of research in the development of individual practitioners, and its place in the profession at large, including how it fits in with counselling psychology's ethos and values. We provide examples of the many kinds of research studies that counselling psychologists might engage with in their professional practice, whether this is psychotherapy, or other domains, such as academia, training, supervision, consultancy, or service development. Through the use of a case example, we illustrate how engaging with research can energise and expand a counselling psychologist's career and employability.

Introduction

It might not have jumped out at you, but if you flip back through these pages, you will notice that *all* of the sections in this book thus far have referred to research. Section 1 emphasises that research is part of the counselling psychology discipline overall. Section 2 discusses how research evidence supports certain ideas that are dear to the heart of counselling psychologists, such as the importance of the therapeutic relationship. Section 3 references research that evidences the effectiveness of particular therapeutic approaches. Section 4 assures you that the practitioner's need for self-care is supported by research. You could argue that the recurring references to research thus far in this book would signify that counselling psychology considers research to be quite important. If we keep mentioning it, we are paying it a certain amount of attention – our field must care about research in some way, or certainly consider it worthy of comment.

On the other hand, you might also notice that while research is frequently mentioned, it is in a rather secondary position to the main event – it shows up at intervals to support clinical practice. Research is rolled in to add weight, to lend authority, to justify or sanction a particular approach or position. Research itself becomes the focal point only now, towards the end of the book. This could be a neutral occurrence – editors have to identify some way of usefully delivering information in an edited book such this – or it could be meaningful. Ten years ago, we might have suggested that the organisation of chapters in this book's table of contents paralleled the way in which research seemed to occupy a secondary, incidental position within counselling psychology itself.

No matter how an aspiring counselling psychologist might feel about research, one thing is certain: if you wish to qualify, you will probably be using it, and you will definitely be doing it! To help you articulate your feelings about that, tackle Piercy et al.'s (2005) reflective exercises in Activity box 12.1.

ACTIVITY BOX 12.1 HOW DO YOU FEEL ABOUT RESEARCH?

1. What five to ten adjectives best capture your experiences of or feelings towards research? How do these compare with the five to ten adjectives that best capture your experiences of or feelings towards working in clinical practice?
2. If you have ever been required to carry out a research study, what metaphor would you use to capture your experience?
3. Please complete one or both of these poems:
   a. Roses are red/Violets are blue/Research is . . .
   b. Violets are blue/Roses are red/Research is . . .

(adapted from Piercy et al., 2005)

Looking at how you responded to the exercises in Activity box 12.1, you might reflect on what research seems to represent to you. Is it a passion, a means to an end, a dread, a curiosity, an excitement, a mix, or something else entirely? Do you see research and clinical practice as different, even opposite kinds of activities, or not? What happens if you change the headings around in Question 1?

As authors, we would like to take a moment to reflect on our own perspectives on research. We are both excited by research and continually engaged in a number of research activities: doing, teaching, and supervising research, reading research and relating it to our therapeutic work, and vice versa. Having observed the changes and developments in the last decade, we believe that the profession is now at an exciting and potentially transformative moment in its relationship with research. We see research and practice becoming increasingly integrated with one another in counselling psychologists' activities, and we believe that this spells significant benefits and opportunities both for individual practitioners and for the profession at large.

This chapter will demonstrate how research and practice can be seen as continually enriching of one another, in a 'virtuous cycle'.

The evolution of the profession, its training, and its research

The humanistic core of counselling psychology

Arguably every applied psychology is defined by the application of knowledge and theories derived from psychological research. In the case of counselling psychology, certain elements of the profession's history may help explain why its relationship with research may be more complicated than in some of the other branches of psychology. Counselling psychology in the UK was inspired by a group of psychologists whose main interest was psychotherapy, and whose main influences were the values and ideas of the humanistic psychology movement. James Bugental's famous 'mission statement' for this movement (1964) proposed that individual human beings are unique, whole, more than the sum of their parts, and not reducible to components.

While these humanistic values still resonate with how many counselling psychologists might want to approach psychotherapy, they also potentially affect how counselling psychologists might evaluate the capacity of research to contribute to practice. If a client is a unique being, the therapist is also a unique being, and the encounter between them one of a kind, how can knowledge derived from one therapeutic situation apply to another? How can any kind of research conducted with participants – from single case studies to large-scale quantitative investigations – apply to a uniquely constituted therapeutic relationship?

Humanistic values are still at the core of counselling psychology today. For instance, the description of the field on the British Psychological Society's website states that counselling psychologists "work with the individual's unique subjective psychological experience" (http://careers.bps.org.uk/area/counselling, n.d.). In the same passage, however, it says that counselling psychologists are "concerned with the integration of psychological theory and research with therapeutic practice" (ibid). The challenge for each of us, and as a field, is to find ways of expressing the values of our profession through our research activity, as a form of "ethics in action" (Cooper, 2009, p. 120). The first time we are called to find this integration is early on in our professional development, as trainees, when we are required to undertake research as a significant part of our journey towards qualification as counselling psychologists.

The changing landscape of research and training

Anyone interested in training as a counselling psychologist will observe that an interest in research and a willingness to carry out a research study are essential (Orlans, 2013). You should be able to see this clearly when you engage in the exercise in Activity box 12.2.

ACTIVITY BOX 12.2 RESEARCH AND QUALIFYING AS A COUNSELLING PSYCHOLOGIST

Go to the BPS website (www.bps.org.uk), locate the search engine for accredited training programmes, and search for counselling psychology. At the time of writing there are 13 approved taught routes to qualification in the UK. Go to the websites for any programmes that interest you.

What do you notice about how the different counselling psychology programmes talk about research? How is research positioned relative to other elements of training (theoretical input, clinical practice, personal development)? Is it presented as a separate element, an integrated one, or both? What do the words used seem to imply about attitudes to and ethos around research?

The university-based taught route is not the only path to qualification. Search for 'society qualifications' on the BPS website to locate the Qualification in Counselling Psychology (QCoP) and look at the Candidate Handbook. How is research positioned there? Use the same questions as above.

You may have noticed interesting differences in how trainings talk about research. However, you will likely have seen reference in all trainings to the multiple research modules you will take, the research supervision you will receive, the number of words your thesis or portfolio might need to be, and details of how you must demonstrate your research skills in order to be admitted in the first place – mini-research proposals, pieces of research you have done before, marks on undergraduate research modules, and so forth.

Research did not always represent such a large proportion of the work of training. Once upon a time, a doctorate was not required in order to become a counselling psychologist; the threshold for qualification was a master's dissertation. In 2006, anticipating eventual statutory regulation of psychologists in the United Kingdom, the Division of Counselling Psychology set doctoral-level training as the expected professional standard for counselling psychology training. That standard went on to become statutory three years later, in 2009, when the Health and Care Professions Council (HCPC) began regulating practitioner psychologists. What did the shift to doctoral level really mean for the kind of research that we need to produce en route to qualification?

What are the essential differences between master's level and doctoral research? From the UK Quality Assurance Agency (QAA, 2008), we know that doctoral research must *extend* its field by making an *original* contribution to knowledge. Reading further into the QAA descriptions of master's and doctoral qualifications, however, is illuminating. True to its name, a master's qualification involves *mastery* of a topic, and of suitable methods for investigating that topic. Part of mastery is being able *to think critically* – to understand that all knowledge comes from people, and that all people have particular perspectives or positions. While some master's dissertations may involve generating new knowledge, the baseline requirement is to unpack, critically examine, and thus master something that already exists in the world.

Holders of doctoral-level qualifications need to do all of this too, but there is an additional requirement, beyond mastery. Here, too, the clue is in the name. A doctor fixes something that needs to be fixed, *identifying a problem that needs to be addressed.* Imagine a patient visiting a medical doctor and presenting him or her with a myriad of health complaints. Particularly in this age of ten-minute, one-symptom-at-a-time appointments, the doctor must decide what is the most important problem to tackle first – at the edge, the forefront of the patient's concerns, and what they know about these. In doing so, the doctor hopes *to help, to make a contribution, and to do some good.* This is also relevant to a doctor in an applied psychology context – having assimilated the state of knowledge in a field, the task is to find the (research) question that needs to be asked, and answered, next. The professional practices of doctors in counselling psychology – whether therapy or research – are oriented towards social action designed to alleviate suffering (Castonguay, 2011). Just as medical doctors contribute to improving patients' health, doctors of counselling psychology must contribute knowledge that advances the field. They take greater responsibility for and ownership of the process and product of their discoveries, and have a stronger remit to put that research into practice in the world, in order to make a difference. This is the moral imperative of counselling psychology research at the doctoral level and beyond: actively considering *who will benefit from your research, and how this benefit will be realised* – 'ethics in action'.

This close connection and relationship between research and practice, or the practical, is further reflected in the fact that all taught routes to counselling psychology qualification in the UK are **professional (or practitioner) doctorates** (abbreviated as DPsych, PsychD, DCounsPsy). Like a PhD, a professional doctorate must produce new knowledge at the forefront of an academic discipline; however, additionally this knowledge must develop individual professional practice and produce knowledge useful to and usable within the wider professional field. Professional doctorates are "normally rooted in an academic discipline *as well as in a profession*" (QAA, 2011, p. 19, our italics).

Lester (2004) suggests that the traditional PhD represents 'mode one knowledge' – an idea of 'pure' abstract knowledge that can be 'applied' to practice in a sequential, linear fashion. In contrast, professional doctorates generate 'mode two knowledge' through a more cyclical relationship between practice and knowledge. This converts doctoral knowledge into a kind of reflective, experiential learning, akin to Aristotle's idea of 'practical wisdom' – which counselling psychologists might gain from and feed back into the busy and complicated environments in which they work. In this context, doctoral counselling psychologists are . . . particularly capable practitioners, with an enhanced ability to improvise and make decisions, in complex, evolving situations (Costley, 2013).

What happens in one's training sets the stage for one's future career, and research is no exception. Counselling psychology professional doctorates not only emphasise research, but promote a dialogical relationship between practice and research, and an ethical commitment to carry out research 'that does good'. We believe that trainees now emerging from programmes are far more likely to continue research engagement in their post-qualification life, and to realise a more intimate, multi-layered connection between their research and practice. The next section considers the kinds of research counselling psychologists might engage with, at doctoral level, and beyond, all of which, in different ways, reflect our suggestions so far about counselling psychology research as ethics in action.

Form and function for counselling psychology research

We live in an era of 'evidence-based everything' (Oakley, Gough, Oliver, & Thomas, 2005). In the UK, bodies such as the National Institute for Health and Care Excellence (NICE) and the Social Care Institute for Excellence (SCIE) determine which health and social care practices are 'evidence-based'. These decisions affect (and to some extent may be determined by) the commissioning of services, the funding of treatments and therapies, and the employment of practitioners. To make these decisions, the outcomes or results of treatments are compared using a hierarchical framework of evidence. The gold standard of evidence is the randomised controlled trial (RCT), a form of experiment that compares the outcomes of one treatment against the outcomes of another under controlled conditions.

Of course, there needs to be some basis, economically, for allocating resources and demarcating services in healthcare settings (McLeod, 2001). However, critics have argued that RCT methods, while perhaps appropriate for drug trials, are not suitable tests for psychotherapy – in therapy, the 'active ingredients' are harder to isolate, and RCT methods cannot reflect, logically or practically, the practices and values of therapy in real world settings (Cartwright, 2007; Rogers, Maidman, & House, 2011). Others have suggested that the hierarchy of evidence has excluded alternative forms of knowledge and encouraged the dissemination of overly prepackaged, protocolised therapeutic practices (Holmes, Murray, Perron, & Rail, 2006).

Midgley (2009) has highlighted the experiences of Archibald Cochrane, one of the formative influences on the evidence-based era in the UK (cf. www.cochranelibrary.com). In his autobiography, Cochrane described his painful experiences as a doctor treating fellow officers for tuberculosis in a prisoner-of-war camp during the Second World War. Cochrane experienced huge uncertainty about what form of treatment to offer, and came away from the experience feeling devastated that the actions he took may inadvertently have contributed unnecessarily to further deaths and suffering. These painful experiences may have left Cochrane with a deep distrust of human judgment.

Indeed, the place of subjectivity or judgment within evidence-based practice seems ambivalent, perhaps even fragile. This is a particular issue for psychotherapy and counselling psychology, arguably more so than for medicine, since psychotherapy is so clearly a dialogical practice, and one that seems to involve uniqueness, intersubjectivity, uncertainty, and complexity, at its heart. As Donald Schön suggested in his book *The Reflective Practitioner* (1987), perhaps there is much about psychotherapy that cannot be fully put into words. Drawing on the example of cookery, Thornton (2006) suggests that even the most detailed recipe books, such as those of the British cookery writer Delia Smith, who prescribes nine steps for making a piece of toast, will never be able to encompass everything we know or need to know at any one time about cooking. For instance, why does the temperature of our hands need to be warm when we make pastry, but not when we make toast? Whatever explicit guidelines or protocols we have to guide our judgments in practice, what will count as correctly following these will always remain to some degree tacit or implicit (Wittgenstein, 1953).

In the light of this apparent dilemma between evidence and practice in psychotherapy, what forms of research might counselling psychologists engage in? How can we take action in the evidence-based world while simultaneously holding onto our humanistic values and philosophy? These kinds of dilemmas can sometimes take the form 'either ors' and lead to anxious 'fight or flight' modes of relating. However, in Table 12.1, I [Isabel] offer an inclusive framework for the kinds of research that counselling psychologists in training and beyond might engage with, and some examples.

You will notice that the framework below is not divided according to qualitative and quantitative methodological distinctions. Counselling psychology tends to eschew methodological divides ('methodolatry') in favour of **methodological pluralism.** In many ways, methodological pluralism in research is similar to client-centredness in therapy – the choice of approach or method is centred around the research question, and both may need to be re-negotiated as time goes on. Just as the needs of the client inform the approach in client-centred work, so in methodological pluralism, the research (topic, question, participants, aims,

TABLE 12.1 Forms of research for counselling psychology

Forms of research	*How these reflect counselling psychology's humanistic values while generating useful 'evidence' – ethics in action*	*Examples*
Research relevant to counselling psychology's professional practices outside psychotherapy (e.g., training, research, supervision, personal and professional development, academia, management, consultancy, social action)	Counselling psychology is a relatively young profession in the UK, but a highly contemporary one, having anticipated many trends in recent years such as the need for reflective practice and personal therapy within training, and the social justice and diversity agenda. Counselling psychology research studies continue to support and develop all areas of practice within the profession.	Rizq & Target (2008) explored the role of personal therapy in developing practitioner competence in counselling psychology. Their participants told them personal therapy had helped them to establish authentic emotional contact with themselves and their clients. Most felt personal therapy should remain obligatory in training. The authors explored these findings in the context of the theory of mentalisation (Fonagy & Target, 1996).
Research which is relevant to psychotherapy but not about psychotherapy	Basic or pure research about experiences, meanings, symptoms, epidemiology, social and cultural contexts, co-factors, discourses, aetiologies or other explanatory frameworks or trajectories, communities, or life-stages. These areas of research can inform counselling psychologists in their psychotherapeutic work, in seeking to help diverse people in diverse contexts.	Josselin & Willig (2015) used a pluralistic research approach to explore chronic self-injury behaviour among women. These researchers found divergent ways of making meaning of this phenomenon, oriented around themes of control, guilt, and relatedness. Their study suggested a need for a careful, exploratory, client-centred approach to working with self-injury to allow space for the multiple, potentially contradictory meanings of self-injury to emerge.
Experimental psychotherapy research (RCTs)	Counselling Psychologist Mick Cooper (2011) has proposed ways of doing RCTs or pilot RCTs that may be more congruent with counselling psychology's values. For instance, therapy manuals might be more descriptive than prescriptive of practice; broader, non-symptom-oriented outcome measures might be conceived; and treatment groups can be non-diagnostically determined. Cooper (2016) argues for collaboration and an outward focus in research, to support the asking of questions that matter to the outside world.	Cooper (2016) has been involved in a programme of research to support and develop counselling in schools in collaboration with the British Association of Counselling and Psychotherapy (BACP) for over ten years. Work began in Glasgow, in a small-scale counselling for schools project funded by the Glasgow NHS. Small-scale mixed methods effectiveness studies followed in 2004 and 2006; a comprehensive review of evidence in 2009; and a pilot RCT in 2010. Cooper subsequently gained funding for a large RCT in 2015.

(Continued)

TABLE 12.1 (Continued)

Forms of research	*How these reflect counselling psychology's humanistic values while generating useful 'evidence' – ethics in action*	*Examples*
Practice-oriented effectiveness studies	Studies of effectiveness in 'real world' settings, which can often be large-scale and use mixed methods. Such studies ask wide-ranging questions not only about outcomes, but about how many sessions are needed (dose-response), long-term longitudinal effects, and mediators and moderators in therapy. Effectiveness studies can generate nuanced 'practice-oriented' data, while at the same time engaging with the terms of NICE's hierarchy of evidence, which allows for some forms of effectiveness research (such as cohort studies).	Barkham (2014) is undertaking a large cohort study across 93 inner-city and rural GP practices in Derbyshire. This mixed method design compares counselling with CBT for depression, and incorporates an RCT, an effectiveness study within routine clinical practice, and qualitative research. The study will answer questions such as, for instance, is therapy that takes place within an RCT context more or less effective than the same therapy in routine services? Do individual therapists make a difference, statistically, to outcomes? How do the most effective therapists talk about their work? Which clients drop out of therapy? What do clients say helped them to change?
Smaller scale accounts of psychotherapy	While less privileged under current NICE guidelines, smaller scale accounts of psychotherapy can be gathered retrospectively from clients, therapists, or both, through data collection techniques such as diaries, interviews, or focus groups. Such studies can be carried out independently or nested within wider research programmes such as RCTs or cohort studies and can focus on different aspects of and contexts for different kinds of therapy. This form of research aims to inform and improve practice by giving voice to the participants of therapy, deepening our understandings of how therapy works, and exploring the interface between therapy, language, and the wider world.	Midgley et al. (2014) explored the hopes and expectations for therapy among 77 moderate to severely depressed young people, who were interviewed using a semi-structured interview schedule. Data was analysed qualitatively using framework analysis. Participants spoke about "the difficulty of imagining what will happen in therapy," "the 'talking cure,' " "the therapist as doctor," "therapy as a relationship," and "regaining the old self or developing new capacities." The study concluded that differing expectations were likely to have implications for how young people engaged with treatment, and failure to identify these expectations could increase the risk of treatment breakdown.

(Continued)

TABLE 12.1 (Continued)

Forms of research	*How these reflect counselling psychology's humanistic values while generating useful 'evidence' – ethics in action*	*Examples*
Case study research	Single case studies or case series research are referenced lower down the NICE hierarchy of evidence, despite their long heritage in psychotherapy. Case studies vary in form from more 'narrative' to more 'systematic' versions. At their best, these studies provide 'evidence' for what works in therapy and how it works, by drawing on multiple sources of data, describing processes and outcomes over time, and describing therapy in context, enabling readers to better judge how useful findings might be to their own situation.	Thurston, McLeod, & Thurston (2013) investigated counselling for a 70-year-old client who had experienced complete, irreversible, post-operative sight loss, in order to understand what was helpful from the client's point of view. A Hermeneutic Single-Case Efficacy Design generated a rich case record that was analysed by a quasi-judicial enquiry team. Results suggested therapy was successful. The client found therapy a helpful opportunity to express emotions around the loss of sight; begin to find a new identity; find ways to cope with fear, loss, dependency, and other people's perceptions; explore the possibility of a positive future without sight; and find new ways to become more socially connected. This study might inform the development of a practice model for an under-researched client group.
Process research	Process research explores the 'interior' of therapy at the micro-level, aiming to identify particular therapy processes, and potentially link these to therapeutic change or outcome. Innovative process research methods have evolved and developed since the 1950s, and include quantitative, narrative, discursive, and dynamic systems approaches. Although process research is not currently admissible in the NICE hierarchy of evidence, this form of research does have the capacity both to reflect the complexities of therapy, to evidence its value or how it works (well), and to be used as a training tool.	Balmforth & Elliott (2012) explored how a particular client disclosure that proved very helpful to the client came about in therapy and what made it important to the client. A bespoke process research method was used called Comprehensive Process Analysis. This analysis showed in detail how the therapist had facilitated the disclosure by careful listening to and following up on the client's hints, trusting the strength of the alliance, and staying close to the client's frame of reference.

Source: Adapted from Midgley (2004)'s rubric for psychotherapy research – a set of concentric circles, zooming in, from broadly relevant areas to the fine detail of therapy work.

contribution) is privileged over the method *per se*, which should not 'come first'. Carl Rogers was a great proponent of methodological pluralism. He argued: "(w)e should realise that there is no special virtue to any one procedure . . . In all instances, the method of testing should be appropriate to the hypothesis, the pattern, the 'vision of reality' " (Rogers, 1968, p. 274). In other words, methodological pluralism suggests that no form of research is better than any other form, and no form should be automatically rejected. Consequently methodological pluralism has been characterised as an egalitarian, ethical, and pragmatic stance towards research – perhaps another form of ethics in action for counselling psychology.

The counselling psychologist researcher

As the doctoral culture intensifies within training programmes, we are also seeing more publications arising from doctoral research. Investment in their own employability, or perhaps a sense of greater commitment to knowledge dissemination, is prompting counselling psychologist-academics to create a stronger culture of expectation around research dissemination. At the time of writing, I (Elaine) have supervisees looking at not just mourning and bereavement online (my own research interest), but at problematic online behaviours after romantic breakup; acculturation in the age of social networking; and body-image construction and evaluation in the context of Instagram. Together, we present symposia at conferences, together we will eventually publish, and together we are co-creating a research cluster that will benefit not just me and my students, but the department, the university, and the audiences for whom we create and disseminate knowledge.

Incorporating research into the portfolio career and increasing employability: A case study

If my own supervisees do become lifelong practitioner-researchers they will be part of a new breed, for research and publication activity has been traditionally been low amongst counselling psychologists (Gordon & Hanley, 2013). However, without question, research engagement can make you far more competitive and employable in today's marketplace. At baseline, research skills increase the number of places you can work, and the number of roles that you can fulfil. A clinician who also has experience in service audit and evaluation and/or outcome research, for example, is a more attractive employment prospect in a service than someone who offers psychological therapy alone. Beyond this, however, when you do doctoral-level research in a particular area, and follow this up by publishing, presenting, and/or developing workshops and trainings in that area, you are seen as an *expert* in that area – in fact, you are often viewed as far more of an expert than you may actually feel yourself to be! One of my trainees, who produced a publication on a particular approach to counselling drug addiction at an earlier stage in training, described to me how easy it subsequently was for her to secure placements in this area.

For individuals with even a passing interest in entering academia and in training the psychologists of the future, research and scholarship can never hurt your career, and increasingly research and scholarship is a *sine qua non* not only for initial employment as a permanent faculty member, but for advancement once there.

Because role models in relation to the above are relatively scarce and published examples few and far between, I offer my own case study below.

CASE STUDY: ELAINE'S RESEARCH JOURNEY

As an undergraduate psychology major in the United States, I associated research with the laboratories where I assisted PhD candidates with a spot of participant recruitment, some data collection, and a lot of data entry. When short of cash, I volunteered in other labs to put my arm in ice water, press buttons in response to stimuli, or rate attractiveness of faces. I was aiming to secure entry onto a clinical psychology postgraduate programme, where I primarily wanted to learn about psychotherapy, but where I knew that I would "have to" do research to get my doctorate.

When I reached that doctoral programme, we were tutored exclusively in quantitative research methods, and I spent three years circumventing research, concentrating on clinical placements and coursework. When I took a break midway through and embarked on a master's degree in counselling psychology in London, I suddenly realised what somehow had not been obvious before: when I identified research questions that mattered to me and to other people, and had a clear application in the world, *I did not feel like avoiding research anymore.*

At that time, the idea of online delivery of mental health services was quite fresh, and the first major book about it had only just come out (Grohol, 2002). Here was a new context that changed or challenged many things about psychotherapy. As-yet-unstudied questions exploded everywhere, like popcorn: What about ethics? What about the relationship? What about the frame? What about risk? Because many practitioners at that time were simultaneously concerned and curious about the possibilities that online mental health resources and interventions presented, there was a lot of interest in my descriptive phenomenological study of the experience of seasoned practitioners conducting therapy online. The multiple existential implications of my findings made *Existential Analysis* (Kasket, 2003a) an ideal journal for my first research article, and I also presented at my first counselling psychology conference (Kasket, 2003b). Four key points are worth noting here: (1) I had stumbled onto an area that was novel and topical; (2) it mattered and was relevant to people's practice; (3) it challenged existing theory; and (4) I felt excited and interested by it as a consequence of 1 through 3.

I returned to my U.S. doctoral programme with renewed motivation. As a doctor's daughter, I had personal reasons for wanting to investigate the physician's experience of patient death, but it was also a topic that coincided with some buzz around functional MRI research on physicians that had recently come out. In publishing and conferencing (Kasket, 2006a, 2006b, 2007b), I at first focused on my usual audience, existential psychotherapists, but quickly realised this was too limited. The field of medical education seemed intensely interested in what I had studied; people from many disciplines were requesting copies of my *Existential Analysis* articles; and references to it were spreading on the Internet. Copyright prevented me from republishing the work elsewhere, so I settled for speaking at my first multidisciplinary event, a conference focused on death and dying (Kasket, 2007a). When a BBC journalist asked to speak with me, having plucked my paper from amongst the press releases from the conference, I realised that I could have an impact *beyond my profession.* Doing work with relevance to multiple disciplines has been a driver for me ever since.

After qualification, no one forced me to continue to research and publish – I found, however, that I *wanted* to. While searching for an old friend on the new social networking site Facebook, I stumbled across the "posthumously persistent" personal page of a similarly named girl and saw how people were continuing to interact with the profile; that inspired my first "degree independent" research study, an intersection of my previously researched areas: the online context, and death/mourning. Since that moment, on this topic, I have lost count of the number of presentations given to bereavement practitioners (e.g., Kasket, 2011); academic articles published (e.g., Kasket, 2012); contributions made to mass-media news and feature articles, TV news spots and documentaries, and radio programmes; and keynote invitations received. I am now considered an expert in this area, and I feed my research back into my own clinical practice with bereaved people. I hit the motherlode: an exciting, current research and scholarship area that feels intellectually stimulating and practically important to (1) me, (2) psychotherapeutic practitioners both in and outside of the counselling psychology field, (3) academics and practitioners in other fields entirely, *and* (4) the lay public.

When I was applying for academic promotion to Principal Lecturer at my university, the thing that the committee cared most about was the extent to which I had engaged in research and scholarly activity, and the ways in which I had shared my knowledge with the world of academics, practitioners, and the rest of the world through publication, conferencing, and public engagement. It also mattered to them that my work was of clear benefit, that it had *impact*. Not only do I take pride in that, but I have taken comfort in the fact that my publication record, relatively modest by some standards but certainly more than respectable in the context of the counselling psychology field, has protected me and will continue to serve as relative job security in a time where things are a bit tough for academics. I also know that it would stand me in good stead if I made a career change. From my point of view, if research is going to help you with job security, you may as well sweeten the pot even further by doing something beneficial to both you and others.

Summary

Partly because of the relatively recent 'doctoralisation' of the counselling psychology profession in the United Kingdom, the discipline is currently engaged in what we think is a fruitful re-examination of its perspective on research, and its engagement in research activity. If you are reading this chapter as someone contemplating a career in counselling psychology, or someone who is in the initial stages of your training, consider this question: How can *what* you research, and *how* you research it, do good in the world? How will it make a difference? In other words: How can your own research turn the humanistic ethos at the heart of counselling psychology into tangible benefits in the real world? Finding meaningful answers to these questions may just turn you into a lifelong researcher.

Learning outcomes

When you have completed this chapter, you should be able to:

- Appreciate the importance of research for your development as a counselling psychologist.

- Understand the relationship between research and practice, values, and ethos in counselling psychology.
- Be familiar with the kinds of research that counselling psychologists might engage with in their professional practice.
- Recognise how engaging with research can not only energise your working life and expand your professional opportunities, but can also benefit the profession at large and the wider world.

Key phrases, concepts and terms

- Methodological pluralism
- Professional doctorate
- Professional practice

Self-test questions

- How can research within counselling psychology strive towards having a 'humanistic ethic' at its core?
- What is the difference between a professional doctorate and a PhD?
- Why might counselling psychology have a conflicted relationship with evidence-based practice?
- What is meant by methodological pluralism?
- What makes it more likely that a practitioner will continue research engagement after professional qualification?

Further reading

Douglas, B., Woolfe, R., Strawbridge, S., Kasket, E., & Galbraith, V. (Eds.). (2016). *Handbook of counselling psychology* (4th ed.). London, UK: Sage.

Vossler, A., & Moller, N. (Eds.). (2014). *The counselling and psychotherapy research handbook*. London, UK: Sage.

Useful weblinks

Division of Counselling Psychology – British Psychological Society: dcop.bps.org.uk/
Health and Care Professions Council: www.hcpc-uk.co.uk
Quality Assurance Agency: www.qaa.ac.uk/

References

Balmforth, J., & Elliott, R. (2012). 'I never talked about, ever': A comprehensive process analysis of a significant client disclosure event in therapy. *Counselling and Psychotherapy Research*, *12*(1), 2–12.

Barkham, M. (2014, May). *The PRaCTICED trial: The arguments, aims and aspirations*. Paper presented at the British Association of Counselling Psychotherapy's annual research conference, London, England.

Bugental, J.F. (1964). The third force in psychology. *Journal of Humanistic Psychology*, *4*(1), 19–26.

Cartwright, N. (2007). Are RCTs the gold standard? *BioSocieties*, *2*, 11–20.

Castonguay, L.G. (2011). Psychotherapy, psychopathology, research and practice: Pathways of connections and integration. *Psychotherapy Research*, *21*(2), 125–140.

Cooper, M. (2009). Welcoming the Other: Actualising the humanistic ethic at the core of counselling psychology practice. *Counselling Psychology Review, 24*(3–4), 119–129.

Cooper, M. (2011). Meeting the demand for evidence-based practice. *Therapy Today, 22*(4), 10–16.

Cooper, M. (2016). *From local evaluation to national impact: Developing a programme of research on school-based counselling*. Keynote paper presented at BACP research conference, 20th May, Brighton, UK.

Costley, C. (2013). Evaluation of the current status and knowledge contributions of professional doctorates. *Quality in Higher Education, 19*(1), 7–27.

Douglas, B., Woolfe, R., Strawbridge, S., Kasket, E., & Galbraith, V. (Eds.). (2016). *Handbook of counselling psychology* (4th ed.). London, UK: Sage.

Fonagy, P., & Target, M. (1996). Playing with reality I. *The International Journal of Psychoanalysis*, 77(2), 217.

Gordon, R., & Hanley, T. (2013). Where do counselling psychologists based in the UK disseminate their research? A systematic review. *Counselling Psychology Review, 28*(4), 7–17.

Grohol, J.M. (2002). *The insider's guide to mental health resources online*. New York: Guilford Press.

Holmes, D., Murray, S. J., Perron, A., & Rail, G. (2006). Deconstructing the evidence-based discourse in health sciences: Truth, power and fascism. *International Journal of Evidence-Based Healthcare, 4*(3), 180–186. doi: 10.1111/j.1479-6988.2006.00041.x

Josselin, D., & Willig, C. (2015). Making sense of self-injury: A pluralistic case-study. *Counselling Psychology Review, 30*(4), 5–15.

Kasket, E. (2003a). Online counselling: Some considerations for existential-phenomenological practitioners. *Existential Analysis, 14*(1), 60–74.

Kasket, E. (2003b, May). *The experience of the online counselling psychologist*. Paper presented at the Division of Counselling Psychology annual conference, Stratford-upon-Avon.

Kasket, E. (2006a). Death and the doctor: Part II. *Existential Analysis, 17*(2), 385–396.

Kasket, E. (2006b). Death and the doctor. *Existential Analysis, 17*(1), 137–150.

Kasket, E. (2007a, September). *Death and the doctor*. Paper presented at the 8th International Conference on the Social Context of Death, Dying and Disposal, Centre for Death and Society, University of Bath, UK.

Kasket, E. (2007b, February). *Death and the doctor: The physician's existential dilemma*. Paper presented at the Society for Existential Analysis Forum, Tavistock Centre, London.

Kasket, E. (2011). *Continuing bonds in the age of social networking*. Paper presented at the 10th International Conference of the Social Context of Death, Dying and Disposal, Nijmegen, the Netherlands.

Kasket, E. (2012). Continuing bonds in the age of social networking. *Bereavement Care, 31*(2), 62–69. doi: 10.1080/02682621.2012.710493

Lester, S. (2004). Conceptualising the practitioner doctorate. *Studies in Higher Education, 29*(6), 757–770.

McLeod, J. (2001). Developing a research tradition consistent with the practices and values of counselling and psychotherapy: Why 'counselling and psychotherapy research' is necessary. *Counselling & Psychotherapy Research, 1*(1), 3–11.

Midgley, N. (2004). Sailing between Scylla and Charybdis: Incorporating qualitative approaches into child psychotherapy research. *Journal of Child Psychotherapy, 30*(1), 89–111.

Midgley, N. (2009). Editorial: Improvers, adapters and rejecters: The link between 'evidence-based practice' and 'evidence-based practitioners'. *Clinical Child Psychology and Psychiatry, 14*(3), 323–327.

Midgley, N., Holmes, J., Parkinson, S., Stapley, E., Eatough, V., & Target, M. (2014). 'Just like talking to someone about like shit in your life and stuff, and they help you': Hopes and expectations for therapy among depressed adolescents. *Psychotherapy Research, 26*(1), 1–11.

Oakley, A., Gough, D., Oliver, S., & Thomas, J. (2005). The politics of evidence and methodology: Lessons from the EPPI-Centre. *Evidence and Policy, 1*(1), 5–31.

Orlans, V. (2013). The nature and scope of counselling psychology. In G. Davey (Ed.), *Applied Psychologies* [Student Companion Site]. Chichester, West Sussex: Wiley.

Piercy, F.P., McWey, L.M., Tice, S., James, E.J., Morris, M., & Arthur, K. (2005). It was the best of times: It was the worst of times: Doctoral students' experiences of family therapy research training through alternative forms of data representation. *Family Process, 44*(3), 363–378.

Quality Assurance Agency. (2008). The framework for higher education qualifications in England, Wales and Northern Ireland. Retrieved August 2, 2014 from www.qaa.ac.uk/Publications/InformationandGuidance/Documents/FHEQ08.pdf

Quality Assurance Agency. (2011). Doctoral degree characteristics. Retrieved August 2, 2014 from www.qaa.ac.uk/Publications/InformationAndGuidance/Documents/Doctoral_Characteristics.pdf

Rizq, R., & Target, M. (2008). 'Not a little Mickey Mouse thing': How experienced counselling psychologists describe the significance of personal therapy in clinical practice and training: Some results from an interpretative phenomenological analysis. *Counselling Psychology Quarterly*, *21*(1), 29–48.

Rogers, C. R. (1968). Some thoughts regarding the current presuppositions of the behavioral sciences. In H. Kirschenbaum & V. L. Henderson (Eds.) (1989), *The Carl Rogers reader* (pp. 263–278). Boston: Houghton Mifflin Company.

Rogers, A., Maidman, J., & House, R. (2011). The bad faith of evidence-based practice: Beyond counsels of despair. *Therapy Today*, *22*(6), 26–29.

Schön, D.A. (1987). *The reflective practitioner: How professionals think in action.* New York: Basic Books.

Thornton, T. (2006). Tacit knowledge as a unifying factor in evidence-based medicine and clinical judgment. *Philosophy, Ethics, and Humanities in Medicine*, *1*(2), 1–10.

Thurston, M., McLeod, J., & Thurston, A. (2013). Counselling for sight loss: Using systematic case study research to build a client informed practice model. *British Journal of Visual Impairment*, *31*(2), 102–122.

Wittgenstein, L. (1953). *Philosophical investigations.* Oxford, UK: Blackwell.

SECTION 6

Developments, training, roles and competencies

13

PROFESSIONAL DEVELOPMENTS IN COUNSELLING PSYCHOLOGY

Helen Nicholas

Chapter overview

The first part of the chapter outlines the importance of belonging to a professional organisation and then goes on to explain how counselling psychologists often choose to affiliate with specific groups, and divisions of counselling psychology. The chapter will focus on what it means to belong to a 'professional home' for psychology and psychologists, and how it provides members with a sense of belonging, support, opportunities to network and other essential professional benefits, such as guidelines, policies and advice. The emphasis will also be on the various regulatory bodies that govern practitioners. Key government policies and particular threats will be described including protected titles that may serve to promote counselling psychology and its unique skills. The chapter will focus on the importance of identifying with core values in the profession and how these overlap greatly within the profession worldwide.

The second part of the chapter will look at developing your professional career path and professional development as counselling psychologists, through continuing professional development, focusing on key values, your own **identity** and career choices. The chapter will highlight the variety in our profession and some of the opportunities afforded to members, such as forming professional connections, and the many transferable skills that counselling psychologists possess. Some suggestions will be made about how you can become more involved within your professional organisation to enhance your professional development as a counselling psychologist.

The importance of belonging to a professional organisation

Many mental health professions have a dedicated body that will act to promote their profession. For psychologists there is the Australian Psychological Society, Canadian Psychological Association, Chinese Psychological Association, American Psychological Association, and the British Psychological Society. These organisations are often responsible for promoting psychology, accrediting training courses, publishing research and play a key part in credentialing and registering psychologists from a variety of specialisms. They also play a key role in ensuring high standards of education, training and practice through their accreditation programmes and learning opportunities, such as courses, annual conferences and working with partner companies to deliver training.

For psychologists in the UK, the **British Psychological Society (BPS)** has been the representative body for psychology and psychologists since 1901 and was granted its Royal Charter in 1965. As a learned society, the BPS is seen as the 'home' of psychologists and psychology, responsible for the development, promotion and application of psychology for the public good. It also promotes the field of psychology and psychologists by ensuring that high standards of professional education and knowledge are adhered to. The BPS aims to:

- Be the learned society and professional body for the discipline;
- Make psychology accessible to all;
- Promote and advance the discipline;
- Be the authoritative and public voice of psychology;
- Determine and ensure the highest standards in all we do.

(www.bps.org.uk)

Many psychological organisations build relationships with each other by signing a memorandum of understanding (MOU). This enables them to set out their shared interest and how they will work together in the future. The BPS in the UK has a number of MOUs with organisations such as the American Psychological Society, and more recently the Russian Psychological Society. These international links help to forge key relationships between countries for the promotion of psychology and the public interest. The APA also has reciprocal partnerships with 18 countries, where it supports its psychologists to attend the annual conferences in other countries, for example, Australia, China, Ireland, Mexico, New Zealand, Spain, Sweden (APA, 2016).

Psychologists may choose to be a member of their professional organisation for a number of reasons. These may include being able to access a wider range of courses, workshops, conferences and continuing professional development opportunities. Some will choose to become more involved in their profession by joining working parties within the psychological association, influencing governmental consultations, and policy development. A sense of **belonging** to a larger community, giving back to the profession and ensuring that their profession is represented at the highest level provides many with a sense of group cohesion.

Membership of your **professional body** is what you make of it and how you choose to engage or not in the organisations, its policies, influences and groups. Volunteering in these professional organisations provides valuable professional development opportunities that can serve to develop your own profession and be a part of the field of psychology, whilst networking with and learning from others.

Professionally affiliating with a division of counselling psychology

For many counselling psychologists, being a member of a professional body does not necessarily bring with it the identity of being a counselling psychologist that many value. Counselling psychologists seek a professional association that is exclusively for **counselling psychology** and counselling psychologists that will acknowledge their core values, historic roots and therapeutic stance.

Most professional bodies have divisions or groups dedicated to the diverse specialty fields within psychology. The historical development of counselling psychology throughout the world often features a division, section or institute that focuses on the specialty of counselling psychology. This is often in the context of a long history and process of seeking their own identity as professional psychologists.

For instance, a small group of scholars developed the section of counselling psychology within the Canadian Psychological Association (Bedi et al., 2016). The Society of Counseling Psychology (DIV 17) of the American Psychological Association began as the Personnel Guidance Psychology, then as the Division of Counseling and Guidance before becoming the Society of Counseling Psychology (Lichtenberg et al., 2016). The growth of counselling psychology as a profession internationally has lent itself to the increased demand for a place where counselling psychologists can network, follow their interests and affiliate with organisations that professionally fulfil their specialism needs.

You will find a **Division of** Counselling Psychology in countries such as Australia, the United States of America and the United Kingdom. Canada has a section of counselling psychology, and South Korea has a division of counselling and psychotherapy. Each division has been formed to highlight the specialist and distinctive training that counselling psychologists receive and the unique skills they bring to the field of psychology.

In the UK, the Division of Counselling Psychology (DCoP) is the third-largest division within the BPS and has over 3,500 members. It began as a section in 1982 and was later recognised as a special group in 1989 and then a division in 1994. The DCoP celebrated its 21st anniversary at a celebratory dinner held in Harrogate during the 2015 DCoP annual conference. The anniversary holds significant meaning to counselling psychology, the history of how it became a division and to the identity of counselling psychologists. The journey to divisional status was an acknowledgement of the status of counselling psychology as an applied psychology and in the space of three decades, counselling psychology has established itself as a specialist applied psychology field, alongside other applied psychology divisions such as clinical, occupational, health and educational. Full individual membership of the Division of Counselling Psychology requires that the person has successfully completed a BPS-accredited programme in counselling psychology or the BPS Qualification in Counseling Psychology and has also maintained their professional subscription with the BPS.

Most of these divisions rely on a voluntary executive committee to carry out the strategic plans of the division and to promote their profession both within their professional body and to the wider society. Committee members may choose to be involved in key roles within their professional bodies and contribute to working groups, practice documents, research, training standards and ethics. Reliance on a voluntary workforce can provide its own unique difficulties; however, committee members tend to engage in this type of work for their own sense of belonging to a group, giving something back to the committee, networking and the varied opportunities these roles bring.

The importance of belonging

As with any voluntary role, individuals' motivation to engage in the field, volunteer their time to something they feel able to contribute to and value is an important part of one's identity. In particular, this can be applied to a professional organisation. Although each will differ in their reasons for volunteering, there are personal as well as professional benefits of doing so. Especially within a close-knit community such as counselling psychology, counselling psychologists have the opportunity to feel a sense of belonging by contributing to their professional organisation.

> **FOCUS BOX 13.1 THE IMPORTANCE OF BELONGING**
>
> Belong to a unique community of counselling psychologists;
> Enhance their networks, personal growth, confidence and skills;
> Gain leadership, mentoring and consultancy opportunities;
> Broaden their knowledge by attending courses, seminars, lectures and the DCoP annual conferences;
> Engage in higher-level policy changes such as consultations (governmental, professional bodies, regulatory bodies etc.);
> Linking to professional networks, such as through the Network and Interest Groups, presenting at conferences, facilitating courses;
> Giving back to the counselling psychology profession;
> Establish a presence with your own specialty and interest;
> Media opportunities; and
> Staying motivated, inspired and engaged.

Unlike general membership of a professional body, membership of a division of counselling psychology provides counselling psychologists with a unique home specific to the values of counselling psychology and plays a key role in our own identity. Given the history of the formation of many divisions, counselling psychologists have had to promote the profession to be acknowledged and valued as an applied science and part of the applied psychology profession. The importance of identity, belonging to the specialism makes this all the more understandable and why it may have been additionally important for counselling psychologists to hold on to divisional membership, their professional community and identity.

The power of professional connections

Networking and being a member of a professional body is much more than just belonging to a professional organisation or like-minded people. There is a sense of connecting with the profession, other professionals, aspiring counselling psychologists, and interested individuals and groups.

The opportunities to connect socially may be through the division special groups or particular network and interest groups. These tend to connect people who have an interest in or specialise in a particular area, such as palliative care, adult mental health, learning disabilities or with a client group such as children and young people, older adults and so on. These groups offer counselling psychologists the opportunity to mentor, lead a team and network with colleagues in a similar field and draw them together to connect professionally. Some offer additional training events, networking opportunities and even a platform to disseminate research relevant to their area. Within divisions, these groups are vital to access the specialists when it comes to feeding into government policy, the professional bodies guidelines and procedures, current issues such as social justice and other political issues that arise.

Defining counselling psychology

Some divisions have sought to define counselling psychology to distinguish the profession from other applied psychology professions. The Institute of Counselling Psychology in New Zealand defines counselling psychology as:

> A psychological specialty that utilises and applies psychological knowledge and research at the individual, group and organisational level. Counselling psychologists enable and empower clients experiencing typical and atypical problems of living to enhance their personal, social, educational and vocational functioning.
>
> *(The New Zealand Psychological Society, 2016, para. 1; see also Du Preez et al., 2016)*

After a consultation process, a definition of counselling psychology was developed, later adopted by the Canadian Psychological Association (CPA-CNPSY, 2016; see also Bedi et al., 2016), which acknowledges counselling psychology as a specialism within psychology.

In South Africa, a government scope of practice set out regulations defining the scope of practice for professions of psychology, including counselling psychology (Government Gazette, 2011, p. 7; see also Bantjes et al., 2016). It states that 'the following acts fall within the scope of practice of counselling psychologists':

(a) Assessing, diagnosing, and intervening in clients dealing with life challenges, and developmental problems to optimise psychological well being; assessing cognitive, personality, emotional and neuropsychological functions in relation to life challenges and developmental problems; assessing developmental processes (e.g. career choice), and adjustment;
(b) identifying psychopathology, and its impact on developmental processes, and adjustment; identifying, and diagnosing disorders of adjustments; applying psychological interventions to clients with developmental challenges, and adjustment problems; performing therapeutic counselling interventions; referring clients to appropriate professionals for further assessment or intervention;
(c) advising on the development of policies, based on various aspects of psychological theory and research; designing, managing and evaluating programmes dealing with developmental, and adjustment problems;
(d) Training, and supervising other registered counselling psychologists in counselling psychology;
(e) Designing, managing, conducting, reporting on, and supervising psychological research; conducting psychological practice, and research in accordance with the Ethical Rules of Conduct for Practitioners registered under the Health Professions Act, 1974; adhering to the scope of practice of counselling psychologists; and
(f) Providing expert evidence and/or opinions.

Definitions of counselling psychology, the work they are entitled to carry out and clarification of competencies are sometimes borne out of distinguishing counselling psychology from other applied psychologists. These topics are still debated in professional organisations and divisions today and at times lend themselves to unnecessary dividing of professions not only in the field of psychology but also within mental health professions.

The BPS partner and accreditation team sets out the standards for doctoral training in counselling psychology and defines counselling psychology as:

> a distinct profession within the field of psychology whose specialist focus is the application of psychological and psychotherapeutic theory and research to clinical practice. Counselling psychology holds a humanistic value base that goes beyond the traditional understanding of human nature and development as passive and linear and views human beings and their experience as inherently dynamic, embodied, and relational in nature. Its aim is to reduce psychological distress and to promote the wellbeing of individuals by focusing on their subjective experience as it unfolds in their interaction with the physical, social, cultural, and spiritual dimensions in living. Counselling psychology takes as its starting point the co-construction of knowledge and as such places relational practice at its centre. The therapeutic relationship is therefore considered to be the main vehicle through which psychological difficulties are understood and alleviated.
>
> *(BPS, 2015, p. 15)*

Regulatory bodies for counselling psychologists

Regulatory bodies are usually set up in accordance with government legislation, with the aim of protecting the public. Statutory regulators hold a list of registrants' details and tend to manage competencies; training and ethical standards; registrant's professional conduct; continuing professional development; and fitness to practice matters. Registration is often a pre-requisite for professional practice. Some regulatory bodies regulate members in a country, whilst others such as Canada and the United States require psychologists to be regulated by individual states through the process of licensure. The process of credentialing differs from country to country; however there are clear guidelines and pathways that counselling psychologist follow to be able to register as a professional. These may include degree specifications, internships, compulsory community service, board examination and/or further studies.

From 1 July 2009 the **Health and Care Professions Council (HCPC)** became the regulatory body for psychologists in the UK. The HCPC is an independent statutory regulator set up to safeguard the 'health and care of persons using or needing the services of its registrants'. Since then, the title '**practitioner psychologist**' has been protected along with clinical psychologist, counselling psychologist, educational psychologist, forensic psychologist, health psychologist, occupational psychologist, sport and exercise psychologist (see Focus box 13.2). The HCPC's main aim is to protect the public by setting (HCPC, 2012) proficiency for a number of health care professions, including practitioner psychologists.

The protection of titles can be seen in other countries. For example, in a survey of 79 counselling psychologists in Canada (Bedi et al., 2016), the authors found that 47.5% of the counselling psychologists used the title 'psychologist', whilst 20.5% used 'therapist or psychotherapist'. In Australia, Belgium, Finland, Greece, Sweden and New Zealand, the title 'psychologist' is protected by law. A contentious issue within the UK psychology field is the decision by the HCPC not to protect the title 'psychologist'. This omission has raised some concerns that individuals who do not meet the requirements for registration under one of the statutory protected titles may describe themselves by using the term 'psychologist' which may lead the public to believe they are delivering the services of a fully qualified psychologist.

For counselling psychologists in the UK, the **protected titles** means that 'Practitioner Psychologist' and 'Counselling Psychologist' can only be used if a practitioner is registered with the HCPC. Furthermore, all recognised training courses in counselling psychology need to be formally approved by the Education and Training Committee of the HCPC, which ensures that graduates can apply to the HCPC for regulation. The HCPC has a formal regulatory framework to which all approved courses need to adhere. This framework includes specific standards of education and training, a set of **Standards of Proficiency** detailing the skills required for the application of knowledge to practice, guidance on conduct and ethics for students as well as standards of conduct, performance, and ethics and standards for continuing professional development for qualified registrants (HCPC, 2012). The Standards of Conduct, Performance and Ethics are the standards set by the HCPC that outline the behaviour and conduct expected from their members. The standards of proficiency for practitioner psychologists list both generic standards as well as more profession-specific standards. Counselling psychologists are required to register with the HCPC and undertake to meet these standards in order to practice 'lawfully, safely and effectively' (HCPC, 2012). In order to be registered to practice, psychologists in the UK need to earn a qualification from an HCPC-approved programme, and demonstrate that they have met the standards set out by the HCPC. The BPS's role in terms of regulation has been to work with the HCPC to promote the specialty, represent members, curriculum frameworks, post-registration education and training and continuing professional development.

The HCPC is also the regulatory body for other health and care professions in the UK, such as art therapists, physiotherapists, radiographers, speech and language therapists – currently a total of 16 professions (www.hcpc-uk.org).

It:

- Sets standards for registrants' education, professional skills and behaviour;
- Keeps a register of professionals who meet those standards;
- Approves programmes that allow students to apply to join their register upon completion of the programme; and
- Takes action when professionals on the register do not meet their standards.

FOCUS BOX 13.2 THE PROTECTED TITLES APPLICABLE TO PSYCHOLOGISTS IN THE UK

Clinical psychologist
Counselling psychologist
Educational psychologist
Forensic psychologist
Health psychologist
Occupational psychologist
Practitioner psychologist
Registered psychologist
Sport and exercise psychologist

Developing your professional career

Chartered membership of the BPS reflects the 'highest standard of psychological knowledge and expertise' (BPS, 2016). Although the BPS no longer holds the regulatory role for psychologists, it still plays a key role in providing members with important professional, research and ethical guidelines. Under the Royal Charter, the title 'Chartered Psychologist' is legally recognised and those who have been deemed eligible to do so are entitled to use the designation 'Chartered Psychologist' and the abbreviation *CPsychol* after their name.

In order to become chartered, a psychologist must be a member of the BPS and have:

a) Achieved a first degree in psychology recognized by the Society as meeting the Graduate Basis for Chartered Membership,
b) Undertaken Society accredited post-graduate qualifications and training, and
c) Agreed to follow the Society's Member Conduct Rules and be guided by the Society's Code of Ethics and Conduct.

By adhering to the BPS's Membership Conduct Rules and Code of Ethics and Conduct, Chartered Psychologists demonstrate to their clients, who may include patients, students, research participants, educational institutions or organisations, that they uphold the highest levels of professional standards and ethics. Counselling psychologists can also apply to be fellows or associate fellows of the BPS, which acknowledges their experience, competence and contribution to the field of psychology.

There are also many other opportunities within professional bodies, regulatory bodies and especially in the network and interest groups in divisions. For example, most divisions of counselling psychology have committees, with a variety of chair, co-chair, group leads and leadership positions available to members. Opportunities to become more involved within the media, to promote counselling psychology are often available to those who would like to put themselves forward for these roles.

Social media is becoming more popular and many counselling psychologists are called upon to put across their viewpoints on a number of issues such as governmental changes, policies, campaigns and social justice. Many will tweet on behalf of their professional body or division and others in their personal capacity. You may want to consider following counselling psychologists on social media and networking in this way. With the increase in popularity of social media, professional and regulatory bodies use this medium to promote key items and it is worth adding them to your 'following' list.

Developing your professional career path

Your journey to becoming a counselling psychologist begins with your interest in taking the undergraduate degree. Counselling psychology is an applied science and within your degree you will be given the chance to experience a range of choices to start your journey.

This will very much depend on your own values, ambitions and interests. For me, this is one of the strengths of counselling psychology as a career path in that the variety, scope and breadth of career choices makes it diverse, unique and personal to you and your choices. There is scope within counselling psychology to create your own unique professional pathways, such as choosing placements and work experience that match your areas of interests and researching areas that you are passionate about and feel can add to the profession.

Counselling psychologists pride themselves as being part of a diverse community and this can be seen in the range of individuals undertaking the doctoral degree in counselling psychology. Some have come into the career later in life, have varied work experience, backgrounds and often other post-graduate degrees. What they will all have in common is a belief in the values of counselling psychology and the understanding of the uniqueness of the profession. As discussed throughout this chapter, the opportunities afforded counselling psychologists are varied and include positions with their professional body, regulatory body, media, interest and network groups, governmental departments, academia, independent private practice and external organisations. Some counselling psychologists forge a portfolio career, where they hold a number of jobs and many include research and independent practice into these roles. The importance of choice, opportunity and your own direction on the journey is fundamental to forging a career in this profession.

Job opportunities, the choices we make and extra curricula activities make us who we are and help us to engage in a lifelong career that will engage, inspire and motivate us. Leadership, mentoring and consultancy work are important in keeping the profession alive. Counselling psychologists embody humanistic values, the importance of relational aspects and the subjective experience. These skills can be applied to building networks outside of the profession as well.

In a recent survey of over 1,200 counselling psychologists from eight countries, Goodyear et al. (2016, p. 14) identified the most frequently cited values and asked participants to 'rate the extent to which each of these values guides your work as a counselling psychologist'. The across-country findings in order of rated importance are:

1. Attention to people's assets, strengths, and resources, regardless of degree of disturbance.
2. A focus on diversity, as well as a consideration of sociocultural context and systematic barriers in making sense of and understanding people's experience.
3. A focus on person-environment interactions rather than exclusively on either the person or the environment.
4. A focus on developmental issues and developmentally appropriate interventions across the lifespan.
5. A focus on social justice and the necessity, when appropriate, to advocate for just causes that promote the welfare of others.
6. Drawing on research to inform practice.
7. An emphasis on both long-term and relatively brief interventions.
8. A focus of preventative interventions.
9. A focus on career-related issues and concerns pertaining to the workplace (e.g. career decision-making, transitions, adjustment, goal-setting.
10. Producing research that adds to knowledge of counselling psychology related topics.

These core values of counselling psychologists globally are a reflection of how counselling psychologists differentiate themselves from other applied psychologists and mental health professionals. The range of therapeutic approaches used by counselling psychologists also set them apart, ranging from humanistic, person-centred approaches to psychodynamic, cognitive-behavioural, and third-wave approaches. Counselling psychologists also engage in diagnosis, assessment, treatment, remediation, prevention, advocacy and psychoeducation. This enables counselling psychologists to work in a variety of settings. For example, in New Zealand, two-thirds of the counselling psychologists surveyed worked in private practice and non-governmental organisations (Du Preez, 2016). In Australia, and the United Kingdom nearly half of the counselling psychologists surveyed work in private practice (Di Mattia & Grant, 2016; Jones Nielsen & Nicholas, 2016).

Developing a personal career path and the journey that this may take is often not a straight path from A to B, especially when it comes to a career in counselling psychology. Counselling psychologists tend to have diverse backgrounds, varied work experience and forge unique career paths. Perhaps you have experienced a few bends or U-turns along your journey that you may choose to reflect upon.

ACTIVITY BOX 13.1 REFLECTION ON YOUR OWN POTENTIAL JOURNEY

Think about your own career journey and reflect on the following questions:

1. What has influenced you to consider counselling psychology as a career?
2. What have you done so far along the path to becoming a counselling psychologist?
3. What do you think you still need to do (e.g. further studies, work experience, voluntary positions)?
4. What have you enjoyed about studying counselling psychology and what are you looking forward to learning more about?
5. What are your values and how do you think they fit with the values of counselling psychology?
6. What are your ambitions for the future?

Developing your leadership, mentoring and consultancy skills

Counselling psychologists can gain leadership and mentoring skills during their doctoral training and build on these once qualified. They have a broad range of transferable skills that will help them with leadership roles. Some of the key personal qualities identified by the NHS leadership competency framework (NHS, 2011) are developing self-awareness, managing yourself, continuing personal development and acting with integrity. One of the first steps in leadership is self-awareness, which counselling psychologists value. This is also something that is threaded throughout the counselling psychology training, together with the importance of personal therapy, reflective practice and analysis of their own processes within therapy. Counselling psychologists are highly skilled to take on leadership roles and mentoring others not only in the field of counselling psychology but also other applied psychologists, allied professionals and health workers. A keen sense of political awareness, learning from one's own and others' experiences and being open to constructive feedback ensure that counselling psychologists continue to be reflective-practitioners and develop professionally throughout their career.

Leadership and mentoring opportunities are often available within the professional bodies, regulatory bodies, government departments and divisions of counselling psychology, and special interest groups. Counselling psychologists are encouraged to get involved in these arenas. Divisions often have a number of incentives investing in and capturing early career psychologists and supporting them in leadership and mentoring roles. For example, divisions often offer funded places each year to attend conferences and events, leadership and development programmes, bursaries and so on. For example, the BPS Division of Counselling Psychology funds places on a leadership and development programme jointly run with the Division of Occupational Psychology. The APA (Div.17) also provides grants to support and enhance the practice of counselling psychology. There are a number of ways counselling psychologists can raise their professional and leadership profile through involvement with government policies, health care systems, charities and media work. These are all opportunities to influence the field of psychology and at the same time for individuals to build professional contacts and reputation.

Counselling psychologists also offer consultancy, advocacy and supervision to professional colleagues, organisations and stakeholders with many engaging in policy at a governmental level. Counselling psychology researchers and academics also add to the knowledge base in the field by applying psychology to a range of practice applicable areas. By forming mentoring relationships with colleagues, peer supervisees and support groups, counselling psychologists utilise their leadership abilities and ensure that the next generation of counselling psychologists have the necessary skills to forge a unique career path for themselves. Leadership is not just about imparting psychological knowledge. It is very much about the mentoring relationship, collaborative working and growth that develops as part of this relationship. Leadership roles may include, for example, providing regular and constructive feedback to supervisees, colleagues and peers as well as motivating them to reflect on their own practice, increase their self-awareness and continue with self-assessment.

The importance of getting involved in your profession lies in the close connections you will make and the development of stronger ties with other applied psychologists, often within your own area of interest and specialism. The division's annual conference offers an opportunity to engage with valuable and valued research applicable to counselling psychologists. Counselling psychologists also present their work and research at other professional conferences around the world and this international dissemination of research, symposiums and workshops is essential to counselling psychologists' sense of belonging and identity. Publications that are dedicated to showcasing the work of counselling psychologists, such as *Counselling Psychology Quarterly*, the *European Journal of Counselling Psychology* as well as in-house publications such as the BPS DCoP *Counselling Psychology Review*, serve to highlight the specialties, competences and areas of interest in the field.

Continuing professional development

The HCPC defines **continuing professional development (CPD)** as:

> a range of learning activities through which health and care professionals maintain and develop throughout their career to ensure that they retain their capacity to practice safely, effectively and legally within their evolving scope of practice.
>
> *(HCPC, 2016, para. 1)*

The key to any professional development is how the professional engages in the continued learning process and personal development. CPD can be both formal and informal. For example, counselling psychologists may complete further training after their doctorate degree specialising in an area of interest or to further their qualifications in a particular field, such as EMDR therapy. They are also required to engage in ongoing CPD activities, to maintain their levels of competency and professional and ethical practice. CPD is a career-long process and essential in the ever-changing profession of psychology where new evidence-based practice, technology and skills are required to enhance personal and professional competencies, knowledge and understanding. Counselling psychologists value this not only as a requirement of their registration but also personally in terms of choice, direction of career, interests and enhancing reflective practice.

CPD can include a wide variety of activities that help to keep counselling psychologists updated in their knowledge, expertise and skills. It may take the form of formal CPD courses through an accredited training programme, external organisation, informal peer discussion, attendance at conferences, group discussions and other professional events. Within many divisions, smaller-interest and specialist groups hold training events and are an ideal way for counselling psychologists to develop their own interests whilst contributing to the group as a whole.

Setting CPD requirements for counselling psychologists also serves to reassure the public through public accountability. Knowing that counselling psychologists are required to update their skills and knowledge throughout their career helps instil confidence in the profession and the professional. In the UK, the regulatory body sets these standards and carries out a random audit (2.5% of professionals) of member's CPD records. The CPD standards state that practitioner psychologists must:

1. Maintain a continuous, up-to-date and accurate record of their CPD activities;
2. Demonstrate that their CPD activities are a mixture of learning activities relevant to current or future practice;
3. Seek to ensure that their CPD has contributed to the quality of their practice and service delivery;
4. Seek to ensure that their CPD benefits the service user; and
5. Upon request, present a written profile (which must be their own work and supported by evidence) explaining how they have met the standards for CPD.

(HCPC, 2016, para.2)

Counselling psychologists are encouraged to engage in a wide variety of CPD opportunities including workshops, conferences, reflective practice groups, seminars and so forth. Self-awareness is key in counselling psychology and as has been explored elsewhere in this book, personal therapy forms an important and compulsory part of the doctoral training in counselling psychology in the UK. Counselling psychologists may choose to continue with personal therapy after their training and this can form part of the ongoing learning process by acknowledging that our own values, beliefs and personal history play a part in the therapeutic relationship.

Professional development cannot be looked at in isolation but rather as part of personal development. As counselling psychologists we relate to clients and others, taking into account their context, subjective experience and relational aspects. Our ability to understand the client's phenomenological experience, exploring their meaning to aspects of their life is an important part of who counselling psychologists are and what we do.

Summary and conclusions

This chapter has provided a broad overview of the importance of belonging to a professional organisation and one that aligns with our own identity as a counselling psychologist. Whilst being registered with the regulatory body is a necessity, belonging to a professional home brings about a sense of belonging and group connection. When choosing to belong, a number of benefits will be afforded but it is inevitably up to the individual to take part, engage with and give something back to the profession. The choices counselling psychologists make along their career path will inevitably shape their experiences and it is hoped, be in line with their own values and that of counselling psychology as a profession. It is therefore important to reflect on your own professional and personal development as well as understanding the professional development of counselling psychology. An exploration of your own journey may help you to understand some of the decisions you have made or will make along the road to either qualification or future career opportunities.

Learning outcomes

When you have completed this chapter you should be able to:

- Identify the importance and benefits of belonging to a professional organisation.
- Identify the key aims of regulatory bodies, which represent counselling psychology and counselling psychologists around the world.
- Critically analyse the importance of continuing professional development.
- Understand what 'sense of belonging' and a professional identity may mean to counselling psychologists.
- Understand some of the key aspects of developing a professional career pathway.
- Reflect on your own professional development and potential career path.

Key concepts and terms

- Belonging
- British Psychological Society (BPS)
- Chartered membership
- Continuing professional development
- Counselling Psychology
- Division of Counselling Psychology
- Health and Care Professions Council (HCPC)
- Identity
- Practitioner psychologist
- Professional body
- Protective title
- Regulatory body
- Standards of proficiency

Sample essay titles

1. Compare and contrast the benefits of belonging to a regulatory body, professional body and a Division of Counselling Psychology.
2. Critically evaluate the reasons for having protective titles for the professional, the profession and the public.
3. Continued professional development can impact upon the career path of a counselling psychologist. Discuss this statement with reference to relevant research.
4. Your journey to becoming a counselling psychologist begins with your interest in taking the undergraduate degree. Evaluate this sentence with reference to your own journey.

Further reading

Books

Goodyear, R.K., & Lichtenberg, J.W. (Eds.). (2017). *A global portrait of counselling psychology*. New York: Routledge.

Douglas, B., Woolfe, R., Strawbridge, S., Kasket, E., & Galbraith, V. (2016). *Handbook of counselling psychology*. London: Sage Publications Limited.

References

American Psychological Association. (2016). *Memoranda of Understanding*. Retrieved from www.apa.org/international/outreach/understanding-memorandum/index.aspx

Bantjes, J., Kagee, A., & Young, C. (2016). Counselling psychology in South Africa. *Counselling Psychology Review*, 29 (2), 171–183.

Bedi, R.P., Sinacore, A., & Christiani, K.D. (2016). Counselling psychology in Canada. *Counselling Psychology Review*, 29 (2), 150–162.

The British Psychological Society. (2015). *Standards for the accreditation of doctoral programmed in counselling psychology*. BPS: Leicester.

The British Psychological Society. (2016). *Chartered member (CPsychol)*. Retrieved from www.bps.org.uk/what-we-do/membership/chartered-member-cpsychol/chartered-member-cpsychol

Canadian Psychological Association. (2016). Counselling Psychology in a Canadian Context:Final Report from the Executive Committee for a Canadian Understanding of Counselling Psychology. Retrieved from www.cpa.ca/docs/File/Sections/Counselling/Readings/CPA-CNPSY-Report-Final%20nov%2009.pdf

Di Mattia, M.A. & Grant, J. (2016). Counselling psychology in Australia: History, status and challenges. *Counselling Psychology Review*, 29 (2), 139–149.

Du Preez, E., Feather, J., & Farrell, B. (2016). Counselling psychology in New Zealand. *Counselling Psychology Review*, 29 (2), 163–170.

Goodyear, R.K., Lichtenberg, J.W., Hutman, H., Overland, E., Bedi, R., Christiani, K., Di Mattia, M., du Preez, E., Farrell, W., Feather, J., Grant, J., Han, Y., Ju, Y., Lee, D., Lee, H., Nicholas, H., Jones Nielsen, J., Sinacore, A., Tu, S., & Young, C. (2016). A global portrait of counselling psychologists' characteristics, perspectives and professional behaviors. *Counselling Psychology Review*, 29 (2), 115–138.

Government Gazette. (2011). *Regulations defining the scope of the profession (No. 34581)*. Retrieved from www.hpcsa.co.za/Uploads/editor/UserFiles/downloads/psych/sept_promulgated_scope_of_practice.pdf

Health and Care Professions Council. (2012). *Standards of conduct, performance and ethics*. Retrieved from www.hpc-uk.org/assets/documents/10003B6EStandardsofconduct,performanceandethics.pdf

Health and Care Professions Council. (2012). *Standards of proficiency: Practitioner psychologists.* Retrieved from www.hcpc-uk.org/assets/documents/10002963SOP_Practitioner_psychologists.pdf

Health and Care Professions Council. (2016). *Our standards for continuing professional development.* Retrieved from www.hpc-uk.org/registrants/cpd/

Jones Nielsen, J. & Nicholas, H. (2016). Counselling psychology in the United Kingdom. *Counselling Psychology Review*, 29 (2), 206–215.

Lichtenberg, J.W., Goodyear, R.K., Hutman, H., & Overland. E.A. (2016). Counselling psychology in the United States. *Counselling Psychology Review*, 29 (2), 216–224.

The New Zealand Psychological Society. (2016). *Institute of counselling psychology.* Retrieved from www.psychology.org.nz/membership/member-groups/institute-of-counselling-psychology/?#.V0xYEmP0jdk

NHS Leadership Academy. (2011). *Clinical leadership competency framework.* NHS Institute for Innovation and Improvement: Coventry.

14

PROFESSIONAL TRAINING IN COUNSELLING PSYCHOLOGY

Nicola Hogan

This chapter aims to provide an overview of both the development and the current status of professional training in counselling psychology in the UK and the processes by which you can qualify as a counselling psychologist today. The, often confusing, issues of **accreditation** and **registration** will be explained and the chapter will include summaries of guidelines and requirements for these processes. All applied psychology trainings share certain core characteristics and requirements but each specialty also has its unique features and specific approaches to the way in which psychological theory is used in real life.

The application and interview stages of the selection process will be explained in detail and some suggestions made for how to prepare for the course interview. A brief summary of the main elements of counselling psychology training will provide a structure and framework to help decide if this is the career for you and give an indication of some of the preparation you will need to do prior to application.

A current trainee from a course route and one from the 'independent route' have shared their motivations to join this profession and their experiences of applying and being selected for each route respectively. Their candid accounts provide a student's perspective on the training process and reveal some of the challenges for the prospective student in beginning this journey.

Counselling Psychology has been evolving rapidly over the last 22 years and there are many exciting developments still to come. Some of the key, contemporary debates in the discipline are mentioned in the concluding section of the chapter to provide you with an opportunity to glance into a future that may become yours.

If you decide this is the career for you, there are a number of things you need to consider in preparing yourself for this move. This preparation involves a certain amount of **research** on the trainings themselves but also some serious **reflection** on your own motivations, suitability and robustness to undertake the programme.

It is not an easy route but it can be an extremely rewarding career. It is hoped that, by the end of the chapter, you will be clearer as to whether this will be your future.

Development of training in counselling psychology

Before we look at the current status of counselling psychology training it may be useful to present a little of the history that has provided the foundations for this training today. The British Psychological Society (BPS) set up a voluntary register for all psychologists in 1987 and the threshold set for entry to the Royal Charter was three years postgraduate study and practice (or part-time equivalent). The external benchmark was doctoral level.

The 'official birth' of counselling psychology was in 1994, when the Special Group in Counselling Psychology was granted permission to become a Division of the British Psychological Society (BPS), and chartered status was granted to counselling psychologists. Many experienced psychologists working as psychotherapists at the time were able to become recognised as chartered counselling psychologists through the Statement of Equivalence or what has become known as 'grand-parenting'. These early pioneers went on to establish the profession and to develop training routes for new entrants.

The original training route, the BPS Diploma in Counselling Psychology, was established in 1994 and has evolved into the **Qualification in Counselling Psychology** (QCoP or just the "Qualification") and is one of the BPS's 'independent routes' to becoming an applied psychologist. At that time some universities offered postgraduate courses in counselling or psychotherapy that were seen as a relevant academic training for counselling psychology. When counselling psychology became a doctoral-level training, many of the Master's-level programmes seized the opportunity to develop into the, relatively new, species of professional or practitioner doctorates.

At the time of writing we have 13 such BPS-accredited and Health and Care Professions Council (HCPC)–approved doctoral programmes offered by Universities in England and Scotland.

Accreditation, registration and chartered status

The story of the regulation of counselling psychology can be a little confusing due to the many changes in recent years in the UK to rules around postgraduate training and the introduction of statutory regulation of psychologists. In essence there are now two bodies with a stake in the accreditation and training of counselling psychologists – the BPS and the HCPC.

The BPS and chartered status

Originally the BPS was the only accrediting body for counselling psychology courses. Programmes wishing to acquire accreditation from the BPS had to apply to, and be scrutinised by, the accreditation teams working for the Training Committee in Counselling Psychology (TCCP). The standards developed by the BPS Division of Counselling Psychology formed the curriculum and structure for all accredited training. These were most recently revised in 2015.

FOCUS BOX 14.1 BPS STANDARDS FOR DOCTORAL PROGRAMMES IN COUNSELLING PSYCHOLOGY (2015)

The key aim of an accredited programme is to produce graduates who will:

1. Be competent, reflective, ethically sound, resourceful and informed practitioners of counselling psychology able to work in therapeutic and non-therapeutic contexts;
2. Value the imaginative, interpretative, personal and collaborative aspects of the practice of counselling psychology;
3. Commit themselves to ongoing personal and professional development and inquiry;
4. Understand, develop and apply models of psychological inquiry for the creation of new knowledge which is appropriate to the multi-dimensional nature of relationships between people;
5. Appreciate the significance of wider, cultural, spiritual, political and economic domains within which counselling psychology operates;
6. Adopt a questioning and evaluative approach to the philosophy, practice , research and theory which constitutes counselling psychology; and
7. Be able to develop and demonstrate communication, influencing, teaching and leadership skills by applying psychological knowledge and skills in a range of professional, clinical, organisational and research contexts.

BPS (October 2015) Standards for the Accreditation of Doctoral Programmes in Counselling Psychology.

When statutory regulation was introduced in 2009 the regulator role passed to the HCPC. However the BPS still plays a part in accreditation of counselling psychologists by way of conferring chartered status (CPsychol) on those who meet the requirements. As a chartered psychologist and HCPC-registered counselling psychologist you are entitled to be a full member of the Division of Counselling Psychology (DCoP). The accreditation teams at the BPS have adopted a new process called, 'Accreditation through Partnership' providing a framework to work with education providers collaboratively and supportively. This allows programmes to work with the Society to enhance counselling psychology provision to the benefit of all, by encouraging diversity, creativity and flexibility within training, leading to a richness that will evolve into a strength as the profession continues to grow. However this must be balanced with the need for standardisation and to this end there is a set of over-arching learning outcomes for all applied psychology doctoral programmes.

FOCUS BOX 14.2 BPS LEARNING OUTCOMES FOR COUNSELLING PSYCHOLOGY PROGRAMMES

Philosophy
Psychological Knowledge and Application
Psychological Assessment and Formulation
Counselling Psychology Practice and Psychological Intervention

Evaluation of Practice
Research and Inquiry
Working with Diversity and Cultural Competence
Personal and Professional Skills and Values
Communication, influencing, teaching and leadership skills

BPS (2015) Standards for the Accreditation *of Doctoral Programmes in Counselling Psychology*

The Health and Care Professions Council (HCPC) and statutory registration

The statutory register for psychologists was set up in 2009 and the Health and Care Professions Council (HCPC) became the regulating body for psychologists. In order to use the title 'registered psychologist' or any of the eight other protected titles (e.g. counselling psychologist) it is required by law to be on the HCPC register. Further details of statutory regulation can be found on both the BPS and HCPC websites (www.hcpc-uk.co.uk; and bps.org.uk).

In order to get on to the register it is necessary to complete an accredited training either via an accredited course route or the independent route. Both of these trainings will have to meet the HCPC Standards of Proficiency (SOPs) and Standards of Education and Training (SETs).

The benchmarks for doctoral training are set by the QAA and all programmes must comply with these.

FOCUS BOX 14.3 QAA DOCTORAL BENCHMARKS

Doctoral degrees are awarded to students who have demonstrated:

i. the creation and interpretation of new knowledge, through original **research** or other advanced scholarship, of a quality to satisfy peer review, extend the forefront of the discipline and merit publication;
ii. a systematic acquisition and understanding of a substantial body of knowledge which is at the forefront of an academic discipline or area of professional practice;
iii. the general ability to conceptualise, design and implement a project for the generation of new knowledge, applications or understanding at the forefront of the discipline, and to adjust the project design in the light of unforeseen problems and
iv. a detailed understanding of applicable techniques for research and advanced academic enquiry.

Typically, holders of the qualification will be able to

- make informed judgements on complex issues in specialist fields, often in the absence of complete data, and be able to communicate their ideas and conclusions clearly and effectively to specialist and non-specialist audiences;
- continue to undertake pure and/or applied research and development at an advanced level, contributing substantially to the development of new techniques, ideas or approaches, and will have

- the qualities and transferable skills necessary for employment requiring the exercise of personal responsibility and largely autonomous initiative in complex and unpredictable situations, in professional or equivalent environments.

Quality Assurance Agency (2014) The Framework for Higher Education Qualifications in England, Wales and Northern Ireland.

Therefore, in summary, to work legally as a psychologist in the UK, you must be on the Statutory Register but, although it is not a legal requirement, you may wish to also become a chartered psychologist in order to benefit from membership of the professional organisation (further detail on this in Chapter 13).

Programmes that are jointly accredited by the BPS and the HCPC will confer graduates with eligibility to join the Register and to be a chartered psychologist.

Elements and competencies of training

Professional training in counselling psychology comprises a number of elements and is assessed according to the demonstration of a number of competencies.

Theory

It is now the case that counselling psychologists must be proficient in one core therapeutic model and have a working knowledge and understanding of a second model. So some courses specialise in a specific model and cover one or even a number of other models to a lesser extent. When you are researching course routes you may wish to consider if their chosen core models fit with your own interests and beliefs. If you are studying via the independent route, then you will need to complete a postgraduate (PG) course in at least two different core models. Often candidates will complete a Master's programme in one approach and then another in training – perhaps a PG certificate or PG diploma level – in another.

Clinical placement

It is a requirement of accreditation that all trainees complete a minimum 450 hours of clinical practice during their training. This work would usually be supervised by a registered clinical or counselling psychologist and is sometimes conducted within an NHS service.

Personal therapy

Personal therapy is another mandatory requirement in training and a minimum of 40 hours must be completed by the end of training. Generally the trainee is responsible for finding a therapist, paying the fee and providing evidence that the hours have been completed. Courses often provide a list of suitable therapists in the area and sometimes rates can be negotiated for trainees.

Personal therapists must be suitably qualified as an accredited member of a therapeutic body such as British Psychological Society (BPS), Health and Care Professions Council (HCPC), United Kingdom Council for Psychotherapy (UKCP), British Association for Counselling and Psychotherapy (BACP).

Research

Counselling psychology is a doctoral-level training and therefore you will be working at this academic level throughout the course. As a practitioner or professional doctorate the degree is awarded for the whole content of the programme rather than just the research element as with a PhD.

For this reason the doctoral thesis is generally shorter in word length than a PhD by research. The length can vary quite significantly between courses and it is worth checking this out. However, independent of the length, you will have to carry out an independent research project which meets doctoral standards.

You may be required to present a research proposal as part of the selection process and even if you are not, it is a good idea to think about the areas of counselling psychology that interest you and to read through some journal articles to get a feel for contemporary research areas in the field and the methodologies currently favoured. Your doctoral thesis must be of publishable standard so this quality of writing is what you are aiming for.

ACTIVITY BOX 14.1 THINKING ABOUT CLINICAL PLACEMENTS

1. Brainstorm the type of clinical work that interests you with reference to these categories:
    - client group
    - type of service
    - therapeutic approach
    - experience you already have
    - experience you wish to gain
    - parameters around payment, hours, location
    - contacts you may have that could help
2. Using the results of your brainstorming, look at the types of **placements** commonly used by trainees and consider what would appeal to you.

Typical placements include:

a) NHS Psychology Services:
- adult services
- child and adolescent services
- forensic services
- learning disability services
- older adult's services
- substance misuse services

b) National Voluntary agencies include:
- Samaritans
- Cruse
- Mind
- Age Concern
- Young Minds
- Refugee Council
- Relate

c) Student Counselling Services
Many Universities and colleges, and even schools, have support services for students so it is worth contacting local institutions if this is an area that interests you.

d) Prison Service
The prison and probation service may provide **placements** for trainee counselling psychologists. Check – HM Prison Service – gov.uk.

More information on all of these can be found by searching the internet.

General eligibility for training

In essence the training to become a counselling psychologist consists of acquiring and demonstrating the competencies which are set out by the HCPC and interpreted by courses in their syllabi and in the Qualification in Counselling Psychology (QCoP) Candidate Handbook (2017).

In order to apply for either a course route or the BPS Qualification you must hold Graduate Basis for Chartered Membership (GBC) of the Society. Most single honours psychology degrees in the UK confer this. If you have a psychology degree that does not confer GBC, you may be able to undertake extra modules to 'top up'. The Society will advise on this. If your degree is in a different subject, you may be able to take a conversion course run by a number of UK Universities to convert your degree to one in psychology.

If English is not your first language, you will be required to have an English Language Testing System (IELT) score of at least 7 and sometimes 8 (for the Qualification and some course routes).

You must gain clearance from the Disclosure and Barring Service (**DBS**), formerly Criminal Records Bureau (CRB). This is a check to see if you have a criminal record. A criminal record will not necessarily preclude you from training but it is important to ensure that individuals who are working with potentially vulnerable people are safe to do so. The Qualification and some course routes require an occupational health clearance statement from a medical practitioner to vouch for your mental health.

Training courses

Counselling psychology is doctoral-level training and most course programmes offer a practitioner or a professional doctorate in counselling psychology, conferring a DPsych award. The specific titles of the award may vary between courses. An accredited route will lead to eligibility to become a Registered Psychologist with the HCPC and also to become a Chartered Psychologist with the BPS.

When the HCPC took on the role of approving the training programmes of all applied psychologies, including counselling psychology, it set up a new approval process. This means that any new programme must apply to this body and be subject to its rigorous process that involves demonstrating, through course documentation, that national standards are complied with and general standards of competence are set. Visits to the programmes are conducted and these may be joint visits with the BPS.

All currently accredited UK training courses can be found listed on the BPS website. All information relating to courses can be found on the relevant University website. On-line application forms are available there. Most courses offer a full-time route, which is around 3 years in duration, and sometimes a part-time route that has a maximum duration of 7 years. Each course will set its fee for the programme and although these vary slightly, the range, at the time of writing, is in the region of £6,500–£10,500 p.a. and can normally be paid in instalments.

Courses do vary in the structure of their programmes so you are advised to gather as much information as possible from websites, literature, open evenings and interview opportunities.

Entry requirements for the course route

The entry requirements for all courses are standard, as they are set by the registering body (HCPC).

They are:

- 2:1 (Hons) degree or higher in psychology with GBC (graduate basis for chartered membership) (or a first degree in another subject and a conversion course).
- Introductory training in counselling to certificate level or equivalent.
- Experience of counselling work (e.g. as support worker, volunteer, trainee in mental health). This generally should involve face-to-face counselling work and not be merely be-friending or caring.

Courses may vary a little in the precise detail of their requirements so always check the course information on the University website.

Personal requirements

Counselling psychology is a profession that involves the use of self. To work therapeutically with clients requires you to be emotionally strong and robust. There are many stories that you will hear which will be harrowing and many clients whose situations are extremely difficult. Some stories may trigger a response from your own experiences and you need to be able to bracket that and not let it interfere with the work. For this reason, it is a requirement of the training that all trainees undergo a minimum of 40 hours of **personal therapy**. This allows you to feel how it is to be a client and also to have an opportunity to work on your own issues that you feel may affect your work as a therapist. The specific number of personal therapy hours differs between courses and can often depend upon the core model of training.

Most programmes will ask for evidence of personal maturity, robustness, stability, self-awareness and reflective capacity and this will be measured in some way during the selection interview. You may be asked to provide evidence from a medical practitioner that you are not suffering from any mental health issues.

As the training is at doctoral level you will be assessed on your potential to work at that level. The QAA doctoral descriptors give an indication of the skills you are aiming for (see Focus box 14.3). Counselling psychologists are often referred to as scientist-practitioners or reflective-practitioners and our work is evidence-based but also relational. Therefore we are scientists working at the level of relationship and there is an expectation that you will work and think within a scientific paradigm (further information on this can be found in Chapter 11).

See Focus box 14.4 for the experiences of one trainee, Raj, on a course route.

FOCUS BOX 14.4 THE COURSE ROUTE – RAJ, 2ND YEAR FULL-TIME TRAINEE

Having completed my degree in psychology I was uncertain what I wanted to do next. My favourite part of the degree had been the clinical modules and I was particularly interested in positive psychology and the area of well-being. Whilst studying for my degree I had worked both as a volunteer on a student help line and also in a psychiatric unit attached to my local hospital and I knew this was the broad area of work that attracted me. There are a couple of counselling psychologists on the team where I work in the unit and through talking with them I began to see that the humanistic philosophy and the approach of working with the client chimed with my values and beliefs about therapy in general.

I knew that there was no subsidy for the training and I would have to find the funds to pay the fees and to support myself for three years. This is sometimes hard, especially as I worked alongside clinical trainees who were receiving government support for their training. However I was fortunate in that the service I had been working for voluntarily recently offered me an assistant's post for the duration of my training. This provides me with a small income, clinical experience, supervised practice and the opportunity to network: something that would be invaluable when I qualified and was looking for a post.

My application to the course was successful and I was called to interview. The selection process was rigorous and quite demanding on applicants. We were asked to give a 15-minute presentation on future challenges for the counselling psychology profession, then take part in a group exercise, followed by an interview. We were also asked to write a research proposal, which we had to submit in advance and this formed part of the interview itself.

The course, to date, has been challenging but rewarding. The skills workshops in the first year were terrifying. Watching our role-play performances on tape and listening to feedback from the rest of the group was one of the most difficult times but I think I learned so much from it and it has made me a more **reflective-practitioner**. **Personal therapy** has been a source of concern to many in my group. It is a course requirement and we have to complete 40 hours in total over the three years of training. Personally I found it an interesting experience to feel how a client must feel in therapy. Overall I would say that this training is not for the faint-hearted. It can be a financial burden, it is emotionally challenging and the workload is heavy but it has never been dull and I think it is the most rewarding career I could have chosen.

The qualification

The BPS also offers a route that has become known as 'the independent route' or 'the qualification' but has the formal title of Qualification in Counselling Psychology.

The BPS qualifications are intended for independent candidates who are not attached to accredited postgraduate training courses and wish to take an independent approach to learning. This route may be preferred by candidates who have some previous, relevant experience for which they can obtain accreditation of existing competence (AEC) for some of the units or for individuals who are unable to commit to regular attendance on a course and prefer the more flexible option of working through the units at their own pace.

Although the Qualification is run by the BPS it is not an education provider and cannot confer academic awards and candidates must put together their own plan of training (POT) with their co-ordinating supervisor (CS). In essence this is a plan to ensure that the trainee will be in a position, by the end of training, to demonstrate all the required competencies for the Qualification.

Appropriate arrangements for access to academic facilities and support throughout the period of training must be made, which may involve arranging library access at local universities and might include buying into modules of training courses. Candidates will have to complete at least one course at Master's level in a core module and a further training in an alternative approach. In addition, 450 hours of clinical practice must be completed, and logged, under the **supervision** of a registered counselling/clinical psychologist. It is necessary to complete 40 hours of personal therapy and it is the responsibility of the candidate to find and pay a suitably qualified therapist. Once all the plans have been made, the candidate, along with the CS, can complete and submit the enrolment portfolio. It is often the case that candidates have previous experience that can be accredited via AEC and these applications are part of the enrolment portfolio.

See Focus box 14.5 for the experiences of a trainee on the independent route.

FOCUS BOX 14.5 THE 'INDEPENDENT ROUTE' VIA THE BPS QUALIFICATION IN COUNSELLING PSYCHOLOGY – CYNTHIA

I came to counselling psychology as a mature student, having worked for many years as a school teacher. My degree was in psychology and although I went into special needs teaching I never lost interest in my degree subject and had put it to good use in my work. A few years before embarking on the qualification I had studied for a counselling certificate at the local college and as a result had taken on some counselling work with a charity for teenagers needing support.

There were no course routes close enough to my home to make that a viable option and I also was not free to commit myself to a full-time programme. Fortunately I had a colleague who was an educational psychologist and she suggested I look at the BPS Qualification. I found most of the information I needed on the BPS website and began to think that this may be a possibility for me. I also contacted the Registrar of the Qualification and she was incredibly helpful in encouraging me and assuring me that some of the qualifications and experience I already had could be accepted for AEC for some of the units. I needed to find a co-ordinating supervisor, a personal therapist, a **placement** and a Master's-level training course. It seemed a lot but once I found a local counselling psychologist from the BPS register I was able to meet with her and carefully work through the programme of training (POT). She was also able to recommend a personal therapist so it all fitted into place. The format of the Qualification was new to me as it is based on competencies but I have just completed a Master's in Cognitive-Behaviour Therapy and have been able to rework some of my assignments to fit the Qualification units. The research project that I am currently completing will also be accepted as evidence of my research competencies.

Although I had hoped to use my charity work as a clinical **placement,** this proved to be unacceptable as there was no qualified supervisor available. However I managed to find an unpaid **placement** with the Child and Adolescent Mental Health Service (CAMHS) at my local NHS Trust where I could work under supervision of a counselling psychologist and log my hours for the Qualification. Although it will take some years on a part-time basis to reach the required 450 hours I am working towards it and the experience has been invaluable. In summary, I think the 'independent route' has been an excellent way of training for me. It has allowed me the flexibility to fit studying in around other aspects of my life, I have been able to go at my own pace, I have had the support of a wide range of colleagues and have been able to use and adapt prior knowledge and skills to this new arena. On the downside I would say that the pressure is on myself to get things done, it can be lonely without the collegiality I would have had with other students on a course route but I had a bit of this on my MSc and that was really helpful.

The application process

To apply for the **independent route** it is necessary to complete the enrolment form on the BPS website and include various documents such as the Plan of Training form. It is therefore essential that you first of all locate an appropriate person who can act as your Co-ordinating Supervisor (CS). They will help you plan your training in accordance with the QCoP regulations and they will be responsible for signing off every aspect of your training. You will also need to find a clinical **placement** and a supervisor who will over-see your clinical practice. Your clinical supervisor must be a Registered counselling/clinical psychologist.

The selection process for a **course route** usually comprises two stages – the application and the interview. Many University courses offer two or three open evening/days throughout the year for prospective students. You can usually register for these on-line on the course website. They provide a valuable opportunity to find out more about the training generally and the particular emphasis of that course in terms of the therapeutic models they teach, attendance requirements, teaching styles, workload, clinical work and so on. You will also meet academic staff and, often, current students too, which allows you to ask questions directly and get a feel for whether the programme suits you.

It is relatively rare that course routes will accept accredited prior learning because it is difficult to vouch for training delivered elsewhere in terms of fitting with the accreditation standards. The exceptions to this are where you may have attended but not completed another accredited counselling psychology training. The credits from the modules completed there may be accepted by the new institution but this would need to be discussed with the course leader.

Once you have decided where you wish to apply for your training you need to complete an application form. Again, this can normally be done on-line and the required documents can be uploaded. You will normally be asked to supply all or some of the following:

- Scanned copies of signed/stamped qualifications (certificates or transcripts) to show how you meet, or expect to meet, the entry requirements
- Evidence of English language level (if English is not your first language)
- A copy of your passport (if you need a visa to study in the UK)
- A personal statement (for non-research programmes)
- A research proposal (for research programmes only) 1,000–1,500 words
- Narrative on becoming a counselling psychologist 1,000–1,500 words
- Contact details of 2 referees who are familiar with your academic and clinical background
- CV
- Evidence of Graduate Basis for **Chartership** (GBC)
- Evidence of **DBS** clearance

The interview process

If your application is successful you will be called to interview. The interview process is normally an intense and thorough process taking most of a full day. In advance of the day itself, you will be required to do some preparation and, possibly, submit some work prior to attending the interview. Some institutions ask for a written research proposal and a personal statement outlining why you want to become a counselling psychologist (both around 1,000–1,500 words long). Others only require one of these but be prepared to have to submit some written work before your interview and definitely have some ideas around your doctoral research topic.

Most courses include a number of activities in the selection process including:

- Individual interviews with staff members
- Specific interview on research
- Specific interview on clinical practice
- Presentation to staff and students on a given topic
- Group exercises
- Role plays
- Reflective exercises on the interview process itself

In addition you may be asked if you have made arrangements for your clinical **placement**. It will make a good impression if you have at least looked into **placement** possibilities. You may also be asked if you have found a personal therapist.

ACTIVITY BOX 14.2 PREPARING FOR INTERVIEW

Experience of helping: Look back over your life experiences and remind yourself of the occasions where you have played the role of helper or mentor or listener. Think what you have learned about yourself from those experiences and be prepared to talk about them.

Clinical placement: Explore clinical **placement** opportunities by contacting local NHS Trusts or voluntary organisations.

Personal therapy: Look through professional registers for a suitably qualified therapist and visit them to see if you feel comfortable having therapy with them. Most therapists will offer a student rate for trainees.

Research: Do some reading around the topic that you would like to research for your thesis and also gain some understanding of methodologies that may be suitable.

Motivation: Prepare a considered response to the question, "why do you want to be a counselling psychologist?" It will almost definitely be asked.

Personal qualities: Unlike many standard interviews, where the aim is to sell yourself, this one also requires you to demonstrate that you are self-aware and reflective, that you are emotionally robust and stable, a good listener and a caring individual. No easy feat!

Recent developments

As with all things, professional training in counselling psychology continues to evolve. There are a number of issues which are currently debated and may determine the way forward for our profession.

In the early days of counselling psychology in the UK we spent a lot of time establishing our identity and explaining who we were and what we did to both the public and other professionals. We needed to make a space for ourselves within the therapeutic world and the health service. It is rewarding that we now have consultant counselling psychologists running NHS departments and taking positions on national and international fora where policy decisions are made. However there is much still to be done and the focus may no longer be inward-looking but broader, deeper and worldwide.

Global perspective

Orlans and Van Scoyoc (2009) give a comprehensive overview of the international situation regarding counselling psychology training. The focus and concept of counselling psychology varies between countries and registration requirements differ also. This can make it difficult to transfer qualifications between countries but counselling psychology is now a member of the International Association of Applied Psychology (IAAP) providing a means to join together with colleagues across the world.

Within Europe we have the European Federation of Psychologists' Associations (EFPA), which is a body representing psychological associations throughout Europe. They feed into the European Commission on matters of training and have set up a qualification known as the EuroPsy by which psychologists can transfer between European states freely.

Pluralism vs specialism

The original syllabus for counselling psychology required trainees to study three therapeutic models in depth. The current revision of the guidelines reduced this to an in-depth knowledge of just one therapeutic model and a working knowledge of another one. Alongside this apparent move towards specialisation there emerged an interest in pluralism and a more social constructionist approach to understanding the human condition. These are philosophical debates that are still to be played out and may provide a spur for the future evolution of the profession.

Integration of theory and practice

Practitioner or professional or clinical doctorates are a relatively new type of research degree in the UK, having originated in the United States as a means by which applied research can be carried out at doctoral level. However the mainstream academic world tends to consider PhD research as blue-sky and the framework and assumptions around this often clash with the philosophy and value system of counselling psychology. Therefore it is important to continue to work on the recognition and acceptance of the exciting and important applied research within the profession, using new methodologies to enhance and change the world of therapeutic practice.

Selling out?

As counselling psychologists have increasingly found employment within the health service the gap between clinical and counselling psychology has lessened or, perhaps, become harder to define. Many managers now refer to 'psychologists' without any adjective and often they will forget if their staff were originally trained in counselling or clinical psychology. This move into what some would define as a medical model environment may appear to be contrary to the humanist foundations of counselling psychology and has come about as a practical need to ensure that young graduates are equipped with the competencies necessary to work within the NHS who, ultimately are the biggest employer. With each review of the standards there is a move further towards concepts and aspects of clinical work that early members of our profession would not have considered within the remit of counselling psychology. Controversial examples include the need to have a knowledge of psychometric testing, psychopharmacology, theories of psychopathology and the requirement to show leadership skills.

On the other side of this argument is the unique approach and training of counselling psychologists which allows us to work across a range of client groups, a range of modalities and a range of settings in a humanistic and relational manner.

Learning outcomes

When you have completed this chapter you should be able to:

- Understand the accreditation and regulation processes of the profession
- Understand the training process in counselling psychology

- Consider if this career is suited to you
- Decide which of the possible trainings would suit you best
- Understand the application process
- Prepare yourself for an interview
- Understand the pressures involved in training to be a counselling psychologist
- Have an awareness of contemporary debates in counselling psychology

Key phrases, concepts and terms

- Accreditation
- Chartership
- DBS
- Personal therapy
- Placement
- Qualification in Counselling Psychology
- Reflection
- Reflective-practitioner
- Registration
- Research
- Scientist-practitioner
- Supervision

Sample essay titles

1. What are the current requirements to work as a counselling psychologist in the UK? Consider the advantages and disadvantages of the training system.
2. Critically evaluate the way in which counselling psychologists are currently trained in the UK with consideration of issues such as accessibility, professionalism, ethos and career development.

Further information

Websites

You will find a lot of information about training in counselling psychology on the Internet.

In particular look at the BPS, HCPC and QAA to give you some information about the professional issues regarding accreditation and registration and also courses.

British Psychological Society www.bps.org.uk
Heath and Care Professions Council www.hcpc-uk.org
International Association of Applied Psychologists www.iaapcounsellingpsychology.org
European Association for Psychotherapy (EAP) www.europsyche.org
European Federation of Psychologists' Associations (EFPA) (1990) Optimal Standards for Professional Training in Psychology. www.efpa.be
The Quality Assurance Agency for Higher Education (QAA) www.qaa.ac.uk

Further Reading

The *Counselling Psychology Review* is the publication of the BPS Counselling Psychology Division and contains a lot of interesting articles written by counselling psychologists on a wide range of relevant topics.

The 2007 issue (22 (1)) focuses on training and careers and, although rather dated now, is still a useful source of information.

Alilovic, K. (2007) 'Practice what you preach': A day in the life of an academic counselling psychologist. *Counselling Psychology Review*, 22 (1), 5–7.

British Psychological Society (2006) *Regulations and Syllabus for the Qualification in Counselling Psychology.* Leicester: BPS.

British Psychological Society (2007) *Summary Report: New Ways of Working for Applied Psychologists in Health and Social Care: Models of Training.* Leicester: BPS.

British Psychological Society (2014) *Division of Counselling Psychology: Professional Practice Guidelines.* Leicester: BPS.

British Psychological Society (2015) *Standards for Doctoral Programmes in Counselling Psychology.* Leicester: BPS.

Carroll, M. (2004) *Counselling Supervision: Theory, Skills and Practice.* London: Sage.

Cooper, M. and McLeod, J. (2007) A pluralistic framework for counselling and psychotherapy: Implications for research. *Counselling and Psychotherapy Research*, 7 (3), 135–143.

Corrie, S. and Callahan, M. (2000) A review of the scientist-practitioner model: Reflections on its potential contribution to counselling psychology within the context of current health trends. *British Journal of Medical Psychology*, 7 (3), 135–143.

Du Plock, S. (2006) Just what is it that makes contemporary counselling psychology so different, so appealing? *Counselling Psychology Review*, 21 (2), 22–32.

Frankland, A. (2007) Counselling psychology: The trade for the portfolio professional. *Counselling Psychology Review*, 22 (1), 41–45.

Galbraith, V.E. (2016) Engaging with Academia and Training Programmes, in B. Douglas, R. Woolfe, S. Strawbridge, E. Kaskett, and V. Galbraith (eds.), *The Handbook of Counselling Psychology.* 4th ed. London: Sage. pp. 74–92.

Galbraith, V.E. and Hart, N.M. (2007) Personal development groups in counselling psychology training: The case for further research. *Counselling Psychology Review*, 22 (4), 49–56.

Georgopoulou, V. (2007) A week in the life of a counselling psychologist in a CAMHS context. *Counselling Psychology Review*, 22 (1), 11–18.

Giovazolias, T. (2005) Counselling psychology and the integration of theory, research and practice: A personal account. *Counselling Psychology Quarterly*, 18 (2), 161–168.

Harding Davies, V., Alred, G., Hunt, K., and Davies, G. (eds.) (2011) *Experiences of Counsellor Training: Challenges, Surprise and Change.* London: Palgrave.

Health and Care Professions Council (July 2015) *Standards of Proficiency: Practitioner Psychologists.* London: Park House.

Helmsley, C. (2013) An enquiry into how counselling psychology in the UK is constructed as a profession within discipline-orientated publications. *Counselling Psychology Review*, 28 (1), 8–23.

Kanellakis, P. and Kinder, A. (2006) Is the independence of counselling psychology training worth the cost? *Counselling Psychology Review*, 21 (2), 49–51.

Lane, D.A. and Corrie, S. (2006) *The Modern Scientist Practitioner: A Guide to Practice in Psychology.* London and New York: Routledge.

Lawrence-Wilks, L. and Ashmore, L. (2014) *The Reflective Practitioner in Professional Education.* Basingstoke: Palgrave-MacMillan.

Lester, S. (2004) Conceptualising the professional doctorate. *Studies in Higher Education*, 29 (5), 750–777.

Martin, P. (2006) Different, dynamic and determined: The powerful force of counselling psychology in the helping professions. *Counselling Psychology Review*, 21 (4), 42–44.
Martin, P. (2010) Training and Professional Development, in R. Woolfe, S. Strawbridge, B. Douglas, and W. Dryden (eds.), *Handbook of Counselling Psychology*. 3rd ed. London: Sage. pp. 547–568.
Milton, M. (2010). *Therapy and Beyond: Counselling Psychology Contributions to Therapeutic and Social Issues*. Chichester: Wiley-Blackwell.
Orlans, V. and Van Scoyoc, S. (2009). *A Short Introduction to Counselling Psychology*. London: Sage.
Quality Assurance Agency (QAA) (2011) *Doctoral Degree Characteristics*. www.qaa.ac.uk
Stefan, E. and Hanley, T. (2013) The power of counselling psychology in an age of powerlessness: A call to action. *Counselling Psychology Review*, 28 (2), 3–7.
Van Skoyoc, S. (2005) The future of our profession: Time to remember our history. *Counselling Psychology Review*, 20 (2), 49–51.

15

WORKING AS A COUNSELLING PSYCHOLOGIST

Ros Howard

Introduction

The purpose of this chapter is to provide an overview and a practical guide to working as a counselling psychologist. The chapter will examine the evolution and practice of counselling psychology, which will guide the reader towards a deeper level of understanding around the philosophy and practice of counselling psychology. The chapter will also examine how counselling psychology includes **self**-awareness, both within oneself and also in the interaction with other people. The use of self-awareness provides a **reflective stance** which needs to be present in all aspects of counselling psychology, such as therapeutic practice, **supervision**, personal therapy, **continued professional development** and discussions with colleagues.

Having qualified as a counselling psychologist, which involves many years of study, often at the expense of leisure time, there begins a new adventure as a fully fledged professional practitioner. There is a sense of accomplishment in achieving a high standard of training. However, the preparation for the period from trainee to qualified counselling psychologist can be over-looked in training. At present there is limited literature about the transition from trainee to qualified counselling psychologist (Palmer & Bor, 2008; Strawbridge, 2006; Martin, 2009), whereas there is notable literature about the professional development of therapists (Ronnestad & Skovholt, 2012; Orlinsky & Ronnestad, 2005).

Working as a counselling psychologist involves a journey dealing with twists and turns both personally and professionally. In managing these twists and turns, it is important to be prepared to defend the position that counselling psychology has a philosophical underpinning (van Deurzen-Smith, 1990) and that counselling psychology promotes an awareness of '**reflective self**', which will be a theme running through this chapter (Ganzer, 2007).

As an overview, recent evidence shows that counselling psychologists are employed in a variety of settings, such as corporate, academic, public, independent, charity and voluntary sectors. Counselling psychologists are trained to work across the age range and can therefore work in any clinical setting, such as working with children, families, adolescents, adults and older adults. There is also evidence that there is an increase in counselling psychologists becoming self-employed practitioners (Knight & Proctor, 2013).

To work as a counselling psychologist requires skills to combine **evidenced-based practice**, to continue with research, to engage in continued professional development, to be **reflective** in practice, supervision and self-care. There will be times when these roles and expectations will be challenged by organisational change, limited time, stress and frustration.

The philosophy and practice of counselling psychology

To work as a counselling psychologist it is important to firstly acknowledge why we have chosen this profession and secondly to acknowledge the evolution of counselling psychology. There will be many times when we have to justify and defend our position as counselling psychologists.

To recap on previous chapters within this text, counselling psychology is born from **humanistic** roots. It has been argued that counselling psychology is underpinned by a humanistic value system and that the most dominant values are based on empathy, acceptance and congruence (Rogers, 1951). Van Deurzen-Smith (1990) describes counselling psychology as having a large subjective element and being located in philosophy rather than science. Orlans & Van Scoyoc (2009) describe counselling psychology as working with the client's subjective experience, facilitating growth and promoting empowerment. It has been argued that counselling psychology bridges the gap between psychotherapy and **evidence-based** science, embraces contrasting methodologies, respects client diversity and addresses the complexity of human distress (Greenfield, 2010). Furthermore, it has been stated that counselling psychology has a focus on establishing a therapeutic relationship. Norcross (2002) reported that the therapeutic relationship is one of the most important contributors to a positive outcome in therapy. In this respect, the counselling psychologist has to be aware of using '**the self**', as an integral part of the psychological process. 'The self' is what we bring into the room. It can be described as self-awareness of personal and interpersonal dynamics, therefore being able to question our values, beliefs and experiences. The dynamics in therapy are affected by 'the self' (Blair, 2010). In relation to gaining greater understanding of 'the self', it can be argued that personal therapy and supervision are conduits towards understanding our role in therapeutic work and how we affect that role.

Counselling psychology takes place in a social, political, economic and **ideological** context (Blair, 2009). Consequently, there is an ethical responsibility for the counselling psychologist to regularly review and question what is changing within these contexts and to review best practice (Blair, 2010). Kottler (2010) argues that the focus of counselling psychology is to promote social justice, human rights and systemic change. Cooper (2009) further argues that counselling psychology acknowledges values. It has been stated that value-based practice is complementary to evidence-based practice and that clients will engage better in therapy that is consistent with their own values and beliefs (Woodbridge & Fulford, 2004).

The practice of counselling psychology involves enabling a helping relationship based in a humanistic value system with a focus on recovery and well-being. It has been argued that counselling psychology is constructional rather than pathological and that it seeks out resilience within a person, thus promoting recovery and well-being (Kagan, 2015). This process requires integrating therapeutic approaches to identify what works for each individual client by modifying interventions and to reformulate for alternative strategies. However, this process is often difficult to apply in a system where there is a different perspective, such as 'the medical model' in the public healthcare system (Blair, 2010). The '**medical model**' is based on scientific enquiry and is the dominant **paradigm** in the healthcare system (Clarkson, 2003; Gelso & Carter, 1994). Counselling psychology is located within humanistic (Rogers, 1951) and philosophical roots (van Deurzen-Smith, 1990), which results in counselling psychology being in conflict with 'the medical model'. In this respect, counselling psychology finds itself situated within roots of competing **ideologies**, frameworks and paradigms (Blair, 2010). It is on this basis that counselling psychology needs to continue to expand research in evidenced-based practice based on humanistic care (Cooper, 2009). Cooper & McLeod (2011) argue that therapy is fluid and that different clients will benefit from different models of therapy at different times in their life. The debate continues to challenge established ways of working in the healthcare system. As counselling psychologists, it is the celebration about counselling psychology being different, acknowledging a deep and varied level of training, which brings added value to the healthcare system (Hammersley, 2009).

The British Psychological Society, Division of Counselling Psychology Professional Practice Guidelines (2005, p. 2) state that, 'It is the responsibility of all Counselling Psychologists to encourage and develop the philosophy of Counselling Psychology'.

FOCUS BOX 15.1

It has been argued that counselling psychology is based on a humanistic value system (Rogers, 1951), having a large subjective element and being located in philosophy rather than science (van Deurzen-Smith, 1990).

Counselling psychology uses 'the self', which is described as self-awareness about personal and interpersonal dynamics (Blair, 2010).

Counselling psychology takes place in a social, political, economic and **ideological** context (Blair, 2009) such that there is an ethical responsibility for the counselling psychologist to review best practice (Blair, 2010).

Counselling psychology is situated within competing ideologies, frameworks and paradigms (Blair, 2010). In this respect, counselling psychology must continue to expand research in evidenced-based practice which is based on humanistic care (Cooper, 2009; Frost, 2012).

Cooper & McLeod (2011) argue that different clients will benefit from different models of therapy at different times in their life.

The debate continues to challenge established ways of working in the healthcare system.

Career development

After many years of hard work and sheer determination, the end result is qualifying with a doctorate in counselling psychology or equivalent. No longer are you bound by trainee restraints; you are now able to launch yourself into the 'working world' as a qualified counselling psychologist.

There are many opportunities for counselling psychologists to develop their career. Finding a job is the first step. Many jobs are advertised on the NHS website. There are also sites such as the British Psychological Society (BPS) website, where *The Psychologist* monthly magazine can be viewed, in which job vacancies are advertised. Plus, there are agencies that can place psychologists in permanent and temporary positions. A major factor in looking for employment is to be creative and persistent. For example, writing an easy-to-read Curriculum Vitae stating your experience, knowledge and skills, including your soft skills, such as communication, resilience and flexibility and then sending your CV to a wide range of employers.

National Health Service settings

History has shown that newly qualified counselling psychologists are eager to find employment within the NHS because of a good starting salary, a steady career structure and **multi-disciplinary** working. To work in multi-disciplinary teams means that information and knowledge can be shared. This way of working offers support to both clinician and 'service user'. A newly qualified counselling psychologist can apply for a Band 7 post if they have Health and Care Professions Council (HCPC, 2016) registration. On average a newly qualified counselling psychologist will remain in a Band 7 post for 2 years and would then apply for a Band 8(a) post. A Band 7 position has been described as an 'internship', enabling a counselling psychologist to gain knowledge, skills, experience and practice, combined with regular supervision. An 8(a) post has more responsibilities, not just in terms of practice, but also in management, service development and clinical governance. An 8(a) post can progress to 8(b) and then 8(c), which is a Consultant post. These job bandings can be viewed on the Department for Health (2004) Agenda for Change website.

The NHS offers a variety of positions for counselling psychologists, such as **Primary Care** and **Secondary Care**. In England, at present, the dominant services are Child and Adolescent Mental Health Services (CAMHS) and Improving Access to Psychological Therapies (IAPT). These services cover both Primary and Secondary Care Services. Typical referrals to the NHS are for Depression and Anxiety Disorders, Psychosis, Obsessive Compulsive Disorders, Post-Traumatic Stress Disorder, Autism Spectrum Disorders, and Dementia.

Child and Adolescent Mental Health Services (CAMHS) offer services for complex, severe or enduring mental health problems. CAMHS is available for 0- to 16-year-olds. Recently, some services are increasing the age up to 25-year-olds. Work within CAMHS will involve assessment and treatment for children and young people who have emotional, behavioural or enduring mental health difficulties. CAMHS is divided into Tiers 1, 2, 3 and 4, which cater for different severity of mental health difficulties. A Tier 4 service is usually an 'in-patient' unit, whereby the young person poses a risk to themselves or to others. Presenting problems referred to CAMHS include difficulties coping with family life, school or the wider world. Problems may manifest as violent or angry behaviour, anxiety, depression, eating disorders, psychosis, complex trauma, conduct disorder, attention deficit hyperactive disorder, self-harm, suicidal behaviour, history of abuse, autism. Within CAMHS there is a multi-disciplinary team of psychiatrists, psychologists, social workers, nurses, support workers, occupational therapists, psychotherapists, family therapists and play therapists.

In England, The Department for Health (2008) introduced Improving Access to Psychological Therapies (IAPT) which provides psychological services involving assessment and treatment for adults of all ages, covering mild to severe symptoms of anxiety or depression. IAPT offers a stepped-care model for **evidenced-based** treatments by primary care organisations. Within IAPT there is a multi-disciplinary **team** of Psychological Well-being Practitioners, High-Intensity Therapists, Cognitive-Behaviour Therapists, Psychotherapists, Clinical and Counselling

Psychologists, Voluntary and Community Sector Workers. A person presenting with complex mental health problems, such as psychosis, may be offered secondary care. Secondary care services are based in hospitals or clinics, whereby a specialist level of intervention and treatment can be provided. Specialist services within CAMHS and IAPT cover, for example, forensic services, learning disability services, older adult services, trauma and neuro-developmental services, eating disorder, drug and alcohol services, dementia, oncology services, Looked After Children (LAC), paediatric services, physical health, pain management and autism services.

The National Institute for Health and Care Excellence (NICE) (2016) develops guidelines based on research, to provide an integrated approach to identification, assessment and treatment of common mental health diagnoses. Multi-disciplinary teamwork is essential to manage different and difficult presenting problems, and to work in accordance with NICE Guidelines. Multi-disciplinary team working enables health professionals to identify gaps and liaise for sign posting to other appropriate agencies, both within and outside the NHS. Outside agencies may be voluntary or charity, such as Relate (relationships), which can be viewed on www.relate.org.uk, Cruse (bereavement), which can be viewed on www.cruse.org.uk, or Mind (mental health charity), which can be viewed on www.mind.org.uk.

Forensic settings – working in prisons or youth offending teams

To work as a counselling psychologist in a forensic setting involves being exposed to high-risk situations. There are physical and emotional considerations for the counselling psychologist. Physical considerations are around security and safety; emotionally, the counselling psychologist will be exposed to arguably the worst elements of human nature. For example, there are prisoners who are intent on harming themselves or others; there are prisoners who have committed serious and heinous crimes, involving violent and sexual crime. Equally, a counselling psychologist working in a Youth Offending Team will be involved in managing vulnerable young people who exhibit high risk and challenging behaviour. The role of the counselling psychologist is to promote positive change for offenders.

It could also be argued that fundamental to counselling psychology philosophy is the belief that human beings can change (Rogers, 1951). In this respect, working within a forensic service may involve managing challenging behaviours, but it may also involve compassion and a belief that this population can reflect on their behaviour, use better coping strategies and therefore reduce the chance of further criminal activity.

The forensic work will involve psychological assessments and formulations which take into account the person's home life, peer group and education. The focus of psychological work is to enable the person to make changes to develop a better future, to understand the consequences of their actions and to prevent re-offending. It could be argued that a person may fall into crime as a result of an experience in early years of poor relationships with their care givers, or experiencing trauma in their life and that criminal behaviour is acting out anger or resentment. Rehabilitation for offenders requires not only compassion and psychological interventions, but also practical assistance which involves working with a multi-disciplinary team including the police, the probation service, social services, health services and other agencies that can support welfare needs such as housing, education or employment.

The essence of working in a forensic setting is predominantly to enable the prevention of re-offending. The counselling psychologist may be challenged professionally and personally by the nature of the forensic population.

Academic or educational settings

There may be employment opportunities in academia such as research, lecturing or teaching. The post may require further training such as Post-Graduate Certificate in Higher Education (PGC in HE). In an academic position, the counselling psychologist can extend their research interests and academic portfolio. Generally, the responsibilities for working in an academic environment will be to support administration procedures, prepare teaching or lecturing programmes, conduct and supervise research, interview and select students and to be available for tutorials.

An interesting way to gain experience with children and young people is to work in a school setting. Some schools offer 'counselling' as part of pastoral care. The school may require an 'ad hoc' service or provide a regular weekly session for appointments or 'drop in'. This may not be 'pure psychology work' but it is a good way of gaining experience with children, staff and parents. Children or young people can struggle with high expectations, academic stress, relationship problems, self-esteem, self-harming behaviours, problems at home, bereavement, bullying to name a few situations that will need compassion and a sympathetic ear. The role requires knowledge of school policies and procedures, plus an in-depth knowledge of Child Protection. The counselling psychologist will also need to be acquainted with agencies that can offer specialist support such as assessments for autism and dyslexia. The benefits of working in this context are that it enables gaining experience in holistic working, networking with other agencies, conflict resolution, mediation and risk assessment.

Developing a portfolio – experience, skills, practice

As discussed previously, an organisation, such as the NHS, can provide a counselling psychologist with good remuneration and a career structure. However, there are many conflicts to endure whilst working in the NHS. It has been argued that counselling psychology is often in conflict with organisational settings and policies (Blair, 2009; Caplan, 1994; Cooper & McLeod, 2011). A newly qualified counselling psychologist may have to adhere to a specific model of therapy, feel overwhelmed by administrative duties, feel constrained by time and session allocation, all of which may create not only stress (Weiss, 2004), but also a sense of conflict in relation to the training and philosophy of counselling psychology. It has been argued that 'ideology governed by philosophy has been juxtaposed with the practicalities of obtaining employment' (James, 2013). However, if the organisation engages with and supports the practice of counselling psychology, this enables the counselling psychologist to work within their own preferred model of therapy (Bilgrave & Deluty, 2002), or to experiment with practice models to promote counselling psychology. On this basis, it could be argued that a thriving healthcare team would integrate counselling psychologists into the workplace.

At present there is a considerable amount of change taking place within the NHS and other public services. This position creates stress due to uncertain job security and changing working conditions, such as loss of personal and professional space and chaotic administrative systems. Plus, there is an ethical stance whereby a counselling psychologist is often challenged by having to work in systems where there are long waiting lists, offering time limited and prescriptive psychological 'treatment'.

Many counselling psychologists, by the nature of their training, are adept in mixing and matching their knowledge and experience in different organisations and contexts. This position not only gives a varied range of opportunity, but also enables the counselling psychologist confidence to find work.

A counselling psychologist, with experience in various settings and organisations, has built up a portfolio of acquired skills and practice. This portfolio provides the individual with transferable skills, which is an asset to any type of employment. Some counselling psychologists know at the beginning of their career where they would like to specialise, others find their way after experiencing different placement or job opportunities.

Many counselling psychologists are taking the opportunity for self-employment and it is interesting to note that recently, there has been a noticeable rise in the number of self-employed and independent counselling psychologists (Burton, 2014; Knight & Proctor, 2013).

Self-employed/independent practitioner

Being self-employed means that you are responsible for creating your own income, so in effect you are running your own business. There are numerous books (Bor & Stokes, 2011; Weitz, 2006) and workshops setting out guidelines for self-employment as a counselling psychologist. Training workshops can be viewed on the BPS website. To create your own income requires a business mindset, which has to overshadow 'being a psychologist'. This position can create ethical conflicts, such as what to charge a client: to charge too high would prohibit affordability for many clients; to charge too low would affect the financial viability and stability of your business. To run a business requires developing a niche in the market – what can you offer that is different or what will complement existing services, looking out for market trends – what is doing well, what is not doing well. An important feature of running a business is to continually assess your own business practice.

There are practicalities to running a business: you will need a business plan and a business bank account. An accountant is a good investment for tax advice and setting up a business. You will need to register with the Information Commissioner's Office (ICO) for Data Protection because you will be keeping confidential information such as client records. You will need to make time for basic business and administrative systems, marketing, advertising and networking. In terms of practice premises you will need to offer an easy-to-reach location, an appropriate therapy room which is quiet and confidential, a reception area or waiting area, toilet facilities, safe parking and ideally, disabled access. You will have to familiarise yourself with basic safety policies and procedures, such as fire safety. You will need to consider boundaries for professional practice such as terms and conditions, contracts detailing payments of fees, late cancellation and non-attendance, confidentiality, storage of notes and professional availability arrangements. If you use a room in your home for psychotherapeutic work, it is important to be aware that there are potential risks associated with being a lone worker, for example, being safe when a client exhibits aggressive or unpredictable behaviour. Plus, clients know where you live and may intrude on your personal space.

However, if you use a room at home for 'office space', this will help to keep costs down. In this respect, there are many practicalities such as convenience, flexibility, minimising travel costs and travel time. However, working from home may hinder the work/life balance, such as business administration and technology overrunning into family and leisure time. It has been argued that modern technology seems to seduce us to being constantly available and not being mindful of boundaries for work and social life (Easton & Van Laar, 2013).

In the current climate, technology is offering new ways of working, such as using Skype, FaceTime, web chat, text and mobile phone. Grover et al. (2002) argue that due to public demand there is now a growing need for on-line access to therapy. Technology arguably provides easy access, flexibility and anonymity. There is information available for practitioners who wish to offer services over the Internet (Evans, 2009; Jones & Stokes, 2009). However, there are discussions against using on-line access to therapy due to physical distance, lack of intimacy, lack of non-verbal communication (Rochlen et al., 2004), plus risks around miscommunication, confidentiality, client's vulnerability and honesty.

Being self-employed opens up many opportunities for diversification, creativity, flexibility and productivity. There are personal and professional benefits in being self-employed. For example, you will have to plan and think for yourself; you can be more creative and adapt to opportunities; you can manage your own working conditions, job satisfaction and well-being, you can work holistically, being confident to use your therapeutic skills and professional judgement (Hammersley, 2009); you can take pride in your work not only in your therapeutic skills but also in your business skills. You can offer choice and flexibility to clients, there is less emphasis on the medical model; you can be more experimental and creative; more ethical and less defensive (Hammersley, 2009).

Equally, there are some disadvantages to being self-employed. For example, having to pay for supervision, continued professional development, books and materials; having to tolerate uncertainty, ebbs and flows in business practice and late payments of accounts; paying attention to personal safety; making time for advertising, marketing and networking; working in isolation. However, there is an opportunity to join other psychologists, some of whom work in a 'company of psychologists'. Links with other counselling psychologists are helpful both personally and professionally. The BPS provides support and links for independent practitioners such as BPS Independent Practitioner's forum, now a Special Group or the Networking Community of Psychologists in Independent Practice, which links psychologists across the United Kingdom (Knight & Proctor, 2013)

Applying the use of 'self'

The self is an intrinsic component in counselling psychology and arguably makes counselling psychology different to other disciplines in psychology. Newly qualified counselling psychologists may struggle to identify 'the self', especially as they often feel overwhelmed with adhering to therapeutic and organisational constraints, which may create a conflict in relation to their training and philosophy of counselling psychology. However, it has been argued that a therapist who is self-aware in their self-doubting would appear to be more effective in their job (Jarrett & Fradera, 2016).

Counselling psychology focuses on the therapeutic relationship; the counselling psychologist is part of the therapeutic relationship, which requires an ability to recognise 'the self'. It has been argued that the therapist's self is recognisable as a component in therapeutic change (Norcross, 2002) and that the counselling psychologist's sense of self contributes to therapeutic outcome. This requires a high level of self-awareness in order not to misuse power in the therapeutic relationship (Omylinska-Thurston & James, 2011). However, recognising the self is often difficult in dynamic relations.

The effective use of self requires self-awareness around complexity of the therapeutic work, different values between the counselling psychologist and the client in terms of racial, cultural, religious values and beliefs. Rawson (2012) argued that being reflective about the self is to be able to understand 'the effect that I have on someone else'. Levine (2007) argued that 'the self' can be shaped by the influence of the other person and can emerge into everyday therapeutic interactions. Furthermore, it has been argued that the self is situated within relational dynamics occurring in the therapeutic situation; the self is not fixed or static but in a state of constant movement (Levine, 2007). However, there is little research on subjective experience in this area (Ganzer, 2007; Arnd-Caddigan & Pozzuto, 2008). Beutler et al. (2004) stated that most research is based on the medical model, ignoring subjectivity, values and meanings, which may result in the self of the therapist being marginalised and overlooked.

ACTIVITY 15.1

Working as a Counselling Psychologist – This is an opportunity to reflect on the self. The reflection may involve examining your own belief and value system. Consider the following questions:

Why do you want to work as a counselling psychologist?
What can you offer to the population?
What can you offer to your team?
How can you promote counselling psychology?
What can you offer politically?

It is also important to identify your own strengths and resources to maintain a healthy balance between the nature of the psychological work and free time for rest and relaxation.

What are your strengths and resources that would enable you to divide your time between work and leisure?

Working as a counselling psychologist – combining research, practice, supervision and continued professional development

Working as a counselling psychologist requires dealing with organisational and contextual stress, plus continuing with research, practice, supervision and continued professional development. The combination of this practice promotes a healthy career portfolio.

Research and practice

In the present political climate there are professional, corporate and government changes which contribute to a feeling of uncertainty. A recent change within the National Health System has been to implement Improving Access to Psychological Therapies (IAPT). There were, and still are, debates discussing the changes that have taken place. For example, IAPT has been criticised for promoting a culture of 'cure' which has failed to acknowledge the real and varied complexities of mental health problems (Fairfax, 2008). This change of emphasis from 'care' to 'cure' firstly belittles the primary task of working therapeutically, and secondly undermines the professionalism of the practitioner (Stokes, 1994). Patterson (2000) argued that human beings are self-conscious and **reflective**, with capacity for choice and personal responsibility rather than being entirely determined by internal and external causes. In support of offering different interventions, Rawson (2012) reported that counselling psychology can be integrated with other approaches and to also experiment with what therapeutic approach works effectively. It is important to offer a range of therapeutic interventions to meet the often complex criteria of evidenced-based and values-based practice. It has been argued that working with complex distress requires models of therapy to respond to individual needs (Cooper & McLeod, 2011). This position may support the need for further scientist-practitioner research. Fairfax (2008) states that IAPT has failed to recognise the complex and often co-morbidity of mental health problems. However, Marzillier & Hall (2009) argue that IAPT has created a debate on the provision of psychological therapies. It is within this culture that counselling psychologists can debate and challenge the zeitgeist of the day.

Psychological therapy takes place in a social, political, economic and **ideological** context (Blair, 2009). As counselling psychologists, we need to be in tune with the undercurrents that drive agendas. It has been argued that counselling psychologists need to have an awareness to promote social justice, human rights and systemic change (Kottler, 2010). Mental health problems need to be understood in the context of societal inequalities such as low income, job insecurity, poor housing, social pressures, poor health and illness that affect well-being. It has been argued that there is a clear link between economic policies and mental health (Blair, 2009; Marmot, 2010). Clients with severe mental health problems may be socially excluded and difficult to reach. Counselling psychology has to speak out for fairer economic and social policies to improve mental health and to challenge the government austerity policies where there are financial cuts to welfare, social education and healthcare. In this respect, counselling psychologists have a voice which can be used to be politically aware and to be involved with agencies and professional bodies, such as the British Psychological Society, who hold forums for debate and promote policy change.

Continued Professional Development (CPD)

The BPS (2005, p. 3) states that every practising counselling psychologist has to provide evidence of Continued Professional Development (**CPD**). The Health and Care Professions Council (HCPC) (2016, p. 7) states that **CPD** is a requirement to keep professional knowledge and skills up to date. Continued professional development can take many forms. It may be engaging in work-based learning, such as supervision and **reflective** practice; professional activity, such as involvement in a professional body; educational, such as writing papers; training, such as learning or updating present or future practice; self-directed learning, such as reading journals, or reviewing books. Continued professional development has to be recorded on a yearly basis and integrated into practice. The procedure of continued professional development is not only mandatory for practice, but also enables knowledge, skills and practice development. This is an opportunity to **reflect** on practice and to record the use of 'self' as a useful learning process. The BPS website is a helpful resource for finding training courses for **CPD**. The site also offers 'myCPD' which is a useful tool for recording and monitoring **CPD**.

Supervision

The mandatory process of supervision is for ethical and professional practice (BPS, 2005, p. 5). The purpose of supervision is to ensure maintenance of good practice in relation to clients, to other people involved in the client's therapy and to the counselling psychologist's professional development. Supervision is a time and place where a counselling psychologist can discuss their work with a colleague. It is a space where a supervisee can share vulnerability and success; it can be used for training and support, for development and reflection.

The practice of supervision within a busy healthcare system is often very different to the theory of supervision. Busy schedules sometimes impact on the supervisor, who may have to cancel supervision, may be distracted by interference from other people, phone calls, or the supervisor may not match the supervisee's therapeutic stance. These are frustrations that may need to be challenged by the supervisee. This position promotes a discussion around self-awareness, professional practice and consequences in challenging an often dysfunctional and overloaded system. Private supervision arrangements are distinctly different in terms of financial arrangements, planning, availability, timing and efficacy of the supervisor/supervisee relationship. The supervisee may feel more empowered to challenge difficulties arising in the supervision contract.

Self-care

Self-care is considered to be an integral part of counselling psychology. It is an ethical duty for all therapists (Norcross & Guy, 2007). The BPS (2005, p. 3) Fitness to Practise Guidelines state that a counselling psychologist has 'to continually monitor and maintain an effective level of personal functioning'. Newly qualified counselling psychologists are arguably more prone to stress (Weiss, 2004). However, any counselling psychologist, despite their experience, may at some point suffer from stress or burnout. In this respect, it is important to acknowledge that we are vulnerable, we are no different to anyone else and sometimes we need help to heal our wounds (Stirzaker, 2014). Personal therapy, supervision and being a reflective-practitioner may help to develop the capacity to tolerate other aspects of ourselves.

Summary

Working as a counselling psychologist requires applying theory and practice, conducting research, engaging in continued professional development, personal therapy and supervision, **reflective practice** and improvement in self-awareness, plus managing challenging workloads, managing organisational stress and looking after yourself. To work in a supportive environment can bring rewards of job satisfaction, a strong sense of professional identity, high levels of accomplishment and efficacy. In this respect, counselling psychologists can promote a dynamic and integrative professional discipline. However, there are frustrations when counselling psychologists encounter competing ideologies, frameworks and paradigms (Blair, 2010), organisational change and targets. It has been argued that despite frustrations within the profession, we need to celebrate why we are different to other psychological disciplines and how we can add value to the healthcare system (Hammersley, 2009).

What does the future hold for counselling psychology? There are concerns that counselling psychology may be subsumed into 'Clinical Psychology' (Giddings, 2009). This position could challenge our humanistic and philosophical roots. It is important to defend our professional status and to be more representative and active on national commissioning bodies around mental health policy (James, 2013).

Learning outcomes

When you have completed this chapter you should be able to:

- Evaluate the inclusion of counselling psychology in multi-disciplinary team work.
- Reflect on 'the self' as an integral part of professional practice and personal development.
- Understand how to build a Counselling Psychology portfolio.
- Evaluate the integral component of research in Counselling Psychology.

Key phrases, concepts and terms

- Continued Professional Development (CPD)
- Evidence-Based Practice
- Humanistic
- Ideologies
- Medical Model
- Multi-Disciplinary
- Paradigms
- Primary Care
- Reflective
- Secondary Care
- Supervision
- The Self

Sample essay titles

1. Based on the evolution of Counselling Psychology, how do you envisage Counselling Psychology to be in 10 years' time?
2. How would you justify your practice as a Counselling Psychologist in a busy organisation where targets are more important than taking time to be reflective on professional practice?
3. In what ways is Counselling Psychology different and similar to Clinical Psychology?
4. How would a Counselling Psychologist make time for reflection on 'the self' both in professional practice and professional development?
5. How can Counselling Psychology promote political change?

Further reading

Books

Orlans, V. & Van Scoyoc, S. (2009). *A Short Introduction to Counselling Psychology.* London: Sage.

Giddings, D. (2009). Counselling psychology and the next 10 years: Some questions and answers. *Counselling Psychology Review, 24* (1), 10.

James, P. (2013). Counselling psychology in the UK: A 30-year passage. *Counselling Psychology Review, 28* (3), 75–79.

The British Psychological Society. *Counselling Psychology Review*. www.bpsshop.org.uk
Hammersley, D. (2009). Counselling psychology: What I see in the crystal ball. *Counselling Psychology Review*, *24* (1), 5–9.
Weitz, P. (2006). *Setting Up and Maintaining an Effective Private Practice: A Practical Workbook for Mental Health Practitioners*. London: Karnac Books.
Bor, R. & Stokes, A. (2011). *Setting Ip in Independent Practice: A Handbook for Counsellors, Therapists and Psychologists*. Basingstoke, UK: Palgrave Macmillan.
Douglas, B., Woolfe, R., Strawbridge, S., Kasket, E., & Galbraith, V. (2016). *The Handbook of Counselling Psychology* (4th Ed.) London: Sage Publications Ltd.
The British Psychological Society. *The Psychologist*. www.thepsychologist.org.uk

Journal articles

Up-to-date topical discussions are available in *The Psychologist* www.thepsychologist.org.uk
The Counselling Psychology Review www.bpsshop.org.uk
The Journal of Counseling Psychology
Burton, M.V. (2014). The stress of being a psychotherapist. *Psychotherapy Section Review*, *52*, 52–57.
Karademas, E.C. (2009). Counselling psychology in medical settings: The promising role of counselling health psychology. *European Journal of Counselling Psychology*, *1* (1), 18–37.

References

Arnd-Caddigan, M. & Pozzuto, R. (2008). Use of self in relational clinical social work. *Clinical Social Work Journal*, *36*, 235–242.
Beutler, L.E., Malik, M.L., Alimohamed, S., Harwood, T.M., Talebi, H., Noble, S., & Wong, E. (2004). Therapist variables. In M.J. Lambert (Ed.), *Handbook of Psychotherapy and Behaviour Change* (2nd Ed.) (pp. 227–306). New York: John Wiley & Sons.
Bilgrave, D. & Deluty, R. (2002). Religious beliefs and political ideologies as predictors of psychotherapeutic orientations of clinical and counselling psychologists. *Psychotherapy Theory, Research, Practice, Training*, *39*, 245–260.
Blair, L. (2009). Psychotherapy and the economic context: Some reflections for practice. *Division of Counselling Psychology Newsletter*, *1* (1), 7–10.
Blair, L. (2010). A critical review of the scientist-practitioner model for counselling psychology. *Counselling Psychology Review*, *25* (4), 19–30.
Bor, R. & Stokes, A. (2011). *Setting Up in Independent Practice: A Handbook for Counsellors, Therapists and Psychologists*. Basingstoke, UK: Palgrave Macmillan.
The British Psychological Society. (2005). *Division of Counselling Psychology Professional Practice Guidelines*. Leicester: BPS.
Burton, M.V. (2014). The stress of being a psychotherapist. *Psychotherapy Section Review*, *52*, 52–57.
Caplan, R.P. (1994). Stress, anxiety and depression in hospital consultants, general practitioners and senior health service managers. *British Medical Journal*, *309* (6964), 1261–1263.
Clarkson, P. (2003). *The Therapeutic Relationship* (2nd Ed.). London: Whurr Publishers.
Cooper, M. (2009). Welcoming the Other: Actualising the humanistic ethic at the core of counselling psychology practice. *Counselling Psychology Review*, *24* (3–4), 119–130.
Cooper, M. & McLeod, J. (2011). *Pluralistic Counselling and Psychotherapy*. London: Sage.
The Department for Health. (2004). *Agenda for Change*. www.healthcareers.nhs.uk/about/careers-nhs/nhs-pay-and-benefits/agenda-change-pay-rates
The Department for Health. (2008). *IAPT National Implementation Plan*. London: DH Publications.
Easton, S. & Van Laar, D. (2013). Evaluation of quality of working life as an outcome for work-based counselling and psychological therapy. *Counselling Psychology Review*, *28* (3), 43–48.
Evans, J. (2009). *Online Counselling and Guidance Skills: A Practical Resource for Trainees and Practitioners*. London: Sage.

Fairfax, H. (2008). CBT or not CBT, is that really the question? Re-considering the evidence base: The contribution of the process research. *Counselling Psychology Review, 23* (4), 27–37.
Ganzer, C. (2007). The use of self from a relational perspective. *Clinical Social Work Journal, 35*, 117–123.
Gelso, C.J. & Carter, J.A. (1994). Components of the counselling relationship: Their interaction and unfolding during treatment. *Journal of Counselling Psychology, 41* (3), 310–312.
Giddings, D. (2009). Counselling psychology and the next 10 years: Some questions and answers. *Counselling Psychology Review, 24* (1), 10.
Greenfield, J. (2010). What's important in psychotherapy? What has been lost in IAPT ? *The Division of Counselling Psychology Newsletter, 2* (1), 4–7.
Grover, F. Jr., Wu, H.D., Blanford, C., Holcomb, S., & Tidler, D. (2002). Computer-using patients want internet services from family physicians. *Journal of Family Practice, 51*, 570–572.
Hammersley, D. (2009). Counselling psychology: What I see in the crystal ball. *Counselling Psychology Review, 24* (1), 5–9.
The Health and Care Professions Council (HCPC). (2016). *Standards of Conduct, Performance and Ethics.* London: HCPC.
James, P. (2013). Counselling psychology in the UK: A 30-year passage. *Counselling Psychology Review, 28* (3), 75–79.
Jarrett, C. & Fradera, A. (2016). The ideal therapist doubts their professional skills, but loves themselves as a person. *The Psychologist, 29* (1), 24.
Jones, G. & Stokes, A. (2009). *Online Counselling: A Handbook for Practitioners.* London: Palgrave Macmillan.
Kagan, C. (2015). Community psychological perspectives and counselling psychology. *Counselling Psychology Review, 30* (3), 12–21.
Knight, A. & Proctor, R. (2013). The silent drift from NHS to private practice. *The Psychologist, 26* (8), 596–599.
Kottler, J.A. (2010). *On Being a Therapist* (4th Ed.). San Francisco, CA: Jossey-Bass.
Levine, S.S. (2007). Nothing but the truth: Self disclosure, self revelation and the persona of the analyst. *Journal of the American Psychoanalytic Association, 55* (1), 81–104.
Marmot, M. (2010). *Fair Society, Healthy Lives: The Marmot Review.* London: The Marmot Review.
Martin, P. (2009). Training and professional development. In R. Woolfe, S. Strawbridge, B. Douglas & W. Dryden (Eds.), *Handbook of Counselling Psychology* (3rd Ed.) (pp. 547–568). London: Sage.
Marzillier, J. & Hall, J. (2009). Alternative ways of working. *The Psychologist, 22* (5), 396–399.
The National Institute for Health and Care Excellence. (2016). www.nice.org.uk/guidance
Norcross, J.C. (Ed.). (2002). *Psychotherapy Relationships That Work: Therapist Contributions and Responsiveness to Patients.* New York: Oxford University Press.
Norcross, J.C. & Guy, J.D. (2007). *Leaving It at the Office: A Guide to Psychotherapist Self-Care.* New York: The Guildford Press.
Omylinska-Thurston, J. & James, P.E. (2011). The therapist's use of self: A closer look at the processes within congruence. *Counselling Psychology Review, 26* (3), 20–33.
Orlans, V. & Van Scoyoc, S. (2009). *A Short Introduction to Counselling Psychology.* London: Sage.
Orlinsky, D.E. & Ronnestad, M.H. (2005). *How Psychotherapists Develop: A Study of Therapeutic Work and Professional Growth.* Washington: APA.
Palmer, S. & Bor, R. (Eds.). (2008). *The Practitioner's Handbook: A Guide for Counsellors, Psychotherapists and Counselling Psychologists.* London: Sage.
Patterson, C.H. (2000). *Understanding Psychotherapy: Fifty Years of Client-Centred Practice.* Ross on Wye, UK: PCCS Books.
Rawson, D. (2012). Ian Florence interviews Don Rawson about combining 'the science of psychology with the art of counselling'. *The Psychologist, 25* (5), 382–385.
Rochlen, A., Zack, J., & Speyer, C. (2004). Online therapy: Review of relevant definitions, debates and current empirical support. *Journal of Clinical Psychology, 60* (3), 269–283.
Rogers, C. (1951). *Client-Centred Therapy: Its Current Practice, Implications and Theory.* London: Constable.
Ronnestad, M.H. & Skovholt, T. (2012). *The Developing Practitioner: Growth and Stagnation of Therapists and Counselors.* New York: Routledge.

Stirzaker, A. (2014). Psychotherapist heal thyself: Is that what we are trying to do? *Psychotherapy Section Review*, *52*, 83–86.

Stokes, J. (1994). Institutional chaos and personal stress. In A. Obholzer & V. Zagier Roberts (Eds.), *The Unconscious at Work: Individual and Organisational Stress in the Human Services* (pp. 121–129). London: Routledge.

Strawbridge, S. (2006). Thoughts on becoming, being and developing as a counselling psychologist. *Counselling Psychology Review*, *21* (1), 27–30.

van Deurzen-Smith, E. (1990). Philosophical underpinnings of counselling psychology. *Counselling Psychology Review*, *5* (2), 8–12.

Weiss, L. (2004). *Therapist's Guide to Self-Care.* New York: Brunner-Routledge.

Weitz, P. (2006). *Setting Up and Maintaining an Effective Private Practice: A Practical Workbook for Mental Health Practitioners.* London: Karnac Books.

Woodbridge, K. & Fulford, K.W.M. (2004). *Whose Values: A Workbook for Values-Based Practice in Mental Healthcare.* London: The Sainsbury Centre for Mental Health.

INDEX